COVID-19

COVID-19

From Bench to Bedside

Edited by

Debmalya Barh

Visiting Full Professor (Titular/Class-E)
Department of Genetics, Ecology and Evolution
Institute of Biological Sciences (ICB)
Federal University of Minas Gerais (UFMG)
Brazil
and
Honorary Scientist
Institute of Integrative Omics and Applied Biotechnology (IIOAB)
India

Kenneth Lundstrom

CEO
PanTherapeutics
Lausanne, Switzerland

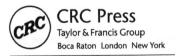

CRC Press
Taylor & Francis Group
Boca Raton London New York

CRC Press is an imprint of the
Taylor & Francis Group, an **informa** business

First edition published 2022
by CRC Press
6000 Broken Sound Parkway NW, Suite 300, Boca Raton, FL 33487-2742

and by CRC Press
2 Park Square, Milton Park, Abingdon, Oxon, OX14 4RN

Library of Congress Cataloging-in-Publication Data
Names: Barh, Debmalya, editor. | Lundstrom, Kenneth H., editor.
Title: COVID-19 : from bench to bedside / edited by Debmalya Barh, Kenneth Lundstrom.
Other titles: COVID-19 (Barh)
Description: First edition. | Boca Raton, FL : CRC Press, 2022. | Includes bibliographical references and index. | Summary: "The COVID-19 pandemic has affected the entire world in an unprecedented way and this book provides an overview of the historical facts as well as ongoing approaches to tackle the COVID-19 pandemic. Experts of the respective domains provide details on anti-SARS-COV-2 drug strategies, including repurposing drugs used for other indications and development of novel drugs looking at different approaches to target virus entry and replication. COVID-19 vaccine development based on inactivated and attenuated live virus, protein subunit and peptide-based vaccines and utilization of vaccine candidates based on viral vectors, DNA and RNA are presented for both preclinical studies and clinical trials"-- Provided by publisher.
Identifiers: LCCN 2021049205 (print) | LCCN 2021049206 (ebook) | ISBN 9781032040622 (paperback) | ISBN 9781032040639 (hardback) | ISBN 9781003190394 (ebook)
Subjects: MESH: COVID-19--drug therapy | COVID-19--diagnosis | COVID-19--prevention & control | Pandemics | COVID-19 Vaccines--therapeutic use
Classification: LCC RA644.C67 (print) | LCC RA644.C67 (ebook) | NLM WC 506 | DDC 616.2/414--dc23/eng/20211101
LC record available at https://lccn.loc.gov/2021049205
LC ebook record available at https://lccn.loc.gov/2021049206

ISBN: 978-1-032-04063-9 (hbk)
ISBN: 978-1-032-04062-2 (pbk)
ISBN: 978-1-003-19039-4 (ebk)

Doi:10.1201/9781003190394

Typeset in Palatino
by SPi Technologies India Pvt Ltd (Straive)

We dedicate the book to all our COVID-19 warriors and the people who are the victims of this pandemic.

Contents

Preface

During 2020–2021 we received information about the devastating COVID-19 pandemic in all possible forms of communication, including written, audio, and visual. We have been overloaded with information related to the origin of SARS-CoV-2, the efficacy of drugs for the treatment of COVID-19, and the safety of the new generation of vaccines developed against SARS-CoV-2.

In our book, *COVID-19: From Bench to Bedside*, we seek to provide the reader with fact-based information on various aspects of SARS-CoV-2 and the COVID-19 pandemic covering basic research to applications, to give the reader a clear overview from bench to bedside. We certainly acknowledge that with the unprecedented resources and effort put into COVID-19 research, and the extraordinary data collection it is impossible to provide the very detailed as well as the absolutely latest information. However, we have attempted to educate the reader with a broad spectrum of topics related to SARS-CoV-2 and COVID-19, and hope to address exciting new discoveries and breakthroughs in future editions of the book.

It is obviously appropriate to start by describing previous coronavirus outbreaks and epidemics, such as SARS and MERS, and place the once-in-a-century COVID-19 pandemic in its correct context (Chapter 1). Where did it start and how did it spread so quickly and widely are important questions. Most relevantly, Chapter 2 is dedicated to the biology of coronaviruses, and particularly to the unsolved origin of SARS-CoV-2.

The three cornerstones of prevention, treatment, and eradication of COVID-19 comprise diagnostics, therapeutics, and vaccines. As no antiviral drugs against SARS-CoV-2 were available at the onset of the pandemic, different approaches have been taken to develop drugs for the treatment of COVID-19 patients, which have been covered in several chapters in the book from different angles. The therapeutic challenges are enormous, which has been laid out in Chapter 3. Therefore, we have dedicated one chapter to prevention and control strategies (Chapter 4) and another to rapid and advanced diagnostic technologies associated with COVID-19 (Chapter 6). To provide an overview on global efforts to encounter COVID-19, we have also introduced a chapter (Chapter 5).

The "fast-and-dirty" approach has been to revisit existing antiviral and antiparasitic drugs to evaluate whether they might be repurposed for COVID-19 treatment. This approach has generated some modest success but also disappointments, as described in Chapter 7. The potential use of convalescent plasma from COVID-19 patients, and the highly promising engineering of monoclonal antibody-based therapy are discussed in Chapter 8. Similarly, the alternative approach of therapeutic interventions based on stem cell and exosome technologies for COVID-19 has generated some exciting results, which are presented in Chapter 9. An insight into host and pathogen-specific drug targets is presented in Chapter 10.

Technology and innovation are essential components in scientific research and development in general. SARS-CoV-2 drug and vaccine development is no exception. It is therefore appropriate to include a description on computational biology and stress its importance in modern drug and vaccine development (Chapter 11). Moreover, nanotechnology and nanomaterials used in various fields of manufacturing have become an essential component in our daily lives, so it is important to highlight how nanotechnology can be implemented for COVID-19 drug development and manufacturing of personal protective equipment (Chapter 12).

Naturally, vaccine development plays a central role in finding a solution to prevent the spread of infectious diseases and to seeing the end of a pandemic. The unprecedented vaccine development against SARS-CoV-2, based on efficient collaboration between academic institutions, pharmaceutical companies and governmental organizations, has allowed several efficacious vaccines to receive Emergency Use Authorization in record time, as described in Chapter 13. The execution of clinical trials on and their limitations for both vaccines and therapeutics are presented in Chapter 14.

Finally, we decided to close the book (Chapter 15) by trying to make a consensus of the whole experience of the COVID-19 pandemic. It is indeed important to try to summarize what has been learned from the pandemic. It is always easy in hindsight to say what should have been done and what should have been left undone. However, we should use all we have learned from COVID-19 to be better prepared for potential emerging pandemics in the future. It is hoped that with the knowledge and novel technologies acquired we might be able to stop future outbreaks reaching pandemic levels.

Debmalya Barh, Ph.D.
Kenneth Lundstrom, Ph.D.

Acknowledgments

We acknowledge the efforts of all our contributors for their generous support and cooperation in completing the book promptly in spite of all the difficulties during this unprecedented COVID-19 pandemic.

Editors

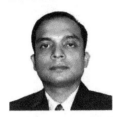 **Dr Debmalya Barh** is an M.Sc. (Applied Genetics), Ph.D. (Biotechnology), Ph.D. (Bioinformatics), Post-Doc (Bioinformatics), and PGDM (Postgraduate in Management). His work has blended both academic and industrial research for decades, and he is an expert in integrative omics-based biomarker and targeted drug discovery, genetic diagnosis, infectious diseases, and precision health. He is currently a Visiting Full Professor (Titular, Grade-E) at the Department of Genetics, Ecology and Evolution, Institute of Biological Sciences (ICB), Federal University of Minas Gerais (UFMG), Brazil. He is also an Honorary Scientist at the Institute of Integrative Omics and Applied Biotechnology (IIOAB), India. Dr Barh has published over 180 research and review articles, 40-plus book chapters, and has edited 25-plus books published by Taylor & Francis/ CRC Press, Elsevier, and Springer. He is an editorial board member of various journals including Frontiers, PeerJ, etc., and frequently reviews articles for Nature publications, Elsevier, AACR journals, NAR, BMC journals, and PlosOne, to name a few.

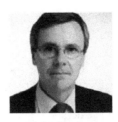 **Dr Kenneth Lundstrom** received his Ph.D. (Molecular Genetics) from the University of Helsinki, Finland and has acquired expertise in molecular biology, virology, gene expression, cancer therapy, vaccine development, and epigenetics from his affiliations with Cetus Corporation (Palo Alto, California), Orion Corporation (Helsinki, Finland), Glaxo Institute of Molecular Biology (Geneva, Switzerland), Glaxo Wellcome (Stevenage, UK), and Roche (Basel, Switzerland). Dr Lundstrom has been involved in applications of alphavirus vectors for drug discovery, neuroscience, gene therapy and vaccine development since the establishment of PanTherapeutics in Lutry (Lausanne), Switzerland. Dr Lundstrom's main interests remain in gene therapy, vaccines (including COVID-19), neuroscience, and epigenetics, and he has published more than 300 scientific research articles and reviews. He has edited two books on G Protein-Coupled Receptors and Structural Genomics, and authored a book on Nutrition and Disease. He serves on editorial boards of various journals including *Biomedicines and Viruses*, and acts as Editor-in-Chief for *Frontiers in Translational Virology*.

Contributors

Parise Adadi
Department of Food Science
University of Otago
Dunedin, New Zealand

Ruchika Agrawal
Department of Ear, Nose & Throat
All India Institute of Medical Sciences
Gorakhpur, India

Mohsen Akbarian
Pharmaceutical Sciences Research Center
Shiraz University of Medical Sciences
Shiraz, Iran

and

Department of Chemistry
National Cheng Kung University
Tainan, Taiwan

Alaa A. A. Aljabali
Faculty of Pharmacy
Department of Pharmaceutics and
  Pharmaceutical Technology
Yarmouk University–Faculty of Pharmacy
Irbid, Jordan

Gajendra Kumar Azad
Department of Zoology
Patna University
Patna, India

Wagner Baetas-da-Cruz
Translational Laboratory in Molecular
  Physiology
Centre for Experimental Surgery
College of Medicine
Federal University of Rio de Janeiro (UFRJ)
Rio de Janeiro, Brazil

Debmalya Barh
Department of Genetics, Ecology and Evolution
Institute of Biological Sciences (ICB)
Federal University of Minas Gerais (UFMG)
Belo Horizonte, Brazil

and

Institute of Integrative Omics and Applied
  Biotechnology (IIOAB)
Purba Medinipur, West Bengal, India

Nicolas G. Bazan
Neuroscience Center of Excellence
School of Medicine
Louisiana State University Health
New Orleans, LA, USA

Aparna Bhardwaj
Indian Institute of Technology Mandi
School of Basic Sciences
VPO Kamand, Mandi, India

Adam M. Brufsky
Department of Medicine
Division of Hematology/Oncology
UPMC Hillman Cancer Center
University of Pittsburgh School of Medicine
Pittsburgh, PA, USA

Yutein Chung
Department of Medicine
Division of Pulmonary
Critical Care and Sleep Medicine
Wayne State University School of Medicine and
  Detroit Medical Center
Detroit, MI, USA

David Connolly
College of Osteopathic Medicine
Michigan State University
East Lansing, MI, USA

Mauricio Corredor
GEBIOMIC Group
FCEN
University of Antioquia
Medellin, CO, USA

Isfendiyar Darbaz
Department of Obstetrics and Gynecology
Faculty of Veterinary Medicine
Near East University
Nicosia, North Cyprus, Turkey

Farzaneh Darbeheshti
Department of Genetics
School of Medicine
Tehran University of Medical Sciences
Tehran, Iran

Shailendra Dwivedi
Department of Biochemistry
All India Institute of Medical Sciences
Gorakhpur, India

Ifeanyichukwu E. Eke
Department of Microbiology and Molecular
  Genetics
Michigan State University
East Lansing, MI, USA

Rajanish Giri
Indian Institute of Technology Mandi
School of Basic Sciences
VPO Kamand
Mandi, India

Sunil Kumar Gupta
Department of Dermatology
All India Institute of Medical Sciences
Gorakhpur, India

Shivani Krishna Kapuganti
Indian Institute of Technology Mandi
School of Basic Sciences
VPO Kamand
Mandi, India

Suleyman Gokhan Kara
Department of Emergency Medicine
Eskisehir City Hospital

and

Cellular Therapy and Stem Cell Production
    Application and Research Centre
ESTEM

and

Department of Stem Cell
Institute of Health Sciences
Eskisehir Osmangazi University
Eskisehir, Turkey

Havva Ö. Kılgöz
Faculty of Dentistry
Eastern Mediterranean University
Famagusta, North Cyprus, Turkey

and

Department of Medical Biology and Genetics
School of Medicine
Marmara University
Istanbul, Turkey

Eymen Ü. Kılıç
Faculty of Arts and Sciences
Department of Biological Sciences
Eastern Mediterranean University
Famagusta, North Cyprus, Turkey

Surekha Kishore
Community Medicine & Family Medicine &
    Executive Director
All India Institute of Medical Sciences
Gorakhpur, India

Anoop Kumar
National Institute of Biologicals (NIB)
Ministry of Health & Family Welfare
Government of India
Noida, India

Ballamoole Krishna Kumar
Nitte (Deemed to be University)
Nitte University Centre for Science Education
    and Research (NUCSER)
Division of Infectious Diseases
Deralakatte, Mangaluru, India

Prashant Kumar
Amity Institute of Virology and Immunology
Noida, India

Prateek Kumar
Indian Institute of Technology Mandi
School of Basic Sciences
VPO Kamand, Mandi, India

Kenneth Lundstrom
PanTherapeutics
Lausanne, Switzerland

Biswajit Maiti
Nitte (Deemed to be University)
Nitte University Centre for Science Education
    and Research (NUCSER)
Division of Infectious Diseases
Deralakatte, Mangaluru, India

Radhieka Misra
Era's Lucknow Medical College and Hospital
Lucknow, India

Sanjeev Misra
Department of Surgical Oncology & Director
All India Institute of Medical Sciences
Jodhpur, India

Tarek Mohamed Abd El-Aziz
Zoology Department
Faculty of Science
Minia University
El-Minia, Egypt

and

Department of Cellular and Integrative
    Physiology
University of Texas Health Science Center at
    San Antonio
San Antonio, TX, USA

Gizem Morris
Department of Marketing
King's Business School
King's College London
London, United Kingdom

Giorgio Palù
Department of Molecular Medicine
University of Padua
Padua, Italy

Pritam Kumar Panda
Condensed Matter Theory Group
Materials Theory Division
Department of Physics and Astronomy
Uppsala, Sweden

Candan Hizel Perry
R&D Pharmacogenetics
OPTI-THREA, Inc.
Montreal, Canada

Praveen Rai
Nitte (Deemed to be University)
Nitte University Centre for Science Education
and Research (NUCSER)
Division of Infectious Diseases
Deralakatte, Mangaluru, India

Amit Ranjan
Department of Physical Medicine &
Rehabilitation
All India Institute of Medical Sciences
Gorakhpur, India

Aakanksha Rawat
Department of Ear, Nose & Throat
All India Institute of Medical Sciences
Gorakhpur, India

Alberto Reale
Department of Molecular Medicine
University of Padua
Padua, Italy

Elrashdy M. Redwan
Department of Biological Sciences
Faculty of Sciences
King Abdulaziz University
Jeddah, Saudi Arabia

Didem Rıfkı
Famagusta State Hospital
Famagusta, North Cyprus, Turkey

Lobelia Samavati
Department of Medicine
Division of Pulmonary, Critical Care and Sleep
Medicine
Wayne State University School of Medicine and
Detroit Medical Center

and

Center for Molecular Medicine and Genetics
Wayne State University School of Medicine
Detroit, MI, USA

Ayla Eker Sariboyaci
Cellular Therapy and Stem Cell Production
Application and Research Centre
ESTEM

and

Department of Stem Cell
Institute of Health Sciences
Eskisehir Osmangazi University
Eskisehir, Turkey

Hülya Şenol
Faculty of Arts and Sciences
Department of Biological Sciences
Eastern Mediterranean University
Famagusta, North Cyprus, Turkey

Ángel Serrano-Aroca
Biomaterials and Bioengineering Lab
Centro de Investigación Traslacional San
Alberto Magno
Universidad Católica de Valencia San Vicente
Mártir
Valencia, Spain

Murat Seyran
Doctoral Studies in Natural and Technical
Sciences (SPL 44)
University of Vienna
Vienna, Austria

Samendra P. Sherchan
Department of Environmental Health Sciences
Tulane University
New Orleans, LA, USA

Shashi Kumar Shetty
Nitte (Deemed to be University)
Medical Imaging Technology
Department of Radiodiagnosis & Imaging
K.S. Hegde Medical Academy
Deralakatte, Mangaluru, India

Kazuo Takayama
Center for IPS Cell Research and Application
Kyoto University
Kyoto, Japan

Murtaza M. Tambuwala
School of Pharmacy and Pharmaceutical
Science
Ulster University
Coleraine, Northern Ireland

Şükrü Tüzmen
Faculty of Dentistry
Eastern Mediterranean University

and

GenBiomics R&D
Eastern Mediterranean University
TechnoPark
Famagusta, North Cyprus, Turkey

Bruce D. Uhal
Department of Physiology
Michigan State University
East Lansing, Michigan

Vladimir N. Uversky
Department of Molecular Medicine and Health
Byrd Alzheimer's Institute
Morsani College of Medicine
University of South Florida
Tampa, FL, USA

and

Department of Biological Sciences
Faculty of Sciences
King Abdulaziz University
Jeddah, Saudi Arabia

Deekshit Vijaya Kumar
Nitte (Deemed to be University)
Nitte University Centre for Science Education
and Research (NUCSER)
Division of Infectious Diseases
Deralakatte, Mangaluru, India

Yong-Hui Zheng
Department of Microbiology and Molecular
Genetics
Michigan State University
East Lansing, MI, USA

Chapter 1   Coronavirus Epidemics and the Current COVID-19 Pandemic

Aparna Bhardwaj, Prateek Kumar, Shivani Krishna Kapuganti, Vladimir N. Uversky, and Rajanish Giri

1.1 EPIDEMIOLOGY OF CORONAVIRUSES

Coronaviruses cause a wide range of diseases such as gastroenteritis, encephalitis, pneumonia-like upper respiratory tract illnesses, and multiple organ failures involving the lungs and kidneys in a number of birds and some mammals [1]. Coronaviruses are enveloped viruses with a positive sense single-stranded RNA genome and club-like spikes that protrude from their surface [1, 2]. They are members of the Nidovirales order, including the Arteriviridae, Coronoviridae, Mesoviridae, and Roniviridae families. Corona-virinae and Torovirinae are subfamilies of the family Coronoviridae [2]. Coronaviridae is further subdivided into four genera: alpha, beta, gamma, and delta coronaviruses. The former two genera affect mammals, and the latter two are mainly responsible for disease in birds and fish, with some exceptions such as porcine deltacoronavirus (PDCoV), which belongs to the deltacoronavirus genus, but infects mammals [2, 3].

The name "coronavirus" was given because of the crown-like appearance of the club-shaped spike (S) protein on the viral surface (see Figure 1.1). Coronaviruses were previously thought to be associated only with mild respiratory illnesses in humans, such as the common cold, that usually resolve on their own and were not considered fatal or a dangerous threat until the SARS outbreak in 2002–2003, MERS in 2012, and recently COVID-19, which has claimed millions of lives worldwide. Currently, the whole world is locked in a pandemic situation. It has been over a year since the declaration of the COVID-19 pandemic by the World Health Organization (WHO) on March 11, 2020 [4, 5], and we are still struggling to find a way out. The first COVID-19 case was reported with diverse pneumonia-like symptoms in December 2019, in Wuhan City, Hubei province, China [4–7]. From its origin, COVID-19 has spread rapidly worldwide since March 2020, with over 170 million cases and over 3.5 million deaths (as of May 28, 2021 Worldmeter Corona cases data) [4, 5]. Further, identification and detailed molecular studies revealed that the causative agent for this disease was a novel virus (hence being named the Novel coronavirus 2019 or nCoV-2019) from the known Coronaviridae family [8]. Five laboratories in China independently performed etiological and sequencing studies for its identification [2, 8]. After taxonomic analysis, the International Committee of Taxonomy of Viruses (ICTV)

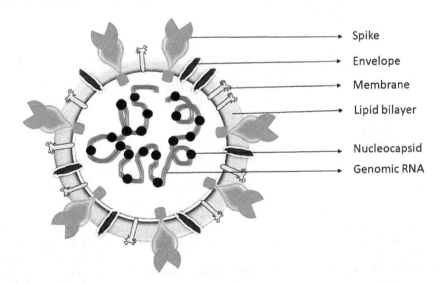

Figure 1.1   Representation of a typical structural model of coronavirus depicting its structural proteins: Spike, Envelope, Membrane, and Nucleocapsid, along with its RNA genome.

DOI: 10.1201/9781003190394-1

later named the virus Severe Acute Respiratory Syndrome Coronavirus-2 (SARS-CoV-2) [5], as the earlier outbreak of another dangerous human coronavirus, SARS-CoV, had occurred in 2002.

SARS-CoV-2 is closely related to SARS-CoV and bat coronaviruses, and more distantly to MERS-CoV. Bats are speculated to be the primary source of SARS-CoV-2, which possibly spread to humans through an intermediate host. As seen so far, the infected cases emerged over a period of months, which put many countries on the back foot. The introduction of travel restrictions, confinement, and lockdowns reduced the spread of SARS-CoV-2, but many countries, such as the USA, Brazil, India, etc. have already witnessed more than one wave of COVID-19. Several SARS-CoV-2 mutations with higher transmissibility have been detected in various countries, which has contributed to the appearance of new waves of COVID-19 with the enhanced risk of claiming more lives.

Early in the pandemic, a D614G variant in the spike (S) protein of SARS-CoV-2 was reported, which showed increased infectivity and replication efficiency. However, there were no significant differences in the pathogenicity of this SARS-CoV-2 variant. Later, the B.1.1.7 variant (alpha) was identified in the UK, which had more than a dozen mutations, most of them in the S protein. This variant reportedly had increased transmissibility [9], and individuals infected with this variant faced increased mortality. In late 2020, the B.1.351 variant (beta) was detected in South Africa. One particular mutation in this variant, E48K in the S protein, showed a reduction in neutralization by antibodies. Therefore, the efficacy of predesigned vaccines may be lowered. The P.1 variant (gamma) is responsible for the chaotic outbreak in Brazil. It has several mutations, including N501Y, E484K, K417T in the S protein [10]. The B.1.617 variant (delta) was first detected in India. It is speculated that this variant is responsible for the onset of the second wave of the pandemic in India and has been listed as a variant of concern (VoC) by the WHO. This variant has two prominent mutations, L452R and E484Q in the S protein, which are responsible for increased transmission and enhanced immune evasion [11].

SARS-CoV-2 spreads from person to person via direct contact, sneezing, coughing, or touching contaminated surfaces. It also shows airborne transmission. SARS-CoV-2 has been detected in respiratory secretions, ocular secretions, excreta, blood, and semen. On average, the virus can be detected in a patient after 18 days from the beginning of symptoms [10]. Furthermore, the transmission of SARS-CoV-2

by asymptomatic people is well documented, even though the resulting infection may be less severe. Risk of re-infection with the variants of concern is high. Typical symptoms include runny nose, sneezing, cough, breathlessness, and fatigue. Nowadays, a black fungal infection called mucormycosis (previously known as zygomycosis) has been increasingly reported in COVID-19 patients [10]. Blood clots and multi-organ failure, especially involving the lungs, kidney and heart, have proved fatal [12].

Because of the high mutation rate in RNA viruses, SARS-CoV-2 has managed to adapt to the environment, making complete eradication of the virus difficult, so far. While both drug repurposing strategies for existing antiviral drugs and vaccine development approaches have been executed, the expected success level has not been reached, at least partly because of new mutations appearing. Therefore preventative strategies such as wearing face masks/shields, maintaining at least a six-foot physical distance from other individuals, regular use of hand sanitizers and washing hands, diligent contact screening and treatment in isolation, and vaccinations are important procedures to keep the pandemic under control and to eradicate SARS-CoV-2 in the near future.

1.2 HISTORY AND EMERGENCE OF COMMON HUMAN CORONAVIRUSES (CoVs)

Human CoVs were first detected in 1965 in respiratory tract samples from patients with colds or respiratory illnesses, by virologists David Tyrrell and Mark Bynoe in Wiltshire, England [13–15]. Many different respiratory infectious viruses were identified, including the first coronavirus of human origin, B814 [14]. Furthermore, after sample fluids were tested in standard tissue cultures, volunteers were intra-nasally infected and showed common cold-like symptoms [14]. At the same time, Dorothy Hamre and John J. Procknow conducted serological studies on samples from medical students with respiratory illnesses at Chicago University [16]. The isolated virus showed a cytopathic effect, unlike effects seen for respiratory viruses of that time. The virus isolated from medical students was named 229E [16]. For the determination of genetic material, the two new strains were subjected to DNA synthesis inhibitors. Neither 5-fluorodeoxyuridine (FUDR) nor 5-iododeoxyuridine (IUDR) inhibited the growth of B814 or 229E strains, indicating that they were RNA viruses [16].

Tyrell and Bynoe, and Hamre and Procknow, independently demonstrated ether lability and sensitivity of the B814 and 229E viruses against

FUDR and IUDR [14, 16]. Since both B814 and 229E viruses were ether-sensitive, it was hypothesized that they needed a lipid-containing coat for infectivity. Morphological characterization of isolated viruses was carried out in 1967 by electron microscopy using negative staining. [17]. The B814 strain isolated by Tyrell and Bynoe, and the 229E strain isolated by Hamre and Procknow were identified. The 229E resembled the avian infectious bronchitis virus (IBV). Also, the B814 viral particles were indistinguishable from the avian IBV and 229E virus particles [17]. They were similar in terms of their pleomorphic shape, the average particle size with a diameter of 800–1200 Å, and 200 Å long surface projections [17]. Furthermore, the two viruses had similar features as the avian IBV virus, including size, resistance to DNA synthesis inhibitors, serological properties, and morphology [17]. After receiving approval from ICTV, Tyrell and Bynoe classified these viruses as coronaviruses. Roughly at the same time, several ether-sensitive viruses from human respiratory tracts were recovered [18], which were grown in organ cultures. These viruses were termed "OC" viruses to indicate passage in organ culture, and under electron microscopy they showed characteristic features of coronaviruses [18]. Unfortunately, many of the clinical samples collected and stored in the 1960s, which were positive for coronavirus-like particles, were subsequently lost [19]. Therefore, until the identification of SARS-CoV in 2003, research on human coronaviruses was limited to

the analysis of HCoV-229E and HCoV-OC43 [20], despite clear evidence of the presence of other strains of HCoVs [21, 22].

So far, seven strains of CoVs are known to infect humans (Figure 1.2). These are HCoV-229E, HCoV-OC43, HCoV-NL63, HCoV-HKU1, SARS-CoV, MERS-CoV, and SARS-CoV-2 [2, 23]. The first four viruses cause mild upper respiratory disease with severe conditions in children, elderly people, and immunocompromised patients [24]. These viruses are prevalent and infect humans repeatedly [24]. On the other hand, the viruses responsible for the recent outbreaks in the past decade (SARS-CoV, MERS-CoV), and SARS-CoV-2 severely attack the upper and lower respiratory tracts in all age groups [23, 25]. The first case of HCoV-NL63 was identified in 2003 [26]. It was isolated from a 7-month-old patient with acute respiratory infection [26]. It is speculated to have evolved from the HCoV-229E strain, as it shares a genome similarity of about 65% [27].

Further, the analysis and characterization of the full genome from patient samples showed that it has evolved from the already present virus. There are two variable regions in the viral genome and multiple recombination sites give its genome a mosaic structure. The variability in the genome of NL63 and analysis of the molecular clock suggested that this virus has been prevalent for decades [27]. HKU1 is another human coronavirus isolated from the nasopharyngeal aspirates of a 71-year-old pneumonia

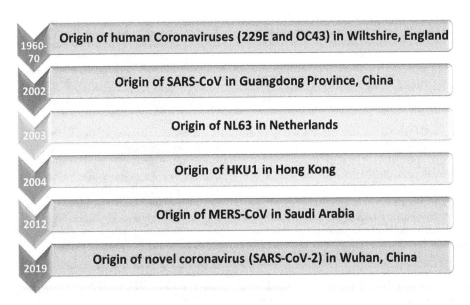

Figure 1.2 Benchmarks in the history of human coronaviruses. The repeated emergence of these coronaviruses has caused epidemics and pandemic-like situations worldwide.

Table 1.1 Some specific features of seven known human CoVs

Causative agent	Origin (Year)	Symptoms	Total Number Infected	Mortality Rate	Country of Origin	Natural and Intermediate Reservoir Host	Status
HCoV-229E	1966	Mild fever, cough, headache, runny nose, sore throat	42.9%–50.0% of children of 6–12 months of age; 65% of children of 2.5–3.5 years of age	—	Wiltshire, England	Bats	Outbreaks
HCoV-OC43	1967	Mild fever, cough, headache, runny nose, sore throat	10%–15% of common cold cases	—	United States	Rodents and cattle	Epidemic
SARS-CoV	2002	Acute respiration problems with cough, fever, and diarrhea	8,098 people infected, 774 deaths	9.6%	Guangdong Province, China	Bats and palm civets	Epidemic
HCoV-NL63	2003	Mild pneumonia-like symptoms	4.7% of common respiratory illnesses	—	The Netherlands	Bats	Outbreaks
HCoV-HKU1	2004	Mild pneumonia-like symptoms	2.6% of respiratory illnesses, mainly during the spring-summer period	—	Hong Kong	Rodents	Outbreaks
MERS-CoV	2012	Severe acute respiratory and renal problems	2,468 laboratory reported cases, 851 deaths	34.5%	Jeddah, Saudi Arabia	Bats and dromedary camels	Epidemic
SARS-CoV-2[a]	2019	Severe acute respiratory symptoms	169,880,483 infected, 3,530,154 deaths	2.1%[a]	Wuhan city, Hubei province, China	Postulated but not confirmed to be bats, pangolins	Pandemic

[a] Details of SARS-CoV-2 are reported as of May 28, 2021.

patient in 2004 who traveled to Hong Kong from Shenzhen, China [28a]. Phylogenetic studies and analysis grouped this virus with OC43 [28b].

SARS-CoV was the first HCoV to break the host species barrier, spreading to humans from the Chinese horseshoe bat in 2002 [29]. MERS-CoV is the second known HCoV of zoonotic origin, in which camels served as the intermediate hosts for the spread of the disease [30]. SARS-CoV-2 is the third HCoV spreading to humans and causing a pandemic [4, 5]. Apart from human CoVs, HKU2-related CoV is of animal origin, which also crossed the species barrier and infected pigs in China, first reported in October 2016 [31]. It was responsible for

the outbreak of swine disease in pig farms of Qingyuan, Guangdong province, China. This Swine Acute Diarrhea Syndrome-Coronavirus (SADS-CoV) is responsible for the death of 24,693 pigs [31]. It shares 98% similarity with the CoV isolated from the horseshoe bat [31]. In this chapter, we shall discuss the three recent human CoV outbreaks, among the seven HCoVs identified since the year 2000 (Table 1.1).

1.3 SEVERE ACUTE RESPIRATORY SYNDROME CORONAVIRUS (SARS-CoV)

The epidemic of SARS-CoV started in the Guangdong Province of China in November

2002 [32, 33]. Later in February 2003, the outbreak spread to Hong Kong [32, 33]. According to WHO, 2,353 cases were detected in April 2003 in Vietnam, at which point it was officially declared an epidemic [33, 34]. This epidemic affected many countries across the globe, including Singapore, Thailand, Vietnam, Taiwan, Hong Kong, Canada, and the USA [33, 35]. There were about 8,000 clinically reported cases, with 7–17% mortality caused by respiratory system failures and major alveolar damage [25, 33]. An International Collaborative group formed by the WHO in March 2003 investigated and identified the causative agent [33]. The name 'Severe Acute Respiratory Syndrome' (SARS) was then given because of its severe respiratory effects [32]. SARS-CoV belongs to lineage b of the betacoronavirus genus. SARS-CoV has a similar genome to all other CoVs, with a positive-sense single-stranded RNA genome [33]. It shares some partial sequence similarity with already known HCoVs, such as 229E and OC43. However, it has a considerable variation that required it to be placed in a different group and be given a unique identity. As a result of technological advancement in serological tests, the virus can be detected in the early stages of the onset of the disease by RT-PCR (Reverse transcription polymerase chain reaction) technique [33]. A virus with 99.8% sequence homology was also isolated from the sample study from animals in Guangzhou. It suggests that this virus might be of animal origin, and affects humans by crossing the species barrier. Civets were identified as natural hosts for SARS-CoV [33]. Surveillance and sample studies from patients revealed that 100% viral infection was attained within 2 weeks. Also, asymptomatic patients were tested positive for viral load by RT-PCR [33].

1.4 MIDDLE EAST RESPIRATORY SYNDROME CORONAVIRUS (MERS-CoV)

Ten years after the 2002 outbreak of SARS-CoV, the first case of MERS-CoV, which is believed to have originated in bats, transmitted to camels, and was reported in a patient in a hospital in Jeddah, Saudi Arabia in June 2012 [36]. According to the 2019 WHO report, since April 2012 (when the first MERS cases were reported), 2,468 laboratory-confirmed cases and 851 deaths are reported in 27 countries, of which 12 countries were in the Eastern Mediterranean region (https://applications.emro.who.int/docs/EMROPub-MERS-SEP-2019-EN.pdf?ua=1&ua=1).

The infection was similar to SARS-CoV. Molecular studies were conducted immediately, and diagnostic tests were developed. The European Centre for Disease Prevention and Control (ECDC) declared the Middle Eastern countries a hotspot, which included Saudi Arabia, Qatar, United Arab Emirates (UAE), Kuwait, Iran, Jordan, and Syria [30]. Moreover, an examination of nasal, lung, and rectal samples from camels in these countries showed positive RT-PCR results for 98%–100% of collected samples [30]. These results supported the fact that MERS-CoV is transmitted from camels to humans [30]. MERS-CoV belongs to lineage c of the betacoronavirus genus. Patients who suffer from MERS had lethal pneumonia and direct renal infections. Lung tissue studies revealed infiltration of macrophages and neutrophils with alveolar oedema [36].

1.5 SEVERE ACUTE RESPIRATORY SYNDROME CORONAVIRUS 2 (SARS-CoV-2)

The current COVID-19 disease caused by the outbreak of SARS-CoV-2 has been responsible for over 3.5 million deaths, as of June 2021. Furthermore, there are over 171.5 million confirmed cases globally [37]. The infection was first detected in a seafood market in Wuhan, China. SARS-CoV-2 bears a close resemblance to bat CoVs, and similar coronaviruses have been identified in pangolins, sold at Chinese seafood markets as food and components of traditional Chinese medication. This prompted the theory that the infection probably began in bats, while pangolins likely acted as intermediate hosts. SARS-CoV-2 quickly spread from one individual to another [38]. Infected individuals show common symptoms such as sore throat, fever, shortness of breath, and pneumonia. Death is caused by multi-organ failure, generally including lungs and kidneys. In the current pandemic, the cases of infections and mortality are much higher than in previous epidemics. Although the mortality rates for SARS, MERS, and COVID-19 are 9.6%, 34.5%, and 2.1%, respectively, the number of infections and deaths are certainly higher for COVID-19 than the two HCoV-related epidemics. Hence it is important to understand the difference between molecular structures of the different viruses. The section below compares the SARS-CoV-2 proteome to the proteomes of other HCoVs.

1.6 PROTEOMIC STRUCTURE OF SEVEN HUMAN CoVs

CoVs are positive-sense, single-stranded RNA viruses with a likely ancient origin, and HCoVs have repeatedly emerged during the past 1,000 years. Table 1.2 presents proteomes of seven HCoVs and shows that despite sharing a similar organization globally (being encoded by

Table 1.2 Some characteristics and major functions of proteins of various HCoVs

		HCoV-229E	HCoV-OC43	SARS-CoV	HCoV-NL63	HCoV-HKU1	MERS-CoV	SARS-CoV-2	Function
ORF1a (polyprotein pp1a)	ORF1ab (polyprotein pp1ab)								
NSP1		111 aa	246 aa	180 aa	110 aa	222 aa	193 aa	180 aa	Leader protein; host 40S ribosome binding, inhibition of the host mRNA translation, induction of the host mRNA degradation
NSP2		768 aa	605 aa	638 aa	788 aa	587 aa	660 aa	638 aa	RNA-binding protein that is accumulated in cytoplasmic inclusions (viroplasms) and is involved in CoV genome replication, binds to PHBs 1, 2
NSP3		1,587 aa	1,899 aa	1,922 aa	1,564 aa	1,979 aa	1,887 aa	1,945 aa	PLpro, papain-like protease responsible for processing the N-terminal region of polyproteins pp1a and pp1ab, generating NSP1, NSP2, and NSP3
NSP4		401 aa	496 aa	500 aa	477 aa	496 aa	507 aa	500 aa	Responsible for membrane rearrangement
NSP5		302 aa	303 aa	306 aa	303 aa	303 aa	306 aa	306 aa	Mpro, main protease or 3C-like proteinase (3CLpro), responsible for processing the C-terminal region of polyproteins pp1a and pp1ab, generating NSP4 through NSP16
NSP6		279 aa	287 aa	290 aa	279 aa	287 aa	292 aa	290 aa	Generates autophagosomes from the endoplasmic reticulum
NSP7		83 aa	89 aa	83 aa	83 aa	92 aa	83 aa	83 aa	Part of the RNA polymerase complex, interacts with NSP8 and NSP12
NSP8		195 aa	197 aa	198 aa	195 aa	194 aa	199 aa	198 aa	Part of the RNA polymerase complex, interacts with NSP7 and NSP12, stimulates NSP12
NSP9		109 aa	110 aa	113 aa	109 aa	110 aa	110 aa	113 aa	Binds to the host DEAD-box RNA helicase 5 (DDX5); important for viral replication
NSP10		135 aa	110 aa	139 aa	135 aa	137 aa	140 aa	139 aa	Stimulates NSP16, interacts 2ith NSP14
NSP11		17 aa	14 aa	13 aa	17 aa	14 aa	14 aa	13 aa	Function unknown

Protein								Function
NSP12	927 aa	928 aa	932 aa	927 aa	928 aa	933 aa	932 aa	RNA-dependent RNA polymerase (RdRp) that copies viral RNA and possesses methylation (guanine) activity
NSP13	597 aa	603 aa	601 aa	597 aa	603 aa	598 aa	601 aa	Possesses nucleoside triphosphatase (NTPase) activity and acts as helicase, possessing 5′-to-3′ RNA and DNA DNA duplex-unwinding activity
NSP14	518 aa	521 aa	527 aa	518 aa	521 aa	524 aa	527 aa	3′ to 5′ exonuclease, S-adenosylmethionine (SAM)-dependent (guanine-N7) methyl transferase (N7-MTase), incorporates the 5′-terminal cap structure to RNA
NSP15	348 aa	375 aa	346 aa	344 aa	374 aa	343 aa	346 aa	EndoRNAse/endoribonuclease that degrade RNA to evade host defense
NSP16	300 aa	299 aa	298 aa	300 aa	299 aa	303 aa	298 aa	2′-O-ribose-methyltransferase, that conducts methylation (adenine), shows 5′-cap RNA activity
Spike	1,173 aa	1,255 aa	1,368 aa	1,355 aa	1,351 aa	1,353 aa	1,273 aa	Surface glycoprotein that mediates attachment of the virus to the host cell via interaction with the human angiotensin-converting enzyme 2 (ACE2) receptor
Membrane	225 aa	221 aa	237 aa	226 aa	223 aa	219 aa	222 aa	An integral membrane protein that plays an important role in viral assembly and can induce apoptosis; interacts with the nucleocapsid protein to encapsulate the RNA genome
Nucleocapsid	389 aa	422 aa	441 aa	377 aa	441 aa	413 aa	419 aa	A structural protein that binds directly to viral RNA and provides stability; inhibits the activity of cyclin-cyclin-dependent kinase (cyclin-CDK) complex; in SARS-CoV-2, can antagonize antiviral RNAi
Envelope	77 aa	84 aa	76 aa	77 aa	82 aa	82 aa	75 aa	A small integral membrane protein that can oligomerize and create an ion channel; plays multiple roles in the viral replication cycle, involved in viral assembly, virion release, and viral pathogenesis
ORF3a	Not present	Not present	274 aa	Not present	Not present	Not present	275 aa	An ion channel protein related to NLRP3 inflammasome activation that interacts with TRAF3
ORF3	Not present	Not present	Not present	Not present	Not present	103 aa	Not present	Located in the host endoplasmic reticulum
Non-structural protein 3b; ORF4a	Not present	Not present	Not present	Not present	Not present	109 aa	Not present	Inhibits the NF-κB function; inhibits IFN regulatory factor 3 (IRF-3)
Non-structural protein 3c; ORF4b	Not present	Not present	Not present	Not present	Not present	246 aa	Not present	Inhibits IFN regulatory factor 3 (IRF-3)

(Continued)

Table 1.2 (Continued) Some characteristics and major functions of proteins of various HCoVs

	HCoV-229E	HCoV-OC43	SARS-CoV	HCoV-NL63	HCoV-HKU1	MERS-CoV	SARS-CoV-2
Non-structural protein 3d; ORF5	Not present	Not present	Not present	Not present	Not present	224 aa	Not present
	Inhibits IFN regulatory factor 3 (IRF-3)						
ORF6	Not present	Not present	63 aa	Not present	Not present	Not present	61 aa
	An accessory protein that related to viral pathogenesis; can interact with NSP8 and promote RNA polymerase activity						
ORF7a	Not present	Not present	122 aa	Not present	Not present	Not present	121 aa
	A type I transmembrane protein acting as an accessory protein						
ORF7b	Not present	Not present	44 aa	Not present	Not present	Not present	43 aa
	An accessory protein that that is localized in the Golgi compartment						
ORF8	Not present	Not present	Not present	Not present	Not present	Not present	121 aa
	Interacts with interferon regulatory factor 3 (IRF3) and inactivates interferon signaling						
ORF8a	Not present	Not present	39 aa	Not present	Not present	Not present	Not present
	Interacts with interferon regulatory factor 3 (IRF3) and inactivates interferon signaling						
ORF8b	Not present	Not present	84 aa	Not present	Not present	112 aa	121 aa
	Interacts with interferon regulatory factor 3 (IRF3) and inactivates interferon signaling						
ORF9b	Not present	Not present	98 aa	Not present	Not present	Not present	Not present
	Plays a role in the inhibition of host innate immune response by targeting the mitochondrial-associated adapter MAVS						
ORF10	Not present	Not present	Not present	Not present	Not present	Not present	38 aa
	A potential viral accessory protein						
Non-structural protein 2a	Not present	278 aa	Not present	Not present	Not present	Not present	Not present
	Shows high degree of sequence similarity to the phosphodiesterases (PDEs) from the mouse hepatitis virus (MHV)						
Non-structural protein 3	Not present	Not present	Not present	225 aa	Not present	Not present	Not present
	Accessory protein: multi-pass transmembrane protein embedded into host membrane						
Non-structural protein 4	Not present	Not present	Not present	Not present	109 aa	Not present	Not present
Non-structural protein 4a	133 aa	Not present	Not present	Not present	Not present	Not present	Not present
	Multi-pass transmembrane protein embedded into host membrane						

Non-structural protein 4b	88 aa	Not present	Not present	Not present	Not present	Not present	Not present	A potential viral accessory protein
Non-structural protein 5a	Not present	109 aa	Not present	Not present	Not present	Not present	Not present	Acts as membrane-anchoring region for structural proteins during virus assembly, or play a role in membrane association of the viral polymerase during replication
Hemagglutinin-esterase	Not present	424 aa	Not present	385 aa	Not present	Not present	Not present	Structural protein that makes short spikes at the surface of the virus; possesses receptor-binding and receptor-destroying activities; serve as a secondary viral attachment protein for initiating infection
Protein I	Not present	207 aa	Not present	205 aa	Not present	Not present	Not present	Structural protein not essential for the viral replication; encoded by a gene included within the N gene (alternative ORF)

exceptionally long non-segmented genomes), they are not identical. In fact, in addition to a set of common proteins found in all these HCoVs, such as polyproteins pp1a and pp1ab (encoded by the large overlapping open reading frames ORF1a and ORF1ab occupying approximately two-thirds of the genome), which are proteolytically cleaved to form 16 nonstructural proteins, (NSP1 to 16) as well as 4 structural proteins, spike (S), envelope (E), membrane (M), and nucleocapsid (N), there are virus-specific sets of accessory proteins. Furthermore, even common proteins, which are assumed to have similar or comparable functions during the viral life cycle are not identical and typically share rather low sequence identity levels. It is likely that the differences between these human HCoVs affect their infectivity and pathogenicity. Moreover, the morbidity and mortality rates are determined by the diversity of accessory proteins and by the dissimilarities of common proteins.

Since HCoVs are RNA viruses, they are characterized by high mutation rates caused either by random replication errors or introduced by RNA editing, which is utilized by the host as one of its defense mechanisms. Both synonymous (when nucleotide substitutions are not associated with changes in the chemical nature of the encoded amino acid) and non-synonymous (nucleotide substitutions that generate amino acid changes) mutations take place on a regular basis in the viral genome. The reported rate of acquired new mutations for SARS-CoV-2 is 0.9×10^{-3} substitutions/site/year, which corresponds to ~26 substitutions per year or ~2 changes per month, or the appearance of a new SARS-CoV-2 mutation every 11–15 days. While this mutation rate corresponds to about a half of the rate of the influenza virus and about a quarter of the HIV rate, it is rather similar to the evolution rates of other HCoVs, 0.80–2.38×10^{-3}, 0.63–1.12×10^{-3}, and 0.43×10^{-3} substitutions/site/year for SARS-CoV, MERS-CoV, and HCoV OC43, respectively.

1.7 THE PROTEOMES OF SARS-CoV AND SARS-CoV-2

SARS-CoV-2 also belongs to the genus beta-coronavirus. The genomic make-up for CoVs has been covered earlier in the chapter. This section delves into this aspect in detail with respect to SARS-CoV and SARS-CoV-2. More than 25 proteins are translated from the huge (~30kb) single-stranded RNA genome of SARS-CoV-2. According to RCSB-PDB, there are 29 proteins in the SARS-CoV-2 proteome. The genomic RNA has ~12 open reading frames (ORFs) which encode multiple nonstructural proteins (NSPs), structural proteins, and accessory proteins. The 16 NSPs are cleaved proteolytically from the two polyproteins, pp1a

(NSP1-11) and pp1ab (NSP12-16). Additionally, four structural proteins are encoded, and accessory proteins are expressed separately from the sub-genomic RNA [39, 40].

1.8 STRUCTURAL AND ACCESSORY PROTEINS OF SARS-CoV AND SARS-CoV-2

The structural and accessory proteins are translation products of ~10 kb from the 3' end one-third of the genome. The genes of these proteins are interspersed along the genome. As mentioned earlier, the structural proteins of SARS-CoV-2 are the S, E, M, and N proteins, and the ORFs code for accessory proteins ORF3a, ORF6, ORF7a, ORF8, ORF9, and ORF10, which are involved in the pathogenesis of the virus [40]. The structural proteins play crucial roles in pathogenesis, replication, viral packaging, and assembly [26]. Docking studies have shown that all four structural proteins interact with each other during their arrangement in the lipid bilayer [41]. The crystal structures of proteins from SARS-CoV and SARS-CoV-2 are presented in Figure 1.3.

The S protein forms homotrimers on the virion surface, as shown in Figure 1.3A. It is a transmembrane glycoprotein possessing subunits S1 and S2. S1 is an extracellular domain that interacts with the host cell receptor, and the S2 domain is involved in the fusion of the viral membrane with the host cell membrane. Thus S2 is known as a fusion peptide, which is further cleaved into S2' to become active and enhances the membrane fusion process. SARS-CoV and SARS-CoV-2 both use ACE2 as the entry receptor [42]. The crystal structure has been resolved for the SARS-CoV and SARS-CoV-2 E protein [43, 44]. In SARS-CoV, it is a single-transmembrane protein forming homo-pentameric ion channel (Figure 1.3B) with poor ionic specificity. The virulence is determined by the transmembrane or the C-terminal domain sequences [43]. Gadhave et al. proved experimentally that the C-terminal domain (CTD) of the E-protein is unstructured in an in vitro environment [45]. As the E protein enters the cellular environment, its conformation changes from disordered to ordered and amyloid state [45]. The SARS-CoV M protein interacts with other structural proteins such as S, E and N, and is involved in viral assembly and budding [46]. It is glycosylated at its ectodomain N-terminal and interacts with the other structural proteins through its C-terminal [41]. It is also responsible for membrane curvature formation and interacts internally with the N protein [46]. Alharbi and Alraefaei used several methods to compare the structures of SARS-CoV, MERS-CoV and SARS-CoV-2 M proteins. Notably, they observed that N-terminal domains of the M proteins of

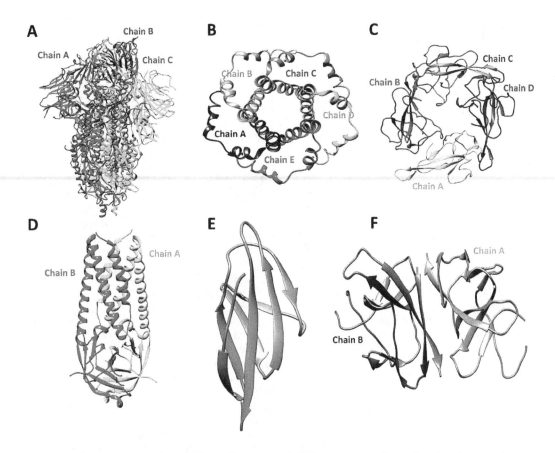

Figure 1.3   Depiction of some three-dimensional (3D) structures of structural and accessory proteins of SARS-CoV and SARS-CoV-2, retrieved from RCSB-PDB. (A) The S protein of SARS-CoV-2 (PDB_ID: 6VYB); (B) The E protein of SARS-CoV (PDB_ID: 5X29); (C) The N protein of SARS-CoV-2 (PDB_ID: 6VYO); (D) The ORF3a accessory protein of SARS-CoV-2 (PDB_ID: 6XDC); (E) The ORF7a accessory protein of SARS-CoV-2 (PDB_ID: 6W37); and (F) The ORF8 accessory protein of SARS-CoV-2 (PDB_ID: 7JTL). The structures are for protein domains, not for full-length proteins. More residual details are found at https://www.rcsb.org/ with PDB_ID of the respective protein.

SARS-CoV and SARS-CoV-2 are translocated (outside) the cell, whereas it is inside (cytoplasmic side) in MERS-CoV. Further, they observed differences in the predisposition of the proteins to intrinsic disorder. In fact, meta-predictor of intrinsic disorder has found two intrinsically disordered regions in the SARS-CoV-2 M protein, residues 1–7 and 205–222, whereas, three intrinsically disordered regions were found in the SARS-CoV M protein, residues 1–6, 207–210, and 216–221. The predicted secondary structure was characterized by three predicted α-helical regions in the M protein of SARS-CoV and SARS-CoV-2 and 4 in MERS-CoV [47]. The N protein binds RNA through its N-terminal domain, which plays a vital role in viral molecular processes. It forms a helical ribonucleoprotein complex with genomic RNA and is involved in

packaging of the viral genome, and in molecular and metabolic pathways of the virus [48]. Yang et al. determined the crystal structure of the SARS-CoV-2 N protein C-terminal domain, which has novel roles in RNA binding and transcription regulation. It was observed that a self-assembled higher order structure of SARS-CoV-2 N-CTD is different from that of the SARS-CoV N-CTD. SARS-CoV N-CTD forms octamers and a twin helix in the crystal structure, whereas SARS-CoV-2 N-CTD packs into a cylindrical shape in the crystal packing [49].

Three putative viroporins are encoded by the genome of SARS-CoV-2: E, ORF3a, and ORF8. These ion channels alter the permeability of the host cell membrane and thus assist in viral assembly [50]. ORFa is a cation (K^+) channel, which has shown inhibition of apoptosis and autophagy in vitro. Figure 1.3D shows the dimeric ORF3a channel [50].

ORF8 is an immune evasion protein that has evolved very rapidly. The ORF8 of SARS-CoV-2 is very distinct from ORF8 of SARS-CoV, with a sequence similarity of less than 20%. ORF8 of SARS-CoV-2 interrupts IFN-I signaling and decreases the level of MHC-I cells [51]. Figure 1.3C presents structures of structural proteins, and Figures 1.3D, 1.3E, and 1.3F show three of the accessory proteins of SARS-CoV and SARS-CoV-2. Two of the accessory proteins of SARS-CoV, ORF3b, and ORF6, have been reported to act as interferon antagonists and inhibit the expression downstream, i.e., signaling for innate immunity in host cells [52]. As interferon antagonists, they block the movement of STAT1 to the nucleus. STAT1 is a signal mediator of both IFN-α and IFN-β and acts as a transactivator. Thus because of viral interference, the IFN pathway is downregulated [53]. ORF7a is a type I transmembrane protein, which induces apoptosis of host cells by inhibition of translation and suppression of the cell cycle [54]. ORF9b is translated from the bicistronic mRNA via leaky ribosome scanning and plays an important role in viral particle packaging [55].

1.9 NON-STRUCTURAL PROTEINS (NSPs) OF SARS-CoV AND SARS-CoV-2

NSPs are translated from ~20 kb (comprising two-thirds of the whole genome) of replicase genes at the 5′ end. The virus has sixteen non-structural proteins, NSP1-16, which are involved in viral RNA synthesis by forming replication transcription complexes (RTCs). The NSPs manage the complex replication process through their enzymatic activities, including papain-like proteinase (PL^{pro}, NSP3), main protease (3CL^{pro}, NSP5), RNA-dependent-RNA polymerase (RdRp, NSP12), RNA helicase (NSP13), guanine-N-7 methyltransferase (NSP14), endoribonuclease (NSP15), and 2′-O-methyltransferase (NSP16) [40].

NSP1 is the cleavage product of the action of PLpro from the divergent 5′ end sequence. The physiological function of SARS-CoV-2 NSP1 is not yet fully understood. Figure 1.4A shows the crystal structure of the NSP1 N-terminal region (polypeptide of residues 13–128) of SARS-CoV [56]. It blocks the translation in the host by binding to the ribosomal 40S subunit. Correlated computational and experimental studies showed the C-terminal of NSP1 as disordered, but it gains helical conformation when provided with organic solvents in its surrounding environment [57]. Much less is known about the NSP2 of SARS-CoV and SARS-CoV-2, but NSP2 has been suggested to suppress the host immune system, such as NSP1, and to

interact with NSP3 [58]. NSP3 is a viral papain-like protease (PLpro) with cysteine in its active site (Figure 1.4B). PLpro cleaves polyproteins for the formation of mature proteins by identifying a specific motif sequence (LXGG) between proteins. It triggers the host innate immunity by its inhibitory action on the production of cytokines and chemokines [59]. It also interacts with NSP4 (predicted to be a transmembrane protein) along with NSP6 (which is also a transmembrane protein) to form a complex to modify the ER into double-membrane vesicles [58]. NSP5 is the main protease (Mpro), also known as 3C-like protease (Figure 1.4C). It is one of the vital enzymes for viral replication and transcription. It cleaves 11 conserved sites on the proteome after its autolytic cleavage from pp1a and pp1ab [60]. These proteases are centrally placed targets for antiviral drugs. However, it was recently reported that viruses mutate at certain hotspots in NSP5, resulting in impaired vaccine efficacy [61]. NSP11 is a small disordered protein of only 13 amino acids, with disordered-like characteristics even in the presence of some natural osmolytes [62].

The main active replication complex consists of the catalytic subunit NSP12 (RdRp), along with accessory subunits NSP8 and NSP7, as shown in Figure 1.4D [63]. The NSP12 is a single subunit polymerase that resembles the right hand: N-terminal domain (fingers), interface domain (palm), and C-terminal domain of RdRp (thumb). The NSP8 and NSP7 bind to the thumb-like domain to function [63]. NSP9 is a dimeric protein when active, with inter-subunit interactions via conserved helical motifs, as shown in Figure 1.4E [64]. Alterations or disruptions of the sequence in this motif leads to a reduction in RNA replication of the virus. This shows its prominent role in RNA binding and replication. It is one of the highly conserved proteins of SARS-CoV-2, which shares 97% similarity with SARS-CoV [64].

Viral RNA translation is improved by methylation of genomic RNA, which also facilitates viruses to trick the host immune system. The methylation is catalyzed by NSP16 and NSP10 (Figure 1.4F), which form a 2′O-methyltransferase complex [65]. The methyl group is donated by the S-adenosyl-L-methionine (SAM) [65]. NSP14 has two domains: the N-terminal for proofreading and the C-terminal for guanine-N7-methyltransferase activity. It is also an important protein linked to viral replication and transcription. NSP13 is the viral RNA helicase, belonging to the helicase superfamily 1 that unwinds the intermediate double-stranded RNA through the nucleotide hydrolysis process. It also has an NTPase activity [39] (Figure 1.4H). NSP10 is a

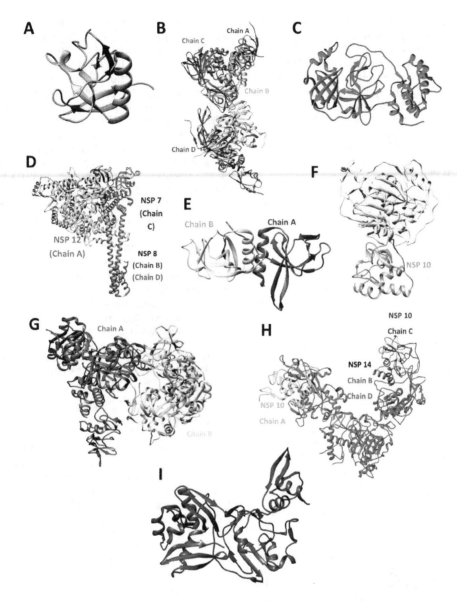

Figure 1.4 Presentation of some of the 3D structures of non-structural proteins (NSPs) of SARS-CoV and SARS-CoV-2, retrieved from RCSB-PDB. (A) NSP1 of SARS-CoV (PDB_ID: 2HSX); (B) NSP3 of SARS-CoV (PDB_ID: 6WUU); (C) NSP5 of SARS-CoV-2 (PDB_ID: 6LU7); (D) Complex of NSP12, NSP8 and NSP7 of SARS-CoV-2 (PDB_ID: 6YYT); (E) NSP9 of SARS-CoV-2 (PDB_ID: 6WXD); (F) Complex of NSP16 and NSP10 of SARS-CoV-2 (PDB_ID: 6WVN); (G) NSP13 of SARS-CoV-2 (PDB_ID: 6ZSL); (H) Complex of NSP 14 and NSP 10 of SARS-CoV (PDB_ID: 5C8S); and (I) NSP 15 of SARS-CoV-2 (PDB_ID: 6WXC). Some of the proteins have truncated structures as full-length structures are not available because of missing electron density for some residues. More residual details are found at https://www.rcsb.org/ with PDB_ID of the respective protein.

co-activator of NSP14 (Figure 1.4H) [66]. NSP15 endoribonuclease, when active, forms three dimers and cleaves specifically at uridine residual sites (Figure 1.4I). The C-terminal domain has catalytic activity with uridine-binding residues. It is capable of cleaving both single and double-stranded RNA and belongs to the highly conserved EndoU family prevalent in all CoVs [67].

1.10 THERAPEUTIC TARGETS OF CoVs

Since the S protein is exposed and involved in the first step of host cell infection, it is the main therapeutic target for neutralizing antibodies [42]. Apart from the S protein, the E protein, and other proteins can be targets for protein-based vaccines or for virus-like particle (VLP) systems. The E protein is essential for the pathogenicity and mortality caused by the virus, as confirmed by studies in animal models [43]. The M protein is complexed with the host immune components like HLA1 and β2-microglobulin, and has also been reported to be a potential target [68]. Three ion channel-forming proteins (E, ORF3a, and ORF8) offer good targets, as these enhance the pathogenicity of the virus by altering the ionic balance in host cells [50]. The active replication complex (NSP12-NSP8-NSP7) is the main target for inhibition of virus growth, as it is the key enzyme for virus survival [63]. The NSP12 is the main target for drugs in this complex, but mutations rendering the virus resistant to drugs have been described [69]. The current antiviral approaches use the S protein and the two proteases, NSP3 (papain-like protease) and NSP5 (3CL protease), as the main targets. However, these strategies can cause severe side effects, as they act non-specifically on host cellular proteases [48]. As NSP15 acts as an endoribonuclease its uridine-binding active site has been used as a drug target because of its effect on host immunity. Tipiracil, a synthesized drug that is a uridine analogue derived from uridine itself, binds to the active site of NSP15 and inhibits its activity [67]. Computational drug screening and simulation studies have been carried out against multiple targets of SARS-CoV and SARS-CoV-2, such as the S protein, proteases, helicases, RdRp, etc. [70, 71]. Moreover, computational methods have been applied for vaccine design targeting multiple epitopes of the structural proteins of SARS-CoV-2 [72].

1.11 CONCLUSIONS AND FUTURE PERSPECTIVES

So far, the human population has faced seven HCoVs,. The recent outbreak of SARS-CoV-2 causing COVID-19 has proved to be very deadly, causing more than 3.5 million deaths worldwide. Unfortunately, the death count increases with every passing day. All developing, as well as developed countries, have been hit extremely hard. The healthcare systems and economy in the world have been stretched to their limits. Therefore, a better healthcare infrastructure and economic system is required, as other outbreaks of CoVs or other viruses may emerge in the future as a result of their adaptive nature and high mutation rates. There are no specific antiviral drugs available for the efficient prevention and treatment of COVID-19. In the past year alone, several vaccines have been developed for SARS-CoV-2, which is a huge milestone achieved by the scientific community. The need of the hour is to develop efficient drugs with minimal side effects, and vaccines that would offer a broad range of immunity against emerging variants and novel mutants. Furthermore, we need to develop a positive attitude with complete awareness of necessary vaccine re-engineering, and well-managed, easily available healthcare systems.

With this book chapter, we wish to express our gratitude and special thanks to healthcare and frontline workers for saving millions of lives by risking their own.

ACKNOWLEDGEMENTS

The authors would like to thank IIT Mandi for providing facilities and would like to acknowledge receiving the following grants: DBT, Government of India (BT/11/IYBA/2018/06); SERB, Government of India (CRG/2019/005603) to RG.

Conflict of Interest: All authors declare that there is no financial competing interest.

REFERENCES

1. Haake, C., Cook, S., Pusterla, N., Murphy, B. (2020). Coronavirus infections in companion animals: Virology, epidemiology, clinical and pathologic features. *Viruses*. 12, 1–22. doi:10.3390/v12091023.

2. Chen, Y., Liu, Q., Guo, D. (2020). Coronaviruses: Genome structure, replication, and pathogenesis. *J. Med. Virol.* 92, 418–423. doi:10.1002/jmv.25681.

3. Jackwood, M.W., Hall, D., Handel, A. (2012). Molecular evolution and emergence of avian gammacoronaviruses. *Infect. Genet. Evol.* 12, 1305–1311. doi:10.1016/j.meegid.2012.05.003.

4. Khanna, R.C., Cicinelli, M.V., Gilbert, S.S., Honavar, S.G., Murthy, G.V.S. (2020). Review article COVID-19 pandemic: Lessons learned and future directions. *Indian J. Ophthalmol.* doi:10.4103/ijo.IJO.

5. Liu, Y., Kuo, R., Shih, S. (2020). COVID-19: The first documented coronavirus pandemic in history. *Biomed. J.* 43, 328–333. doi:10.1016/j.bj.2020.04.007.

6. Van Damme, W., Dahake, R., Delamou, A., Ingelbeen, B., Dossou, P., Wouters, E., Vanham, G., Van De Pas, R., Bloom, G., Van Engelgem, I., Ali, M., Ahmed, A., Kiendrébéogo, J.A., Verdonck, K., De Brouwere, V., Bello, K., Kloos, H., Aaby, P., Kalk, A. (2020). The COVID-19 pandemic: Diverse contexts; different epidemics — How and why? *BMJ Global Health* 1–16. doi:10.1136/bmjgh-2020-003098.

7. Pitlik, S.D. (2020). COVID-19 compared to other pandemic diseases. *Rambam Maimonides Med. J.* 11, 1–17. doi:10.5041/RMMJ.10418.

8. Tao, Z., Tian, J., Pei, Y.-Y., Yuan, M.-L., Zhang, Y.Y.-Z.Y.-L., Dai, F.-H., Wu, F., Zhao, S., Yu, B., Chen, Y.-M., Wang, W., Song, Z.-G., Hu, Y., Tao, Z., Tian, J., Pei, Y.-Y., Yuan, M.-L., Zhang, Y.Y.-Z.Y.-L., Dai, F.-H., Liu, Y., Wang, Q.-M., Zheng, J.-J., Xu, L., Holmes, E.C., Zhang, Y.Y.-Z.Y.-L. (2020). A new coronavirus associated with human respiratory disease in China. *Nature.* 579, 265–269. doi:10.1038/s41586-020-2008-3.

9. Graham, M.S., Sudre, C.H., May, A., Antonelli, M., Murray, B., Varsavsky, T., Kläser, K., Canas, L.S., Molteni, E., Modat, M., Drew, D.A., Nguyen, L.H., Polidori, L., Selvachandran, S., Hu, C. (2021). Changes in symptomatology, reinfection, and transmissibility associated with the SARS-CoV-2 variant B.1.1.7: An ecological study. *Lancet Public Health.* doi:10.1016/s2468-2667(21)00055-4.

10. Pöhlmann, S.P., Hoffmann, M., Arora, P., Groß, R., Kleger, A., Münch, J. (2020). SARS-CoV-2 variants B.1.351 and P.1 escape from neutralizing antibodies. *Cell* 84, 2324–2393. doi:10.1016/j.cell.2021.03.036.

11. Vaidyanathan, G. (2021). Coronavirus variants are spreading in India — What scientists know so far. *Nature.* doi:10.1038/d41586-021-01274-7.

12. Mokhtari, T., Hassani, F., Ghaffari, N., Ebrahimi, B., Yarahmadi, A., Hassanzadeh, G. (2020). COVID-19 and multiorgan failure: A narrative review on potential mechanisms. *J. Mol. Histol.* 51, 613–628. doi:10.1007/s10735-020-09915-3.

13. Mahase, E. (2020). COVID-19: Coronavirus was first described in The BMJ in 1965. *BMJ* 369, m1547. doi:10.1136/bmj.m1547.

14. Tyrrell, D.A., Bynoe, M.L. (1966). Cultivation of viruses from a high proportion of patients with colds. *Lancet.* 1, 76–77. doi:10.1016/s0140-6736(66)92364-6.

15. Kahn, J.S., McIntosh, K. (2005). History and recent advances in coronavirus discovery. *Pediatr. Infect. Dis. J.*24, 223–227. doi:10.1097/01.inf.0000188166.17324.60.

16. Hamre, D., Procknow, J.J. (1962). A new virus isolated from the human respiratory tract. *Cureus* 190–193. doi:10.3181/00379727-121-30734.

17. Tyrrell, D.A.J., Almeida, J.D. (1967). The morphology of three previously uncharacterized human respiratory viruses that grow in organ culture. Department of Medical Microbiology, St Thomas's Hospital Medical School. *J. Gen. Virol.* 175–178. doi:10.1099/0022-1317-1-2-175.

18. McIntosh, K., Dees, J.H., Becker, W.B., A.Z. Kapikian, R.M. Chanock (1967). Recovery in tracheal organ cultures of novel viruses from patients with respiratory disease. *Proc. Natl. Acad. Sci. USA* 57, 933–940.

19. Berry, M., Gamieldien, J., Fielding, B.C. (2015). Identification of new respiratory viruses in the new millennium. *Viruses.* 7, 996–1019. doi:10.3390/v7030996.

20. McIntosh, K. (2005). Coronaviruses in the limelight. *J. Infect. Dis.* 191, 489–491.

21. McIntosh, K., Kapikian, A.Z., Hardison, K.A., Hartley, J.W., Chanock, R.M. (1969). Antigenic relationships among the coronaviruses of man and between human and animal coronaviruses. *J. Immunol.* 102, 1109–1118.

22. Lee, N., Hui, D., Wu, A., Chan, P., Cameron, P., Joynt, G.M., Ahuja, A., Yung, M.Y., Leung, C., To, K.F. (2003). A major outbreak of severe acute respiratory syndrome in Hong Kong. *N. Engl. J. Med.* 348, 1986–1994.

23. Su, S., Wong, G., Shi, W., Liu, J., Lai, A.C.K., Zhou, J., Liu, W., Bi, Y., Gao, G.F. (2016). Epidemiology, genetic recombination, and pathogenesis of coronaviruses. *Trends Microbiol.* 24, 490–502. doi:10.1016/j.tim.2016.03.003.

24. Liang, Y., Wang, M.L., Chien, C.S., Yarmishyn, A.A., Yang, Y.P., Lai, W.Y., Luo, Y.H., Lin, Y.T., Chen, Y.J., Chang, P.C., Chiou, S.H. (2020). Highlight of immune pathogenic response and hematopathologic effect in SARS-CoV, MERS-CoV, and SARS-Cov-2 infection. *Front. Immunol.* 11, 1–11. doi:10.3389/fimmu.2020.01022.

25. Kin, N., Miszczak, F., Lin, W., Ar Gouilh, M., Vabret, A., Consortium, E. (2015). Genomic analysis of 15 human coronaviruses OC43 (HCoV-OC43s) circulating in France from 2001 to 2013 reveals a high intra-specific diversity with new recombinant genotypes. *Viruses.* 7, 2358–2377. doi:10.3390/v7052358.

26. Van Der Hoek, L., Pyrc, K., Jebbink, M.F., Vermeulen-Oost, W., Berkhout, R.J.M., Wolthers, K.C., Wertheim-Van Dillen, P.M.E., Kaandorp, J., Spaargaren, J., Berkhout, B. (2004). Identification of a new human coronavirus. *Nat. Med.* 10, 368–373. doi:10.1038/nm1024.

27. Pyrc, K., Dijkman, R., Deng, L., Jebbink, M.F., Ross, H.A., Berkhout, B., van der Hoek, L. (2006). Mosaic structure of human coronavirus NL63, one thousand years of evolution. *J. Mol. Biol.* 364, 964–973. doi:10.1016/j.jmb.2006.09.074.

28a. Woo, P.C.Y., Lau, S.K.P., Chu, C., Chan, K., Tsoi, H., Huang, Y., Wong, B.H.L., Poon, R.W.S., Cai, J.J., Luk, W., Poon, L.L.M., Wong, S.S.Y., Guan, Y.,

Peiris, J.S.M., Yuen, K. (2005). Characterization and complete genome sequence of a novel coronavirus, coronavirus HKU1, from patients with pneumonia. *J. Virol.* 79, 884–895. doi:10.1128/jvi.79.2.884-895.2005.

28b. Chaillon, A. Li, X., Zai, J., Zhao, Q., Nie, Q., Li, Y., Foley, B.T. (2020). Evolutionary history, potential intermediate animal host, and cross-species analyses of SARS-CoV-2.pdf. *J. Med. Virol..* doi:10.1002/jmv.25731.

30. Al-Osail, A.M., Al-Wazzah, M.J. (2017). The history and epidemiology of Middle East respiratory syndrome corona virus. *Multidiscip. Respir. Med.* 12, 1–6. doi:10.1186/s40248-017-0101-8.

31. Zhou, P., Fan, H., Lan, T., Yang, X.L., Shi, W.F., Zhang, W., Zhu, Y., Zhang, Y.W., Xie, Q.M., Mani, S., Zheng, X.S., Li, B., Li, J.M., Guo, H., Pei, G.Q., An, X.P., Chen, J.W., Zhou, L., Mai, K.J., Wu, Z.X., Li, D., Anderson, D.E., Zhang, L.B., Li, S.Y., Mi, Z.Q., He, T.T., Cong, F., Guo, P.J., Huang, R., Luo, Y., Liu, X.L., Chen, J., Huang, Y., Sun, Q., Zhang, X.L.L., Wang, Y.Y., Xing, S.Z., Chen, Y.S., Sun, Y., Li, J., Daszak, P., Wang, L.F., Shi, Z.L., Tong, Y.G., Ma, J.Y. (2018). Fatal swine acute diarrhoea syndrome caused by an HKU2-related coronavirus of bat origin. *Nature.* 556, 255–259. doi:10.1038/s41586-018-0010-9.

32. Chan-Yeung, M., Xu, R., Sinha, M., Pande, B., Sinha, R., Zhou, Y., Macgeorge, E.L., Myrick, J.G., Morin, C.M., Carrier, J., Bastien, C., Godbout, R., Choi, E.P.H., Hui, B.P.H., Wan, E.Y.F., O'Connor, R.C., Wetherall, K., Cleare, S., McClelland, H., Melson, A.J., Niedzwiedz, C.L., O'Carroll, R.E., O'Connor, D.B., Platt, S., Scowcroft, E., Watson, B., Zortea, T., Ferguson, E., Robb, K.A., Pierce, M., Hope, H., Ford, T., Hatch, S., Hotopf, M., John, A., Kontopantelis, E., Webb, R., Wessely, S., McManus, S., Abel, K.M., Ingram, J., Maciejewski, G., Hand, C.J. (2003). SARS: Epidemiology. *Respirology* 8, S9–S14.

33. Poon, L.L.M. (2003). Sars and other coronaviruses in humans and animals, 457–462.

34. Drosten, L.L.M., Günther, S., Preiser, W., van der Werf, S., Brodt, H.-R., Becker, S., Rabenau, H., Panning, M., Kolesnikova, L., Fouchier, R.A.M., Berger, A., Burguière, A.-M., Cinatl, J., Eickmann, M., Escriou, N., Grywna, K., Kramme, S., Manuguerra, J.-C., Müller, S., Rickerts, V., Stürmer, M., Vieth, S., Klenk, H.-D., Osterhaus, A.D.M.E., Schmitz, H., Doerr, H.W. (2003). Identification of a novel coronavirus in patients with severe acute respiratory syndrome. *N. Engl. J. Med.* 348, 1967–1976. doi:10.1056/nejmoa030747.

35. Kumar, D. (2020). Corona virus: A review of COVID-19. doi:10.14744/ejmo.2020.51418.

36. Zumla, A., Hui, D.S., Perlman, S. (2015). Middle East respiratory syndrome. *Lancet* 386, 995–1007. doi:10.1016/S0140-6736(15)60454-8.

37. World Health Organization (2021). COVID-19 weekly epidemiological update 22. *World Heal. Organ.* 1–3.

38. Zhang, T., Wu, Q., Zhang, Z. (2020). Probable pangolin origin of SARS-CoV-2 associated with the COVID-19 outbreak. *Curr. Biol.* 30, 1346–1351. doi:10.1016/j.cub.2020.03.022.

39. Lubin, J.H., Zardecki, C., Dolan, E.M., Lu, C., Shen, Z., Dutta, S., Westbrook, J.D., Xie, L., Venkatachalam, T., Arnold, S. (2020). Evolution of the SARS-CoV-2 proteome in three dimensions (3D) during the first six months of the COVID-19 pandemic. *bioRxiv.* doi:10.1101/2020.12.01.406637.

40. Bojkova, D., Klann, K., Koch, B., Widera, M., Krause, D. (2020). Proteomics of SARS-CoV-2-infected host cells reveals therapy targets. *Nature.* 583. doi:10.1038/s41586-020-2332-7.

41. Kumar, A., Kumar, P., Garg, N., Giri, R. (2020). An insight into SARS-CoV-2 Membrane protein interaction with Spike, Envelope, and Nucleocapsid proteins. *bioRxiv.* doi:10.1101/2020.10.30.363002.

42. Walls, A.C., Park, Y.J., Tortorici, M.A., Wall, A., McGuire, A.T., Veesler, D. (2020). Structure, function, and antigenicity of the SARS-CoV-2 spike glycoprotein, *Cell* 181, 281–292. doi:10.1016/j.cell.2020.02.058.

43. Surya, W., Li, Y., Torres, J. (2018). Structural model of the SARS coronavirus E channel in LMPG micelles. *Biochim. Biophys. Acta Biomembr.* 1860, 1309–1317. doi:10.1016/j.bbamem.2018.02.017.

44. Mandala, V.S., McKay, M.J., Shcherbakov, A.A., Dregni, A.J., Kolocouris, A., Hong, M. (2020). Structure and drug binding of the SARS-CoV-2 envelope protein transmembrane domain in lipid bilayers. *Nat. Struct. Mol. Biol.* 27, 1202–1208. 10.1038/s41594-020-00536-8.

45. Gadhave, K., Kumar, A., Kumar, P., Kapuganti, S.K., Garg, N., Vendruscolo, M., Giri, R. (2020). Environmental dependence of the structure of the c-terminal domain of the SARS-CoV-2 envelope protein. *bioRxiv.* doi:10.1101/2020.12.29.424646.

46. Arndt, A.L., Larson, B.J., Hogue, B.G. (2010). A conserved domain in the coronavirus membrane protein tail is important for virus assembly. *J. Virol.* 84, 11418–11428. doi:10.1128/JVI.01131-10.

47. Alharbi, S.N., Alrefaei, A.F. (2021). Comparison of the SARS-CoV-2 (2019-nCoV) M protein with its counterparts of SARS-CoV and MERS-CoV species. *J. King Saud Univ. Sci.* 33. doi:10.1016/j.jksus.2020.101335.

48. Kang, S., Yang, M., Hong, Z., Zhang, L., Huang, Z., Chen, X., He, S., Zhou, Z., Zhou, Z., Chen, Q., Yan, Y., Zhang, C., Shan, H., Chen, S. (2020). Crystal structure of SARS-CoV-2 nucleocapsid protein RNA binding domain reveals potential unique drug targeting sites. *Acta Pharm. Sin. B* 10, 1228–1238. doi:10.1016/j.apsb.2020.04.009.

49. Yang, M., He, S., Chen, X., Huang, Z., Zhou, Z., Zhou, Z., Chen, Q., Chen, S., Kang, S. (2021). Structural insight into the SARS-CoV-2 nucleocapsid protein C-Terminal domain reveals a novel recognition mechanism for viral transcriptional

regulatory sequences. *Front. Chem.* 8. doi:10.3389/fchem.2020.624765.

50. Brohawn, S.G., Kern, D.M., Sorum, B., Mali, S.S., Hoel, C.M., Sridharan, S., Remis, J.P., Toso, D.B., Kotecha, A., Bautista, D.M. (2021). Cryo-EM structure of the SARS-CoV-2 3a ion channel in lipid nanodiscs. *bioRxiv* 1–43. doi:10.1101/2020.06.17.156554.

51. Flower, T.G., Buffalo, C.Z., Hooy, R.M., Allaire, M., Ren, X., Hurley, J.H. (2020). Structure of SARS-CoV-2 ORF8, a rapidly evolving coronavirus protein implicated in immune evasion. *bioRxiv* 1–6. doi:10.1101/2020.08.27.270637.

52. Kopecky-Bromberg, S.A., Martínez-Sobrido, L., Frieman, M., Baric, R.A., Palese, P. (2007). Severe acute respiratory syndrome coronavirus Open Reading Frame (ORF) 3b, ORF 6, and nucleocapsid proteins function as interferon antagonists. *J. Virol.* 81, 548–557. doi:10.1128/jvi.01782-06.

53. Frieman, M., Yount, B., M. Heise, Kopecky-Bromberg, S.A., Palese, P., Baric, R.S. (2007). Severe acute respiratory syndrome coronavirus ORF6 antagonizes STAT1 function by sequestering nuclear import factors on the rough endoplasmic reticulum/Golgi membrane. *J. Virol.* 81, 9812–9824. doi:10.1128/jvi.01012-07.

54. Huang, C., Ito, N., Tseng, C.-T.K., Makino, S. (2006). Severe acute respiratory syndrome coronavirus 7a accessory protein is a viral structural protein. *J. Virol.* 80, 7287–7294. doi:10.1128/jvi.00414-06.

55. Xu, K., Zheng, B.J., Zeng, R., Lu, W., Lin, Y.P., Xue, L., Li, L., Yang, L.L., Xu, C., Dai, J., Wang, F., Li, Q., Dong, Q.X., Yang, R.F., Wu, J.R., Sun, B. (2009). Severe acute respiratory syndrome coronavirus accessory protein 9b is a virion-associated protein. *Virology.* 388, 279–285. doi:10.1016/j.virol.2009.03.032.

56. Almeida, M.S., Johnson, M.A., Herrmann, T., Geralt, M., Wüthrich, K. (2007). Novel β-barrel fold in the nuclear magnetic resonance structure of the replicase nonstructural protein 1 from the severe acute respiratory syndrome coronavirus. *J. Virol.* 81, 3151–3161. doi:10.1128/jvi.01939-06.

57. Kumar, A., Kumar, A., Kumar, P., Garg, N., Giri, R. (2020). SARS-CoV-2 NSP1 C-terminal region (residues 130–180) is an intrinsically disordered region. *bioRxiv.* doi:10.1101/2020.09.10.290932.

58. Mariano, G., Farthing, R.J., Lale-Farjat, S.L.M., Bergeron, J.R.C. (2020). Structural characterization of SARS-CoV-2: Where we are, and where we need to be. *Front. Mol. Biosci.* 7, 344. doi:10.3389/fmolb.2020.605236.

59. Rut, W., Lv, Z., Zmudzinski, M., Patchett, S., Nayak, D., Snipas, S.J., El Oualid, F., Huang, T.T., Bekes, M., Drag, M., Olsen, S.K. (2020). Activity profiling and crystal structures of inhibitor-bound SARS-CoV-2 papain-like protease: A framework for anti–COVID-19 drug design. *Sci. Adv.* 6, 1–13. doi:10.1126/sciadv.abd4596.

60. Jin, Z., Du, X., Xu, Y., Deng, Y., Liu, M., Zhao, Y., Zhang, B., Li, X., Zhang, L., Peng, C., Duan, Y., Yu, J., Wang, L., Yang, K., Liu, F., Jiang, R., Yang, X., You, T., Liu, X., Yang, X., Bai, F., Liu, H., Liu, X., Guddat, L.W., Xu, W., Xiao, G., Qin, C., Shi, Z., Jiang, H., Rao, Z., Yang, H. (2020). Structure of Mpro from SARS-CoV-2 and discovery of its inhibitors. *Nature* 582, 289–293. doi:10.1038/s41586-020-2223-y.

61. Padhi, A.K., Tripathi, T. (2021). Targeted design of drug binding sites in the main protease of SARS-CoV-2 reveals potential signatures of adaptation. *Biochem. Biophys. Res. Commun.* 555, 147–153. doi:10.1016/j.bbrc.2021.03.118.

62. Gadhave, K., Kumar, P., Kumar, A., Bhardwaj, T., Garg, N., Giri, R. (2020). NSP 11 of SARS-CoV-2 is an intrinsically disordered protein. *bioRxiv.* doi:10.1101/2020.10.07.330068.

63. Hillen, H.S., Kokic, G., Farnung, L., Dienemann, C., Tegunov, D., Cramer, P. (2020). Structure of replicating SARS-CoV-2 polymerase. *Nature.* 584, 154–156. doi:10.1038/s41586-020-2368-8.

64. Littler, D.R., Gully, B.S., Colson, R.N., Rossjohn, J. (2020). Crystal structure of the SARS-CoV-2 nonstructural protein 9, Nsp9. *iScience* 23, 101258. doi:10.1016/j.isci.2020.101258.

65. Rosas-Lemus, M., Minasov, G., Shuvalova, L., Inniss, N.L., Kiryukhina, O., Brunzelle, J., Satchell, K.J.F. (2020). High-resolution structures of the SARS-CoV-2 2′-O-methyltransferase reveal strategies for structure-based inhibitor design. *Sci. Signal.* 13, 1–12. doi:10.1126/scisignal.abe1202.

66. Ma, Y., Wu, L., Shaw, N., Gao, Y., Wang, J., Sun, Y., Lou, Z., Yan, L., Zhang, R., Rao, Z. (2015). Structural basis and functional analysis of the SARS coronavirus nsp14-nsp10 complex. *Proc. Natl. Acad. Sci. USA* 112, 9436–9441. doi:10.1073/pnas.1508686112.

67. Kim, Y., Wower, J., Maltseva, N., Chang, C., Jedrzejczak, R., Wilamowski, M., Kang, S., Nicolaescu, V., Randall, G., Michalska, K., Joachimiak, A. (2021). Tipiracil binds to uridine site and inhibits Nsp15 endoribonuclease NendoU from SARS-CoV-2. *Commun. Biol.* 4, 1–11. doi:10.1038/s42003-021-01735-9.

68. Liu, J., Sun, Y., Qi, J., Chu, F., Wu, H., Gao, F., Li, T., Yan, J., Gao, G.F. (2010). The membrane protein of severe acute respiratory syndrome coronavirus acts as a dominant immunogen revealed by a clustering region of novel functionally and structurally defined cytotoxic T-lymphocyte epitopes. *J. Infect. Dis.* 202, 1171–1180. doi:10.1086/656315.

69. Padhi, A.K., Shukla, R., Saudagar, P., Tripathi, T. (2021). High-throughput rational design of the remdesivir binding site in the RdRp of SARS-CoV-2: Implications for potential resistance. *iScience* 24. doi:10.1016/j.isci.2020.101992.

70. Kumar, P., Bhardwaj, T., Kumar, A., Gehi, B.R., Kapuganti, S.K., Garg, N., Nath, G., Giri, R. (2020). Reprofiling of approved drugs against

SARS-CoV-2 main protease: An in-silico study. *J. Biomol. Struct. Dyn.* 1–15. doi:10.1080/07391102.2 020.1845976.

71. Zhang, L., Linm D., Sun, X., Curth, U., Drosten, C., Sauerhering, L., Becker, S., Rox, K., Hilgenfeld, R. (2020). Crystal structure of SARS-CoV-2 main protease provides a basis for design of improved α-ketoamide inhibitors. *Science*. doi:10.1126/science.abb3405.

72. Kalita, P., Padhi, A.K., Zhang, K.Y.J., Tripathi, T. (2020). Design of a peptide-based subunit vaccine against novel coronavirus SARS-CoV-2. *Microb. Pathog.* 145, 104236. doi:10.1016/j.micpath.2020.104236.

Chapter 2   Biology of Coronaviruses and Predicted Origin of SARS-CoV-2

Giorgio Palù, Alberto Reale, Nicolas G. Bazan, Pritam Kumar Panda, Vladimir N. Uversky,
Murat Seyran, Alaa A. A. Aljabali, Samendra P. Sherchan, Gajendra Kumar Azad,
Wagner Baetas-da-Cruz, Parise Adadi, Murtaza M. Tambuwala, Bruce D. Uhal,
Kazuo Takayama, Ángel Serrano-Aroca, Tarek Mohamed Abd El-Aziz, Adam M. Brufsky,
and Kenneth Lundstrom

2.1 INTRODUCTION

The Coronavirus Disease 19 (COVID-19) pandemic has had a global impact, and has also highlighted the importance of the Severe Acute Respiratory Syndrome-Coronavirus-2 (SARS-CoV-2), and coronaviruses (CoVs) in general. It is therefore appropriate to dedicate a chapter to the biology of CoVs, and to reflect on the origin of SARS-CoV-2 to be better prepared for potential emerging outbreaks or future pandemics. CoVs were first described in 1969 based on their pleomorphic, circular, 80–160 nm in diameter shape with 15-nm club-shaped projections (so-called spike glycoproteins) that resemble a crown (*corona* in Latin) [1]. SARS-CoV-2 is the seventh coronavirus known to infect humans, but the first and only one to cause a pandemic [2, 3]. The first human pathogenic coronavirus HCoV-229E was identified in 1962 in Chicago and possibly originated from African Sundevall's roundleaf bat CoVs around 200 years ago, via zoonotic transmission from the alpaca [2, 4–6]. The second human pathogenic CoV HCoV-OC43, detected in 1964 in Maryland, possibly originated from Norway Rat CoVs, around 120 years ago via zoonotic transmission from the cow [2, 7, 8]. The third human pathogenic CoV, SARS-CoV detected in 2002 in Foshan, China possibly originated from Chinese horseshoe bat CoV 35 to 20 years ago via zoonotic transmission from the civet [2, 9–11]. The fourth human pathogenic CoV, HoV-HKU1 detected in 2002 in Hong Kong, possibly originated from Norway Rat CoV, 70 years ago via zoonotic transmission from the rodent [2, 12, 13]. The fifth human pathogenic CoV, HCoV-NL63 was first isolated in 1988 and identified in 2004 in Rotterdam (The Netherlands) that possibly originated from African trident bat CoV, 563–822 years ago via an unknown zoonotic host [2, 6, 14]. The sixth human pathogenic CoV, MERS-CoV, detected in 2012 in the Kingdom of Saudi Arabia (KSA), possibly originated from South African Bat CoV, around 14 years ago via zoonotic transmission from the camel [2, 8, 15]. Finally, SARS-CoV-2 was first detected in 2019 in Wuhan, China, and possibly originated from a recombination event in an ancestor of SARS-CoV-2, a horseshoe bat CoV, around 11 years ago via zoonotic transmission from the pangolins [16–18].

In 2003, the previously mentioned SARS-CoV caused an epidemic of viral pneumonia in humans in China and Hong Kong [19]. As zoonotic pathogens, coronaviruses have a wide range of hosts such as, birds, bats, mice, and humans, and they mainly affect the respiratory tract, the gastrointestinal tract, and the heart. Coronaviruses are a broad group of viruses that typically cause mild to severe illnesses in the upper respiratory tract. Since the millenium, SARS-CoV, MERS-CoV, and SARS-CoV-2 have arisen from animal sources to cause severe respiratory disease and high mortality in humans.

2.2 BIOLOGY OF CORONAVIRUSES

2.2.1 Classification of Coronaviruses (CoVs)

The family Coronaviridae is one of three RNA virus families within the order Nidovirales, with two subfamilies known as Coronavirinae and Torovirinae. CoVs are divided into four genera (Table 2.1). The human coronavirus (HCoV-229E), HCoV-NL63, and several animal viruses belong to the Alpha-coronavirus genus. Beta-coronaviruses comprise the prototype mouse hepatitis virus (MHV), the HCoV-OC43, the SARS-CoV, and HCoV-HKU1 variants. Alpha-coronaviruses and Beta-coronaviruses mainly infect mammals, while Gamma-coronaviruses and Delta-coronaviruses infect birds [20, 21]. CoVs have been associated with respiratory tract infections, including the common cold, and more severe manifestations such as pneumonia in humans. Because of the broad range of host organisms infected by CoVs, diseases such as gastroenteritis, renal diseases, and respiratory infections have affected livestock, causing significant losses in the cattle and poultry industries (Table 2.1) [22, 23]. Wildlife can also be infected by CoVs. A novel CoV, SW1 was isolated from a deceased Beluga whale, which had suffered from a respiratory disease and acute liver failure [24]. According to phylogenetic analysis, the SW1

Table 2.1 Examples of coronaviruses and coronavirus genera

Alpha-corona

Virus	Disease/Species	Effect
TGEV	Gastroenteritis in pigs	High morbidity, high mortality
PEDV	Gastroenteritis in pigs	High morbidity, high mortality
FCoV	Enteric infection in cats	Mild or asymptomatic disease in cats
FIPV	Peritonitis in cats	Lethal peritonitis in cats
HCoV-229E	Respiratory infection	15%–30% of the annual common cold
HCoV-NL63	Respiratory infection	Associated with croup

Beta-corona

Virus	Disease/Species	Effect
PHEV	Enteric infection	Diarrhea, encephalitis in pigs
BCoV	Respiratory tract infection	Losses in the cattle industry
RCoV	Respiratory tract infection in rat	Useful model for studies on innate immune responses
MHV	Respiratory infection, enteritis	
Bat CoV HKU4	Respiratory tract infection	Severe respiratory infection, encephalitis in mice
Bat CoV HKU5	Respiratory tract infection	
GD Pangolin CoV	Potential natural reservoir	Potential threat of epidemics
GX Pangolin CoV	Potential natural reservoir	Potential threat of epidemics
HCoV-OC43	Respiratory infection	Potential threat of emergence of novel coronaviruses
HCoV-HKU1	Respiratory infection	Potential threat of emergence of novel coronaviruses
SARS-CoV	SARS	15%–30% of the annual common cold
MERS-CoV	MERS	15%–30% of the annual common cold
SARS-CoV-2	COVID-19	8,098 cases, 774 deaths in 2002–2003 855 cases, 333 deaths in 2013 142.8 million cases, > 3 million deaths 2019–2021

Gamma-corona

Virus	Disease/Species	Effect
IBV	Respiratory infection, renal disease	Losses in the poultry industry
BWCoV-SW1	Respiratory, acute liver failure	Isolated from Beluga whale
TCoV	Enteric disease in turkeys	Highly contagious in turkeys, closely related to IBV

Delta-corona

Virus	Disease/Species	Effect
PDCoV	Diarrhea in pigs	Co-infections with PEDV
BuCoV HKU11	Natural reservoir	Potential spread to poultry
ThCoV HKU12	Natural reservoir	Potential spread to poultry
MunCoV HKU13	Natural reservoir	Potential spread to poultry
WECoV HKU16	Natural reservoir	Potential spread to poultry
SpCoV HKU17	Natural reservoir	Potential spread to poultry
WiCoV HKU20	Natural reservoir	Potential spread to poultry
CMCoV HKU21	Natural reservoir	Potential spread to poultry

Abbreviations: BCoV, bovine coronavirus; BuCoV HKU11, bulbul coronavirus; BWCoV-SW1, Beluga whale coronavirus SW1; CMCoV HKU21, common moorhen coronavirus; FCoV, feline enteric coronavirus, FIPV, feline infectious peritonitis virus; IBV, infectious bronchitis virus; MERS-CoV. Middle East Respiratory Syndrome-Coronavirus; MHV, murine hepatitis virus; MunCoV HKU13, munia coronavirus; PDCoV, porcine deltacoronavirus; PEDV, porcine epidemic diarrhea virus; PHEV, porcine hemagglutinating encephalomyelitis virus; SARS-CoV. Severe Acute Respiratory Syndrome-Coronavirus; SpCoV HKU17, sparrow coronavirus; TCoV, turkey coronavirus; TGEV, transmissible gastroenteritis virus; ThCoV HKU12, thrush coronavirus; WECoV HKU16, white-eye coronavirus; WiCoV HKU20, wigeon coronavirus.

belongs to the group of Gamma-coronaviruses. Moreover, wild birds such as the bulbul act as reservoirs for a number of Delta-coronaviruses (BuCoV HKU11), common moorhen coronavirus (CMCoV HKU21), thrush coronavirus (thCoV HKU13), wigeon coronavirus (WiCoV HKU20) and others (Table 2.1) [25].

Several human CoVs such as HCoV-229E, HCoV-OC43, and HCoV-HKu1 have been associated with self-limiting infections responsible for

15%–30% of annual common cold cases [4, 26]. The first major outbreak was caused by the SARS-CoV, which resulted in the SARS epidemic of 2002–2003 [27], followed a decade later by the Middle East Respiratory Syndrome (MERS) caused by the MERS-Coronavirus (MERS-CoV) [28]. Both the SARS and MERS epidemics were contained relatively quickly and never reached pandemic proportions. SARS-CoV spread to 27 countries in 2002–2003 with 8,096 cases, 774 deaths, and a fatality rate of 10%, but disappeared in 2004 [9]. The MERS-CoV was found to be less human-to-human transmissible compared to the SARS-CoV, and cases have been detected in the Kingdom of Saudi Arabia (KSA), Jordan, the UK, and South Korea since 2012 [9]. The MERS-CoV epidemic has recorded 2,494 cases and caused 858 deaths. The SARS-CoV-2 has a lower fatality rate (2%–3%) compared to MERS-CoV (34.4%) and SARS-CoV (10%) despite its pandemic spread [9]. Both SARS and MERS epidemics were contained relatively quickly and never reached pandemic proportions. In contrast, the recent SARS-CoV-2 outbreak causing the COVID-19 pandemic has reached an unprecedented scale with 240 million infections and more than 4.9 million deaths (as of October 14, 2021) with devastating global social and economic consequences.

2.2.2 Genome Organization and Structure of SARS-CoV-2 Particles

The SARS-CoV-2 genome showed approximately 88% similarity to those of two bat viruses, bat-SL-CoVZC45 and bat-SL-CoVXC21, but it was much lower for the SARS-CoV (79%) and the MERS-CoV (50%), respectively [29]. CoVs have three main structural proteins: a very large (200 kDa) S glycoprotein (spike) forming the bulky (15–20 nm) peplomer on the virus surface, an irregular transmembrane glycoprotein (M) and an internal, phosphorylated nucleocapsid protein (N). There is also a small transmembrane envelope protein (E), and a few members of the CoV family contain a further envelope protein with both esterase and hemagglutinin functions. The approximately 30 kb genome of CoVs is a non-segmented, single-stranded RNA (ssRNA) molecule with a positive-sense polarity [30] with a capped 5′ end and polyadenylated 3′-end. As a consequence of heterologous RNA recombination, extensive rearrangements can occur. At the 5′ end of the genome is located an untranslated region (UTR) of 65–98 nucleotides. The 3′ end of the RNA genome contains a poly (A) tail with another UTR sequence of 200–500 nucleotides. For the regulation of RNA replication and transcription, both UTRs are essential [31].

Two-thirds of the genome contain the replicase genes rep1a and rep1b, which encode the non-structural proteins (NSP1-16), and one third is represented by the structural genes (S, E, M, and N), and various accessory genes (ORF3a, ORF6, ORF7a, ORF7b, ORF8, and ORF10) (Figure 2.1). The accessory genes have been suggested to play a role in virulence, infectivity, ion channel activity, increased replication, virus particle assembly and release, and down-regulation of the interferon pathway. Moreover, the SARS-CoV-2 ORF8 and ORF10 are both unique among CoVs and have been postulated to affect virus spread and the degradation of antiviral proteins, respectively [32, 33].

The structure of SARS-CoV-2 particles has been determined by cryo-electron tomography and microscopy, which identified approximately 125 nm spherical particles with prominent club-shaped spike proteins [34]. The helically symmetrical N protein enwraps the RNA genome, the triple-spanning membrane M protein binds to the N protein, while the small E protein, with a postulated transmembrane structure and ion channel activity, is associated with the assembly and release of viral particles. Furthermore, the E protein has been identified as an essential virulence factor in other CoVs, including SARS-CoV [35]. Specifically, the PDZ-binding motif (PBM) of the E protein, a domain involved in protein–protein interaction, plays a role in pathogenicity [36]. In the human OC43 coronavirus, this protein has also been linked to neurovirulence [37]. The S protein mediates the attachment to the host cell angiotensin-converting enzyme 2 (ACE2) receptor. In the case of SARS-CoV-2, a host cell furin-like protease cleaves the S protein into S1 and S2 polypeptides. There is evidence that both ACE2 as well as transmembrane protease serine 2 (TMPRSS2) may be segregated in membrane microdomains and the SARS-CoV-2 entry might be facilitated by tetraspanins, transmembrane proteins clustered in membrane microdomains [38]. These microdomains are not lipid rafts as they lack glycosyl-phosphatidylinositol (GPI)-linked proteins, caveolin and Src-kinases [39].

As with other viral proteins, one of the characteristic features of CoV proteins is their multifunctionality. This capability to execute multiple, diverse functions is determined by the capability of viral proteins to be engaged in a broad range of interactions with a multitude of viral and host partners, which, at least in part, can be explained by the presence of intrinsically disordered protein regions (IDPRs). In fact, three SARS-CoV-2 proteins, N, NSP8, and ORF6, are highly disordered, and the remaining proteins also contain functional IDPRs. For example, cleavage sites in the

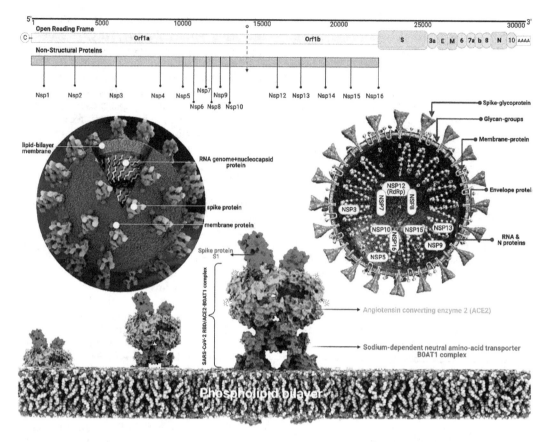

Figure 2.1 The SARS-CoV-2 genome. The general organization of the SARS-CoV-2 genome with ORFs and the corresponding proteins (top), a view of the viral surface (middle, left), a cross-sectional view of the virion (middle, right) and the interaction of the S1 domain of SARS-CoV-2 with its receptor ACE2 on the cellular surface (bottom).

replicase 1ab polyprotein are found to be highly disordered, and almost all SARS-CoV-2 proteins contain molecular recognition features (MoRFs), which are the disorder-based protein–protein interaction sites that are capable of folding at interaction with specific partners, and are commonly utilized by proteins for target binding [40].

2.2.3 Life Cycle of SARS-CoV-2

The first step in the life cycle of SARS-CoV-2 is the initial attachment of the viral particle by the receptor-binding domain (RBD) in the S1 region to the ACE2 receptor on bronchial epithelial cells and alveolar pneumocytes to downregulate the receptor expression, which leads to severe acute respiratory failure (Figure 2.2) [41]. The virus tropism is determined by the location of the RBD and the target receptor. For example, the RBD is located at the N-terminus of the S protein in the murine hepatitis virus (MHV), but at the C-terminus of

the S1 region in SARS-CoV. Furthermore, carcinoembryonic antigen-related adhesion molecule-1 (CEACAM1) is the receptor for MHV [42], while MERS-CoV targets dipeptidyl-peptidase 4 (DPP4) [43] and SARS-CoV, HCoVNL63, and SARS-CoV-2 attach to ACE2 [44].

Following the initial attachment, the S protein is cleaved by cathepsin or another protease. Then fusion takes place in endosomes or at the plasma membrane, and the viral RNA is released into the cytoplasm. Expression of non-structural proteins (NSPs) generates the replicase-transcriptase complex, and initiates synthesis of genomic and subgenomic RNA and translation of structural and accessory proteins. Specifically, while NSPs are transcribed directly from the genomic RNA, transcription of all other viral proteins is mediated by nested, subgenomic RNAs located at the 3′ end. This is a shared feature of all viruses of the Nidovirales order (from Latin *nidus*, "nest").

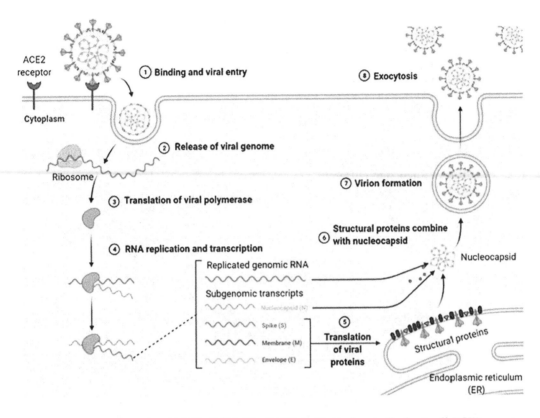

Figure 2.2 The life cycle of SARS-CoV-2. The SARS-CoV attaches to the host cell ACE2 receptor, its RNA is released into the cytoplasm where genome replication and translation of structural and accessory protein occurs. After assembly, mature viral particles are released by exocytosis (see text for details).

Source: Created with BioRender.com.

The structural proteins are transported to the endoplasmic reticulum (ER) and further to the ER-Golgi intermediate compartment (ERGIC), where the RNA is enwrapped by the N protein, and assembled into viral particles with S, E, and M proteins. Mature virions are transported to the plasma membrane in vesicles and released by exocytosis.

2.3 ORIGIN OF SARS-CoV-2

2.3.1 Homology to Other Coronaviruses

Sequence comparisons between bat, snake, and pangolin CoVs and SARS-CoV-2 from infected patients aim to identify potential animal carriers of SARS-CoV-2. The sialic acid–binding domain of the SARS-CoV-2 S protein has a flat and non-sunken N-terminal domain (NTD), which is a unique feature compared to other CoVs [45]. Furthermore, the structure of the NTD of the SARS-CoV-2 S protein is similar to human galectins, galactose-binding lectins, and contributes to evading host immune recognition by mutant versions sinking beneath the surface according to the Canyon hypothesis [46, 47].

The alteration pattern of the depression of the NTD of the S protein has been validated experimentally for MERS-CoV, HCoV-OC43, and HCoV-HKU1 [47, 48].

Another unique aspect of the SARS-CoV-2 host tropism relates to recombination, which has enabled the S protein to be cleaved by furin protease. The RNA recombination pattern in CoVs has been explained by a template-switching (copy-choice) mechanism [45, 49]. During translation, CoV RNAs show discontinuous and non-progressive replication in host cells, with replication pauses at specific RNA sites, creating free RNA blocks This could allow recombination with other CoVs, leading to novel recombinant CoV strains [45, 49]. For example, the NTD sialic acid–binding domain in the MHV S protein has been suggested to have originated from recombination with human galectin RNA sequences [45, 49].

On the other hand, as the S1/S2 site in the SARS-CoV-2 S protein corresponding to the furin recognition motif does not exist in other Beta-coronaviruses such as the Pangolin-CoV and bat RaTG13, it seems that the S1/S2 site is not a hot spot or RNA termination site [45, 49]. Moreover, based on clinical isolates of SARS-CoV-2 S, recombination does not occur in this area, indicating that the insertion of the furin recognition motif represents a one-time event of particular recombination. However, this does not exclude other CoV host tropism events, which supports the urgent need to investigate the host tropism from samples collected from the sarbecovirus subgenus in Southeast Asia [50].

2.3.2 Scientific Evaluation of Different Theories of the Origin of SARS-CoV-2

SARS-CoV-2 was first detected in Wuhan, China in December 2019 and has been postulated to have originated naturally from wild animals at the Huanan market in Wuhan and spread by person-to-person transmission, causing the COVID-19 pandemic [51]. However, an intermediate host has still to be found as the pandemic virus has lost its ability to infect bat cells from which RaTG13, the most likely progenitor, has derived. In addition, the SARS-CoV-2 S protein has gained peculiar structural features among which a polybasic amino acid sequence in a region unlikely to undergo recombination events. Such a feature is also shared by influenza type A viruses grown in tissue culture for several passages [52]. Recently, a delegation from the WHO inspected the Wuhan Institute of Virology in China for a possible laboratory leak of SARS-CoV-2 and stated that "all available evidence suggested its natural animal origin and not being manipulated in the laboratory" [53]. Furthermore, the WHO has pledged to collaborate with experts, member states, and other partners to identify the source of origin of the SARS-CoV-2. However, before definite proof is available the debate of the natural or engineered origin of the SARS-CoV-2 strain goes on.

2.4 CONCLUSION

The biology of CoVs and the origin of SARS-CoV-2 provide essential information for a better understanding of CoVs, facilitating the development of drugs and vaccines against SARS-CoV-2, preparation for emerging novel viruses, and the prevention of future spill-over events and outbreaks. Comparison of genomic structures and sequence homologies between SARS-CoV-2 and other human CoVs, especially SARS-CoV and MERS-CoV, facilitate the development of COVID-19–specific therapeutics and vaccines. Moreover, investigating the origin of SARS-CoV-2 is of utmost importance, not only for determining where and from what species SARS-CoV-2 originated but also for being prepared for any emerging outbreaks.

REFERENCES

1. Bradburne, A.F., Tyrrell, D.A. (1969). The propagation of "coronaviruses" in tissue-culture. *Arch. Gesamte Virusforsch.* 28, 133–150.

2. Forni, D., Cagliani, R., Clerici, M., et al. (2017). Molecular evolution of human coronavirus genomes. *Trends Microbiol.* 25, 35–48.

3. Steffens, I. (2020). A hundred days into the coronavirus disease (COVID-19) pandemic. *Euro Surveill.* 25, 2000550.

4. Hamre, D., Procknow, J.J. (1966). A new virus isolated from the human respiratory tract. *Proc. Soc. Exp. Biol. Med.* 12, 190–193.

5. Corman, V.M., Baldwin, H.J., Tateno, A.F., et al. (2015). Evidence for an ancestral association of human coronavirus 229E with bats. *J. Virol.* 89, 11858–11870.

6. De Sabato, L., Lelli, D., Faccin, F., et al. (2019). Full genome characterization of two novel Alphacoronavirus species from Italian bats. *Virus Res.* 260, 60–66. doi:10.1016/j.virusres.2018.11.007.

7. McIntosh, K., Becker, W.B., Chanock, R.M. (1967). Growth in suckling-mouse brain of "IBV-like" viruses from patients with upper respiratory tract disease. *Proc. Natl. Acad. Sci. USA* 58, 2268–2273.

8. Lau, S.K., Lee, P., Tsang, A.K., et al. (2011). Molecular epidemiology of human coronavirus OC43 reveals evolution of different genotypes over time and recent emergence of a novel genotype due to natural recombination. *J. Virol.* 85, 11325–11337.

9. de Wit, E., van Doremalen, N., Falzarano, D., et al. (2016). SARS and MERS: Recent insights into emerging coronaviruses. *Nat. Rev. Microbiol.* 14, 523–534. doi:10.1038/nrmicro.2016.81.

10. Hu, B., Ge, X., Wang, L.F., Shi, Z. (2015). Bat origin of human coronaviruses. *Virol. J.* 12, 221.

11. Ge, X.Y., Li, J.L., Yang, X.L., et al. (2013). Isolation and characterization of a bat SARS-like coronavirus that uses the ACE2 receptor. *Nature* 503, 535–538.

12. Woo, P.C., Lau, S.K., Huang, Y., et al. (2005). Phylogenetic and recombination analysis of coronavirus HKU1, a novel coronavirus from patients with pneumonia. *Arch. Virol.* 150, 2299–2311.

13. Lau, S.K., Woo, P.C., Li, K.S., et al. (2015). Discovery of a novel coronavirus, China Rattus coronavirus HKU24, from Norway rats supports the murine origin of Betacoronavirus and has implications for the ancestor of Betacoronavirus lineage A. *J. Virol.* 89, 3076–3092.

14. Fouchier, R.A., Hartwig, N.G., Bestebroer, T.M., et al. (2004). A previously undescribed coronavirus associated with respiratory disease in humans. *Proc. Natl. Acad. Sci. USA* 101, 6212–6216.

15. Ithete, N.L., Stoffberg, S., Corman, V.M., et al. Close relative of human Middle East respiratory

syndrome coronavirus in bat. *South Africa. Emerg. Infect. Dis.* 19, (10) 2013 1697–1699.

16. Patiño-Galindo, J.Á., Filip, I., AlQuraishi, M., et al. Recombination and convergent evolution led to the emergence of 2019 Wuhan coronavirus. *bioRxiv.* preprint doi:10.1101/2020.02.10.942748.

17. Zhou, P., Yang, X.L., Wang, X.G., et al. (2020). A pneumonia outbreak associated with a new coronavirus of probable bat origin. *Nature* 579, 270–273.

18. Ren, L.L., Wang, Y.M., Wu, Z.Q., et al. (2020). Identification of a novel coronavirus causing severe pneumonia in human: A descriptive study. *Chin. Med. J.* 133, 1015–1024.

19. Poutanen, S.M., Low, D.E., Henry, B., et al. (2003). Identification of severe acute respiratory syndrome in Canada. *N. Engl. J. Med.* 348, 1995–2005.

20. Woo, P.C.Y., Lau, S.K.P., Lam, C.S.F., et al. (2012). Discovery of seven novel Mammalian and avian coronaviruses in the genus deltacoronaviruses supports bat coronaviruses as the gene source of alphacoronaviruses and betacoronaviruses and avian coronaviruses as the gene source of gammacoronavirusesso and deltacoronaviruses. *J. Virol.* 86, 3995–4008. doi:10.1128/JVI.06540-11.

21. Lundstrom, K. (2020). Coronavirus pandemic: Therapy and vaccines. *Biomedicines* 8, 109. doi:10.3390/biomedicines8050109.

22. Amer, H.M. Bovine-like coronaviruses in domestic and wild ruminants. *Anim. Health Res. Rev.* 19 2018 113–124.

23. Perlman, S., Netland, J. Coronaviruses post-SARS: Update on replication and pathogenesis. *Nat. Rev. Microbiol.* 7 2009 439–450.

24. Mihindukulasuriya, K.A., Wu, G., St Leger, J., Nordhausen, R.W., Wang, D. Identification of a novel coronavirus from a Beluga whale by using a panviral microarray. *J. Virol.* 82 2008 5084–5088.

25. Wille, M., Holmes E.C. (2020). Wild birds as reservoirs for diverse and abundant gamma- and deltacoronaviruses. *FEBS Microbiol. Rev.* 44, 631–644.

26. Bradburne, A.F., Bynoe, L.M., Tyrell, D.A.J. (1967). Effects of a "new" human respiratory virus in volunteers. *Br. Med. J.* 3, 767–769. doi:10.1136/bmj.3.5568.767.

27. Cherry, J.D. (2004). The chronology of the 2002–2003 SARS mini pandemic. *Paediatr. Resp. Rev.* 5, 262–269.

28. Aleanizi, F.S., Mohmed, N., Alqahtani, F.Y., et al. (2017). Outbreak of the Middle East respiratory syndrome coronavirus in Saudi Arabia: A retrospective study. *BMC Infect. Dis.* 17, 23.

29. Lu, R., Zhao, X., Li, J. (2020). Genomic characterisation and epidemiology of 2019 novel coronavirus: Implications for virus origins and receptor binding. *Lancet* 395, 565–574.

30. Naqvi, A.A.T., Fatima, K., Mohammad, T., et al. (2020). Insights into SARS-CoV-2 genome structure, evolution, pathogenesis and therapies. Structural genomics approach. *Biochim. Biophys. Acta Mol. Basis Dis.* 1866, 165878.

31. Dokland, T. (2010). The structural biology of PRRSV. *Virus Res.* 154, 86–97.

32. Hassan, S.S., Aljabali, A.A.A., Kumar Panda, P., et al. (2021). A unique view of SARS-CoV-2 through the lens of ORF8 protein. *Comp. Biol. Med.* doi:10.1016/j.compbiomed.2021.104380.

33. Hassan, S.S., Attrish, D., Ghosh, S., et al. (2021). Notable sequence homology of the ORF10 protein introspects the architecture of SARS-CoV-2. *Int. J. Biol. Macromol.* 181, 801–809.

34. Wang, M.-Y., Zhao, R., Gao, L.J., et al. (2020). SARS-CoV-2: Structure, biology, and structure-based therapeutics development. *Front. Cell. Infect. Microbiol.* 10, 587269.

35. DeDiego, M.L., Nieto-Torres, J.L., Jimenez-Guardeno, J.M., et al. (2014). Coronavirus virulence genes with main focus on SARS-CoV envelope gene. *Virus Res.* 194, 124–137.

36. Jimenez-Guardeno, J.M., Nieto-Torres, J.L., DeDiego, M.L., et al. (2014). The PDZ-binding motif of severe acute respiratory syndrome coronavirus envelope protein is a determinant of viral pathogenesis. *PLoS Pathog.* 10 8, e1004320.

37. Stodola, J.K., Duboi, G., Le Coupanec, A., et al. (2018). The OC43 human coronavirus envelope protein is critical for infectious virus production and propagation in neuronal cells and is a determinant of neurovirulence and CNS pathology. *Virology* 515, 134–149. doi:10.1016/j.virol.2017.12.023.

38. Hantak, M.P., Qing, E., Earnest, J.T. (2019). Tetraspanins: Architects of viral entry and exit platforms. *J. Virol.* 93, e01429-17.

39. Laude, A.J., Prior, I.A. (2004). Plasma membrane microdomains: Organisation, function and trafficking. *Mol. Membr. Biol.* 21, 193–205.

40. Giri, R., Bhardwaj, T., Shegane, M., et al. (2021). Understanding COVID-19 via comparative analysis of dark proteosomes of SARS-CoV-2, human SARS and bat SARS-like coronaviruses. *Cell Mol. Life Sci.* 78, 1655–1688.

41. Kubo, H., Yamada, Y.K., Taguchi, F. (1994). Localization of neutralizing epitopes and the receptor binding site within the amino-terminal 330 amino acids of the murine coronavirus spike protein. *J. Virol.* 68, 5403–5410.

42. Cheng, P.K., Wong, D.A., Tong, L.K., et al. (2004). Viral shedding patterns of coronavirus in patients with probable severe acute respiratory syndrome. *Lancet* 363, 1699–1700.

43. Nedellec, P., Dveksler, G.S., Daniels, E., et al. (1994). Bgp2, a new member of the carcinoembryonic antigen-related gene family, encodes an

alternative receptor for mouse hepatitis viruses. *J. Virol.* 68, 4525–4537.

44. van Doremalen, N., Miazgowicz, K.L., Milne-Price, S., et al. (2014). Host species restriction of Middle East respiratory syndrome coronavirus through its receptor dipeptidyl peptidase 4. *J. Virol.* 88, 9220–9232.

45. Seyran, M., Takayama, K., Uversky, V.N., et al. (2020). The structural basisof accelerated host cell entry by SARS-CoV-2. *FEBS J.* doi:10.1111/febs.15651.

46. Li, F. (2015). Receptor recognition mechanisms of coronaviruses: A decade of structural studies. *J. Virol.* 89, 1954–1964. doi:10.1128/JVI.02615-14.

47. Hulswit, R.J., de Haan, C.A., Bosch, B.J. (2016). Coronavirus spike protein and tropism changes. *Adv. Virus Res.* 96, 29–57. doi:10.1016/bs.aivir.2016.08.004.

48. Hulswit, R.J.G., Lang, Y., Bakkers, M.J.G., et al. (2019). Human coronaviruses OC43 and HKU1 bind to 9-O-acetylated sialic acids via a conserved receptor-binding site in spike protein domain A.

Proc. Natl. Acad. Sci. U.S.A. 116(7), 2681–2690. doi:10.1073/pnas.1809667116.

49. Makino, S., Keck, J.G., Stohlman, S.A., Lai, M.M. (1986). High-frequency RNA recombination of murine coronaviruses. *J. Virol.* 57(3), 729–737. doi:10.1128/JVI.57.3.729-737.1986.

50. Seyran, M., Hassan, S.S., Uversky, V.N. et al. (2021). Urgent need for field surveys of coronaviruses in Southeast Asia to understand the SARS-CoV-2 phylogeny and risk assessment for the future outbreaks. *Biomolecules* 11, 398.

51. Yang, Y. et al. (2020). The deadly coronavirus: The 2003 SARS epidemic and the 2020 novel coronavirus epidemic in China. *J. Autoimmun.* 109, 102434.

52. Seyran, M., Pizzol, D., Adadi, P. et al. Questions concerning the proximal origin of SARS-CoV-2. *J. Med. Virol.* 93(3), 2021 1204–1206. doi:10.1002/jmv.26478.

53. WHO Origin of SARS-CoV-2. The WHO report, Document number WHO-2019-nCoV-FAQ-Virus_origin-2020.1

Chapter 3   Therapeutic Challenges in COVID-19

Alaa A. A. Aljabali, Murtaza M. Tambuwala, Debmalya Barh, and Kenneth Lundstrom

3.1 INTRODUCTION

The current COVID-19 pandemic has resulted in more than 240 million infections, more than 4.9 million deaths globally, and generated socio-economic destruction [1]. In addition to unpreparedness for a global pandemic related to hospital equipment and personal protection awareness, no efficient antiviral drugs or vaccines against SARS-CoV-2 were available at the beginning of the pandemic. Because of the high stakes, significant financial and scientific investments were allocated to the research and development of drugs and vaccines against COVID-19 [1]. The urgent demands brought together unprecedentedly global resources, leaving no stone unturned and exploring all possible avenues, including repurposing existing antiviral drugs, and a search for novel types of drugs to target SARS-CoV-2 (Table 3.1). Drugs showing efficacy against other viruses, parasites, and neurological disorders were retested for drug efficacy against SARS-CoV-2 in preclinical animal models, and further in clinical trials in COVID-19 patients [2]. The drug discovery process and in particular the search for new drug molecules and the exploration of novel signaling pathways have received strong support from computational biology, structural biology, and screening programs [3]. While vaccine development has been visualized as the ultimate game-changer in preventing the spread of SARS-CoV-2, and the best option for ending the COVID-19 pandemic [4], the focus of the chapter will be solely on antiviral therapeutics as vaccines, and monoclonal antibodies against SARS-CoV-2 will be described in other chapters of the book. The focus will also be on the reasons behind the failures to develop antiviral drugs against SARS-CoV-2, and the challenges researchers face to achieve success. This chapter will also address issues related to comorbidity, personalized and asymptomatic management of COVID-19, and the challenges related to treatment at home, in homes for the elderly, and in intensive care units (ICUs).

3.2 SUMMARY ON ANTIVIRAL COVID-19 DRUGS

Two major strategies have been pursued for COVID-19 drug development. In one approach, existing approved drugs for other indications, such as viral and parasitic infections, have been repurposed for targeting SARS-CoV-2 infections. The apparent benefits of this strategy are the swift production and approval of these products for human use. The drawbacks are the unclear consequences on SARS-CoV-2 of the repurposed medications, and any negative effects caused to COVID-19 patients. The other strategy has been to developed novel antiviral pharmaceutical products based on computational biology, structural biology, and high-throughput screening, targeting signaling pathways, and exploring new viral inhibitors for cellular entry and replication. Examples of COVID-19 drugs are summarized in Table 3.1. Chloroquine (CQ) and hydroxychloroquine (HCQ) were developed primarily for malaria treatment and initially received much attention as prominent candidates for the treatment of COVID-19 patients [2, 3]. Initial excitement related to reduced viral load in COVID-19 patients treated with HCQ [6] quickly disappeared when it was revealed that the clinical study design was inadequate, and the obtained results were not reliable [7]. Moreover, a systematic review and meta-analysis based on twelve observational studies and three randomized clinical trials in 10,659 COVID-19 patients treated with HCQ showed no significant reduction in mortality, time to fever resolution, clinical deterioration, and development of acute respiratory distress syndrome (ARDS) [8]. In contrast, patients treated with HCQ posed a greater risk of ECG abnormalities and arrhythmia.

RNA-dependent RNA polymerase (RdRp) inhibitors have previously shown efficacy against different viruses such as influenza virus, hepatitis C virus (HCV), and Zika virus (ZIKV), and are therefore potential targets as antiviral drugs against COVID-19 [9]. Molecular docking studies showed high binding affinity of remdesivir (RDV) [15], ribavirin (RBV), favipiravir (FPV), sofosbuvir, galidesivir, and tenofovir to SARS-CoV-2, indicating their potency as antiviral drugs for COVID-19 patients [10]. Moreover, RDV has demonstrated antiviral activity in human cell lines and primary cell lines against HCoV-229E, HCoV-OC43, SARS-CoV, and MERS-CoV [11] and reduction in SARS-CoV and MERS-CoV viral loads in mice and rhesus macaques, respectively [12]. RDV has been evaluated for safety and efficacy in a randomized, placebo-controlled clinical trial in 1,062 COVID-19 patients [13]. Intravenous

DOI: 10.1201/9781003190394-3

Table 3.1 Examples of drugs (excluding monoclonal antibodies) for COVID-19 treatment

Drug	Function	Findings	References
HCQ	Lysosomal enzyme inhibition	No clinical benefits and no decrease in mortality rates of HCQ based on a meta-analysis of 15 trials	[8]
		Higher arrhythmia risk of HCQ	[8]
RDV	RdRp inhibitor	Reduced recovery time in hospitalized COVID-19 patients	[13]
		RDV approved for the treatment of hospitalized COVID-19 patients	[56]
FPV	RdRp inhibitor	Fewer adverse events, shorter viral clearance in phase I	[16]
		Superior recovery rates compared to umifenovir	[17]
		Clinical improvement in a retrospective observational trial in Thailand	[18]
		Reduced time of fever duration	[19]
		Approval of FPV in Russia, Bangladesh, Pakistan, Egypt, Jordan, and Saudi Arabia	[58]
RBV	RdRp inhibitor	SARS-CoV-2 inhibition in Vero E6 cells	[20]
		Recovery time reduced from 12 to 7 days	[21]
		RBV not associated with improvement in negative conversion time or mortality rate	[22]
Sofosbuvir	RdRp inhibitor	Shorter hospital stays (5 days) and lower mortality rate (6%) compared to RBV (9 days, 33%)	[23]
		Improved clinical recovery (88%) compared to standard care (67%), shorter hospitalization (6 days versus 8 days)	[24]
		No reduction in hospital stays, ICU admissions, or deaths compared to standard care	[25]
Galidesivir	RdRp inhibitor	Inhibition of SARS-CoV-2 in molecular docking studies	[26]
		No clinical benefit compared to placebo in phase I	[27]
EIDD-2801	RdRp inhibitor	Inhibition of SARS-CoV-2 in vitro and in vivo	[28]
		Reduced viral load in SARS-CoV-2 infected ferrets	[29]
		Safe and tolerable drug administration in phase I	[30]
		Recruiting in progress for phase II	[31]
Azvudine	RdRp inhibitor	Potential shorter time of first NANC	[32]
Ivermectin	3CLPro inhibitor	90% reduced viral RNA in SARS-CoV-2 infected Vero cells	[34]
		No clinical benefit compared to placebo in phase I study	[35]
		No reduction in recovery time or mortality based on a meta-analysis of 12 clinical trials	[36]
Naphthalene-based L10	PLpro inhibitor	Inhibition of SARS-CoV-2 replication in Vero E6 cells	[39]
Nafamostate mesylate	TMPRSS2 inhibitor	The combination of nafamostate mesylate and FPV resulted in improvement of critically ill COVID-19 patients	[46]
		Nafamostate mesylate therapy improved condition in elderly	[47]
Dexamethasone	Corticosteroid	Lower 28-day mortality compared to standard care	[49]
		Increase in ventilator-free days of COVID-19 patients	[50]

Abbreviations: 3CLPro, 3-chymotrypsin-like protease; EIDD-2810, nucleotide analogue; FPV, Favipiravir: HCQ, Hydroxychloroquine; ICU, intensive care unit; RBV, Ribavirin; RDV, remdesivir; TMPRSS2, transmembrane protease serine 2.

administration of RDV significantly reduced the recovery time from 15 to 10 days in hospitalized patients. However, interim results from the WHO Solidarity Trial indicated that RDV, HCQ, lopinavir (LPV), and interferon regimens had minor or no effect on hospitalized COVID-19 patients based on overall mortality, the start of ventilation, and length of hospital stay [14]. In clinical evaluations, it was demonstrated that RDV was associated with significantly enhanced recovery, with a 62% reduced odds of death compared to standard care [4].

Combination therapy of FPV and interferon-α (IFN-α) showed fewer adverse events, shorter clearance time of virus, and improved chest CT scans compared to LPV/ritonavir (RTV) treatment in a phase I study [16]. FPV did not show improvement in clinical recovery in other clinical trials but provided superior relief in pyrexia and cough compared to umifenovir [17]. Moreover, clinical improvement was observed in studies in Thailand [18] and reduced time to fever reaction in Japan [19].

RBV has been shown to inhibit SARS-CoV-2 replication in Vero E6 cells [20]. In an open-label, randomized, phase II trial, the triple combination RBV, IFN-β-1b, and LPV/RTV was compared to treatment with LPV/RTV, IFN-β-1b, and RBV alone, which resulted in the reduction of time from the start of treatment to a confirmed negative nasopharyngeal swab test to 7 days for the triple combination compared to 12 days for LPV/RTV therapy [21]. In another study, patients with severe COVID-19 received intravenous RBV together with supportive care in a retrospective cohort study [22]. The outcome was that RBV therapy did not improve the negative conversion time for SARS-CoV-2 testing and was not associated with an improved mortality rate.

Other RdRp inhibitors such as sofosbuvir [23–25], galidesivir [26, 27], and EIDD-2801 [28–31] have all been subjected to preclinical evaluations and clinical trials on COVID-19 patients, showing some benefits related to a shortened hospital stay and lower mortality rates for sofosbuvir and EIDD-2801, as summarized in Table 3.1. Moreover, preliminary results indicated that azvudine might shorten the time of the first nucleic acid negative conversion (NANC) in mild and common COVID-19 patients [32].

As proteases such as 3-chymotrypsin-like protease (3CLPro) play a role in SARS-CoV-2 replication, inhibitors such as ombitasvir, paritaprevir, tipranavir, ivermectin, and micafungin have been suggested as potential antiviral drugs for the treatment of COVID-19 patients [33]. Ivermectin, characterized for its anti-parasitic

and antiviral activities, has demonstrated a 90% reduction in viral RNA levels in SARS-CoV-2 infected Vero E6 cells [34]. When subjected to clinical evaluation, ivermectin showed no superiority to placebo in non-severe COVID-19 patients in a pilot study [35]. Furthermore, a systematic review and meta-analysis of 15 clinical trials did not show reduced mortality or shortened recovery time in COVID-19 patients receiving ivermectin compared to the control group subjected to standard care [36]. The mega-analysis further revealed that the clinical trials were badly designed, biased, and provided low certainty of evidence. The papain-like protease (PLpro) is another potential target because of its involvement in viral replication [37]. Computational biology identified 147 potential SARS-CoV-2 inhibitors from the screening of FDA-approved drugs [38]. For example, the naphthalene-based PLpro inhibitor L10 inhibited coronavirus replication in Vero E6 cells [39]. The SARS-CoV-2 helicase has also been evaluated as a target for COVID-19 therapy [40]. In addition to lumacaftor, cepharatine, and bananin, flavonoid phytomedicines such as caflanone, equivir, hesperitin, quercetin, and myricetin can inhibit SARS-CoV helicase [41, 42]. The 99.8% homology between SARS-CoV and SARS-CoV-2 suggests that helicase inhibitors could be potential COVID-19 therapeutics [40].

Herbal medicines have also been investigated for the treatment of COVID-19 patients. In this context, the combination of glycyrrhizic acid (GA) from the Chinese herb *Glycyrrhizae radix* and vitamin C has been approved for clinical trials in COVID-19 patients in China [43]. Moreover, Chinese traditional medicines like Huoxiang Zhengqi (HXZQ), Jinhua Qinggan Granules (JHQG), Xuebijing, and Huashi Baidu (HSBD) have been used for relieving severe symptoms in COVID-19 patients [44].

The involvement of the transmembrane protease serine 2 (TMPRSS2) in SARS-CoV-2 S protein priming, and S protein-driven cell entry has made it a target for COVID-19 drug development [45]. For example, nafamostat mesylate, in combination with FPV, allowed the removal of seven critically ill COVID-19 patients from mechanical ventilation, the release of nine patients from the ICU, and only one death among eleven patients treated [46]. Improvement was also detected in three elderly COVID-19 patients treated with nafamostat mesylate [47].

Dexamethasone, an abundant and cheap steroid, was approved by the FDA as a broad-spectrum immunosuppressor in 1958 and has been repurposed for COVID-19 treatment [48]. However, while short-term treatment with dexamethasone could be beneficial in seriously ill intubated COVID-19 patients, it can be dangerous during recovery because of the prevention of protective antibody production. In a recent clinical trial in hospitalized COVID-19 patients, 2,104 individuals received dexamethasone, and 4,321 were given standard care [49]. Overall, 482 (22.9%) patients died within 28 days in the dexamethasone group, compared to 1,110 (25.7%) individuals in the control group. Dexamethasone treatment showed lower 28-day mortality compared to the control group in patients subjected to invasive ventilation or receiving oxygen alone, However, no difference was observed in patients receiving no respiratory support. In the CoDEX randomized clinical trial, use of intravenous dexamethasone and standard care in COVID-19 patients with moderate or severe ARDS generated statistically significant increase in the number of ventilator-free days over 28 days compared to standard care alone [50].

3.3 CHALLENGES IN DRUG DEVELOPMENT AGAINST COVID-19

While mass vaccinations with several COVID-19 vaccines are in full swing, there is high demand for novel COVID-19 drugs. Despite the many different attempts at repurposing drugs developed and approved for other indications, the success rate has been modest. In contrast to the impressively fast COVID-19 vaccine development, which targeted the viral surface, particularly the S protein, antiviral drugs aim at targeting the SARS-CoV-2 replication representing a more complicated level of action. Therefore there are several challenges in developing drugs against coronaviruses. In the first place, coronaviruses are single-stranded RNA viruses, which are prone to mutate, generating potentially novel drug and vaccine-resistant variants [51]. Second, as many drug candidates show a high EC_{50}/C_{max} ratio, they are likely to develop severe side effects such as hemolytic anemia, neutropenia, and cardiopulmonary distress, as seen for high doses of RBV [52]. Viral research can often be incredibly challenging and requires high biosafety levels (BSL3-4) to conduct experiments with lethal viral pathogens in cell cultures and animal models. Bioinformatics and genomics have been essential for establishing several screening models for SARS-CoV and MERS-CoV based on inhibitors of nucleic acids, proteases, and polymerases. So far, the efficacy of broad-spectrum antiviral medicines against coronaviruses has been modest. Further additional research is needed to obtain more efficacious drugs and address potential toxic side effects [5].

Another challenge comprises the transfer of in vitro activity to in vivo proof-of-concept. In this context, though SARS-CoV, MERS-CoV, and HCoV-OC43 have demonstrated sensitivity to RBV in vitro, the doses needed for inhibition in vivo exceed the tolerance of humans [53]. Another issue is that while several flavonoids have demonstrated high binding affinity against SARS-CoV helicase, their poor bioavailability has limited in vivo applications [54]. However, this shortcoming has been addressed by engineering nanoparticles for improved delivery and bioavailability [55].

3.4 FDA APPROVED DRUGS

There are only a few examples of drugs approved for the treatment of COVID-19 so far. For example, RDV has been approved by the FDA for the treatment of hospitalized adults and children with COVID-19 [56]. Recently, the European Commission granted conditional marketing authorization in the EU countries for RDV. Moreover, though mortality rates were not reduced by RDV treatment, the European Medicines Agency (EMA) approved RDV for adults and children over 12 years of age with severe COVID-19 who are suffering from pneumonia and need oxygen supplementation [57]. Despite the uncertainty of therapeutic benefits, FPV has been approved by the Indian Drug Regulator for the treatment of mild-to-moderate COVID-19 under restricted emergency use [58]. Moreover, FPV has also been commercialized in Russia, Bangladesh, Pakistan, Jordan, Egypt, and Saudi Arabia for COVID-19 therapy [58]. In contrast, the FDA has not approved ivermectin for the prevention and treatment of COVID-19 patients because of insufficient certainty and poor quality of evidence.

3.5 COMORBIDITY AND PERSONALIZED COVID-19 DRUGS

The major challenges in COVID-19 management are the yet unknown origin as well as the biology of SARS-CoV-2 and the lack of a gold standard COVID-19 drug. The third important concern is the existing comorbid conditions of COVID-19 patients. Comorbid conditions are directly associated with the disease's severity and outcomes of COVID-19. Recent reports suggest that hypertension (28%–32%) is the most prevalent comorbid condition followed by obesity (25%), diabetes (14%–18%), cardiovascular disease (CVD) (12%–16%), and chronic kidney disease (5%) [59, 60]. Further, the severity and mortality of COVID-19 disease are associated with pre-existing chronic kidney diseases (51% and 44%), cerebrovascular accidents (43% and 44%), and cardiovascular disease (44% and 40%), respectively [60].

However, obesity may not correlate with mortality in COVID-19 [61]. It has also been reported that geographic differences or ethnicity are associated with the prevalence of comorbidities, and COVID-19 severity and mortality. The European and Latin American COVID-19 patients ($\geq$65 years and mostly male) with any comorbid condition show the highest mortality rate. Severe COVID-19 with any comorbid condition was detected in Asians, and the highest prevalence of comorbidities in COVID-19 patients was found in Americans [60]. Apart from these factors, host genetic factors have also been associated with COVID-19 susceptibility, severity, and resistance. The homozygous mutation in the *IFITM3* gene (rs12252) correlates with disease severity [62]. Genetic variations in human leukocyte antigen (HLA) genes are associated with COVID-19 susceptibility. The ****HLA-A*25:01*, *-B*15:27*, *-B*46:01*, *-C*01:02*, an-*C*07:29* alleles correlate with COVID-19 susceptibility, and *HLA-A*02:02*, *-B*15:03*, and -*C*12:03* may have a protective role. Genetic polymorphisms that affect ACE2 and TMPRSS2 expression also increase the risk of infection, and variations in cytokine genes such as *IL6*, *ILR*, *TNF* etc. could be associated with cytokine storm affecting disease severity. In the GWAS (Genome-Wide Association Study), two loci are found associated with COVID-19 severity. These are 3p21.31 harboring genes such as *FYCO1*, *SLC6A20*, *CCR9*, *LZTFL1*, *XCR1*, and *CXCR6*, and 9q34.2, where the *ABO* genes are located [63]. It has also been reported that people with blood group A are more susceptible to SARS-CoV-2 infections [64]. Furthermore, inborn errors of type I IFN immunity are associated with very severe COVID-19 [65].

Therefore it is evident that pre-existing comorbidity, ethnicity, and patient genotype are associated directly with susceptibility, disease severity, and outcomes of COVID-19. Since no effective drug against SARS-CoV-2 is available and most COVID-19 patients are managed based on the symptoms they develop, it is necessary to identify the COVID-19 phenotype based on the genetic makeup of the patient to be able to personalize management of the disease. To achieve this goal, the global COVID-19 Host Genetics Initiative has been initiated [66]. In this context, in a recent study, targets and approved drugs have been predicted for the first time for COVID-19 patients with specific pre-existing conditions as well as a combination of comorbid conditions, using a multi-omics approach [67]. Drugs and their targets need to be validated by applying all necessary caution to evaluate drug efficacy in personalized COVID-19 management. Among several predicted targets and drugs, interferon-α (IFN-α) therapy has recently been approved by the Drugs Controller General of India (DCGI) to treat moderate COVID-19 infections. However, IFN-α therapy could be more beneficial if it is used for COVID-19 patients with kidney diseases.

Another issue relates to the disproportionately high number of immunosuppressed patients, including solid organ transplant recipients (SOTR) impacted by COVID-19 [68]. The mortality among SOTR has been estimated to be as high as 20.5%. Vaccination has been considered as an option to reduce COVID-19 morbidity and mortality [69]. In a recent study, SOTRs showed poor immunogenicity against SARS-CoV-2 after receiving two doses of the BNT162b2 mRNA vaccine [70]. In a retrospective, observational study SOTRs were subjected to vaccinations with the adenovirus-based ChAdOX1 nCoV-19 and Ad26.COV2.S vaccines, and the mRNA-based BNT162b2 and mRNA-1273 vaccines, and only 9 (1.6%) of fully vaccinated individuals tested positive [69]. These findings strongly encourage the vaccination of SOTRs.

3.6 MANAGEMENT OF COVID-19 PATIENTS

In the initial phase of the COVID-19 pandemic, panic struck the healthcare systems around the world. There were no antiviral drugs or vaccines against SARS-CoV-2, but more strikingly, the world was not prepared for a pandemic of this extent. Hospitals, healthcare centers, and retirement homes showed an alarming shortage of basic materials such as personal protection equipment (PPE). Ventilators and other sophisticated equipment for treating seriously ill COVID-19 patients were not available in sufficient quantities, and clinicians were forced to make awkward decisions about who would have access to respirators and who would be left to die. Moreover, many first-line responders among the healthcare personnel were infected by SARS-CoV-2, and more than 3,000 healthcare professionals have died of COVID-19 [70]. It is therefore no surprise that a full-blown crisis was encountered.

After half a year of experience of COVID-19 management, it seemed that the clinicians were still perplexed about how to treat COVID-19 patients, as stated in a publication by Wiersinga and co-workers in August 2020 [71]:

As of July 1, 2020, more than 10 million people worldwide had been infected with SARS-CoV-2. Many aspects of transmission, infection and treatment remain unclear. Advances in prevention and effective management of COVID-19 will require basic and clinical investigation and public health and clinical interventions.

Despite the success in developing several vaccines against SARS-CoV-2 and the approval of some repurposed drugs such as RDV [56, 57] and FPV [58], the management and treatment of COVID-19 still mainly aims at reducing mortality [72]. In the early phases of the pandemic, attention was paid to the significant abnormality of coagulation function, which triggered intravenous administration of immunoglobulins and low molecular weight heparin anticoagulation therapy [73]. Multi-organ evaluation and treatment were also recommended in severe and critically ill COVID-19 patients, in addition to supportive respiratory treatment [74]. Moreover, in a systematic review of full articles published between December 1, 2019, and March 26, 2020, of the 449 identified articles, 41 were included [74]. According to the findings, corticosteroid treatment was most frequently used, followed by lopinavir and oseltamivir.

Nutrition also plays an essential role in stimulating the immune system, and nutritional therapy should be implemented as a first-line treatment into the standard practice of COVID-19 patients [75]. In the case of seriously ill patients, guidelines have been published for nutritional management. As several natural bioactive compounds interact with ACE2 and can also reduce inflammatory responses induced by SARS-CoV-2, nutritional management of COVID-19 patients should not be overlooked.

Finally, COVID-19 management must also deal with post-COVID-19 complications, the so-called long COVID-19 phenomenon, and organ injuries. In the context of the potential for a post-viral syndrome that might manifest after SARS-CoV-2 infection, it was discovered that some patients, especially healthcare workers, developed an illness similar to chronic fatigue syndrome/myalgic encephalomyelitis (CFS/ME) [76]. Based on experience, a subgroup of remitted COVID-19 patients is expected to experience long-term adverse events, long COVID-19, resembling CSF/ME symptoms including persistent fatigue, widespread muscle pain, depression, and non-restorative sleep, which prevent normal activities and return to work for periods up to 20 months [76, 77]. Moreover, in a follow-up study on COVID-19 patients in France, patients experiencing a mild disease complained about relapse with persistent muscle pain, intense fatigue, shortness of breath, tachycardia, headaches, and anxiety [78]. SARS-CoV-2 might trigger a similar immune response as seen for autoimmune diseases. For this reason, patients with post-COVID-19 complications should be tested for antinuclear antibodies in order to rule out any possible underlying autoimmune disease. It has also been suggested that long COVID can be related to the virus- or immune-based disruption of the autonomic nervous system, which might trigger orthostatic intolerance syndromes [79].

In the management of COVID-19, it is important to acknowledge that, in addition to causing pneumonia, damage has been detected in other organs such as the heart, liver, and kidneys [80, 81]. Moreover, the blood and the immune system are also affected. As COVID-19 patients die of multiple organ failure, attention should be paid to protecting and treating multi-organ injuries.

3.7 CONCLUSIONS

At the beginning of the outbreak of SARS-CoV-2, no antiviral drugs or vaccines were available for the treatment and prevention of COVID-19, and more than 3 million lives have been lost. Today, the severity of disease and reduced hospital stays have been possible as a result of advancements in restriction of the spread of SARS-CoV-2, improved knowledge of treatment, and the application of several repurposed drugs. A limited number of drugs have been approved by national authorities for treatment of COVID-19 patients. For example, RDV has been approved by the FDA, and FPV by the EMA and national drug administrations in Russia and other countries. Though not the topic of this chapter, the approval of several vaccines has had a significant impact on seeing light at the end of the tunnel. However, the recently discovered, more transmissible and potentially more deadly SARS-CoV-2 variants/mutants and rare cases of vaccine-induced thrombotic thrombocytopenia (VITT) has added pressure to develop efficacious novel COVID-19 therapeutics and potentially personalized vaccines.

REFERENCES

1. Global Health Policy. Available online: https://www.google.com/covid19-map (accessed on June 4, 2021).

2. Yousefi, H., Mashouri, L., Okpechi, S.C., et al. (2021). Repurposing existing drugs for the treatment of COVID-19/SARS-CoV-2 infection: A review describing drug mechanisms of action. *Biochem. Pharmacol.* 183, 114296.

3. Lam, S., Lombardi, A., Ouanounou, A. (2020). COVID-19: A review of the proposed pharmacological treatments. *Eur. J. Pharmacol.* 886, 173451.

4. Lundstrom, K. (2020). The current status of COVID-19 vaccines. *Front. Genome Edit.* 2, 579297.

5. Krogstad, D.J., Schlesinger, P.H. (1987). The basis of antimalarial action: Non-weak base effects of chloroquine on acid vesicle pH. *Am. J. Trop. Med. Hyg.* 36, 213–220.

6. Gautret, P., Lagier, J.-C., Parola, P., et al. (2020). Hydroxychloroquine and azothromycin as a treatment of COVID-19: Results of an open-label non-randomized clinical trial. *Int. J. Antimicrob. Agents* 56, 105949.

7. Lundstrom, K. (2020). Coronavirus pandemic: Therapy and vaccines. *Biomedicines* 8, 109.

8. Elavarasi, A., Prasad, M., Seth, T., et al. (2020). Chloroquine and hydroxychloroquine for the treatment of COVID-19: A systematic review and meta-analysis. *J. Gen. Intern. Med.* 35, 3308–3314.

9. Wang, Y., Anirudhan, V., Du, R., et al. (2021). RNA-dependent RNA polymerase of SARS-CoV-2 as a therapeutic target. *J. Med. Virol.* 93, 300–310.

10. Elfiky, A.A. (2020). Ribavirin, Remdesivir, Sofosbuvir, Galidesivir, and Tenofovir against SARS-CoV-2 RNA dependent RNA polymerase (RdRp): A molecular docking study. *Life Sci.* 253, 117592.

11. Sheahan, T.P., Sims, A.C., Graham, R.L., et al. (2017). Broad-spectrum antiviral GS-5734 inhibits both epidemic and zoonotic coronaviruses. *Sci. Transl. Med.* 9, eaal3653.

12. de Wit, E., Feldmann, F., Cronin, J., et al. (2020). Prophylactic and therapeutic remdesivir (GS-5734) treatment in the rhesus macaque model of MERS-CoV infection. *Proc. Natl. Acad. Sci. USA* 117, 6771–6776.

13. Beigel, J.H., Tomashek, K.M., Dodd, L.E., et al. (2020). Remdesivir for the treatment of COVID-19: Final report. *N. Engl. J. Med.* 383, 1813–1826.

14. Pan, H., Peto, R., Henao-Restrepo, A.M., et al. (2021). Repurposed antiviral drugs for COVID-19: Interim WHO solidarity trial results. *N. Engl. J. Med.* 384, 497–511.

15. Gandhi, R.T. (2020). The multidimensional challenge of treating coronavirus disease 2019 (COVID-19): Remdesivir is a foot in the door. *Clin. Infect. Dis.* doi:10.1093/cid/ciaa1132.

16. Cai, Q., Yang, M., Liu, D., et al. (2020). Experimental treatment with Favipiravir for COVID-19: An open-label control study. *Engineering* 6, 1192–1198.

17. Chen, C., Zhang, Y., Huang, J., et al. (2020). Favipiravir versus arbidol for COVID-19: A randomized clinical trial. *medRxiv* doi:10.1101/2020.03.17.

18. Rattanaumpawan, P., Jirajariyavej, S., Lerdlamyong, K., et al. (2020). Real-world experience with favipiravir for treatment of COVID-19 in Thailand: Results from a multicenter observational study. *medRxiv*. doi:10.1101/2020.06.24.20133249.

19. Doi, Y., Hibino, M., Hase, R., et al. (2020). A prospective, randomized, open-label trial of early versus late Favipiravir therapy in hospitalized patients with COVID-19. *Antimicrob. Agents Chemother.* 64, e01897–20.

20. Morra, M.E., Van Thanh, L., Kamel, M. G., et al. (2018). Clinical outcomes of current medical approaches for Middle East respiratory syndrome: A systematic review and meta-analysis. *Rev. Med. Virol.* 28, e1977.

21. Unal, M.A., Bitirim, C.V., Summak, G.Y., et al. (2020). Ribavirin shows antiviral activity against SARS-CoV-2 and downregulates the activity of TMPRSS2 and activity of ACE2 in vitro. *bioRxiv*. doi:10.1101/2020.12.04.410092.

22. Hung, I.F., Lung, K.C., Tso, E.Y., et al. (2020). Triple combination of interferon beta-1b, lopinavir-ritonavir, and ribavirin in the treatment of patients admitted to hospital with COVID-19: An open-label, randomised, phase 2 trial. *Lancet* 39, 1695–1704.

23. Eslami, G., Mousaviasl, S., Radmanesh, E., et al. (2020). The impact of sofosbuvir/daclatasvir or ribavirin in patients with severe COVID-19. *J. Antimicrob. Chemother.* 75, 3366–3372.

24. Sadeghi, A., Ali Asgari, A., Norouzi, A., et al. (2020). Sofosbuvir and daclatasvir compared with standard of care in the treatment of patients admitted to hospital with moderate or severe coronavirus infection (COVID-19): A randomized controlled trial. *J. Antimicrob. Chemother.* 75, 3379–3385.

25. Abbaspour Kasgari, H., Moradi, S., Shabani, A.M., et al.(2020). Evaluation of the efficacy of sofosbuvir plus daclatasvir in combination with ribavirin for hospitalized COVID-19 patients with moderate disease compared with standard care: A single-centre, randomized, controlled trial. *J. Antimicrob. Chemother.* 75, 3373–3378.

26. Ataei, M., Hosseinjani, H. (2020). Molecular mechanisms of Galidesivir as a potential antiviral treatment for COVID-19. *J. Pharmaceut. Care* 8, 150–151.

27. BioCryst Sops COVID-19 work to target other viral R&D. www.ncbiotech.org (accessed on June 3, 2021).

28. Sheahan, T.P., Sims, A.M., Shuntai, Z., et al. (2020). An orally bioavailable broad-spectrum antiviral inhibits SARS-CoV-2 in human airway epithelial cell cultures and multiple coronaviruses in mice. *Science Transl. Med.* 12, 5883.

29. Cox, R.M., Wolf, J.D., Plemper, R.K. (2021). Therapeutically administered ribonucleoside analogue MK-4482/EIDD-2801 blocks SARS-CoV-2 transmission in ferrets. *Nat. Microbiol.* 6, 11–18.

30. Painter, W.P., Holman, W., Bush, J.A., et al. (2021). Human safety, tolerability and pharmacokinetics of Molnupiravir, a novel broad-spectrum oral antiviral agent with activity against SARS-CoV-2. *Antimicrob. Agents Chemother.* doi:10.1128/AAC.02428-20.

31. The safety of molnupiravir (EIDD-2801) and its effect on viral shedding of SARS-CoV-2

(END-COVID). Available online: https://clinical-trials.gov/ct2//show/NCT04405739 (accessed on June 3, 2021).

32. Ren, Z., Luo, H., Yu, Z., et al. (2020). A randomized, open-label, controlled clinical trial of azvudine tablets in the treatment of mild and common COVID-19: A pilot study. *Adv. Sc.* 7, 2001435.

33. Moody, V., Ho, J. (2021). Identification of 3-chymotrypsin like protease (3CLPro) inhibitors as potential anti-SARS-CoV-2 agents. *Commun. Biol.* 4, 93.

34. Caly, L., Druce, J.D., Catton, M.G., et al. (2020). The FDA-approved drug ivermectin inhibits the replication of SARS-CoV-2 in vitro. *Antiviral Res.* 178, 104787.

35. Chaccoura, C., Casellasa, A., Blanco-Di Matteo, A., et al. (2021). The effect of early treatment with ivermectin on viral load, symptoms and humoral response in patients with non-severe COVID-19: A pilot, double-blind, placebo-controlled, randomized clinical trial. *EClinicalMedicine* doi:10.1016/j.eclinm.2020.100720.

36. Castañeda-Sabogal, A., Chambergo-Michilot, D., Toro-Huamanchumo, C.J., et al. (2021). Outcomes of ivermectin in the treatment of COVID-19: A systemic review and metanalysis. *medRxiv* doi:10.1101/2021.01.26.21250420.

37. Klemm, T., Ebert, G., Calleja, D.J., et al. (2020). Mechanism and inhibition of the papain-like protease, PLpro, of SARS-CoV-2. *EMBO J.* 39, e106275.

38. Kouznetsova, V.L., Zhang, A., Tatineni, M., et al. (2020). Potential COVID-19 papain-like protease PLpro inhibitors: Repurposing FDA-approved drugs. *PeerJ.* 8, e9965.

39. Bhati, S. (2020). Structure-based drug designing of naphthalene based SARS-CoV PLpro inhibitors for the treatment of COVID-19. *Heliyon* 6, e05558.

40. White, M.A., Lin, W., Cheng, X. (2020). Discovery of COVID-19 inhibitors targeting the SARS-CoV-2 Nsp13 helicase. *J. Phys. Chem. Lett.* 11, 9144–9151.

41. Lee, C., Lee, J.M., Lee, N.R., et al. (2009). Chong, investigation of the pharmacophore space of Severe Acute Respiratory Syndrome coronavirus (SARS-CoV) NTPase/helicase by dihydroxychromone derivatives. *Bioorg. Med. Chem. Lett.* 19, 4538–4541.

42. Ma, C., Sacco, M.D., Hurst, B., et al. (2020). Boceprevir, GC-376, and calpain inhibitors II, XII inhibit SARS-CoV-2 viral replication by targeting the viral main protease. *Cell Res.* 30, 678–692.

43. Sun, Z.-G., Zao, T.-T., Lu, N., et al. (2019). Research progress of glycirrhizic acid on antiviral activity. *Mini Rev. Med. Chem.* 19, 826–832.

44. Zhao, Y.S., Hou, X.Y., Gao, Z.H., et al. (2020). Research on medication for severe type of COVID-19 based on Huashi Baidu prescription. *Chin. Arch. Tradit. Chin. Med.* 21, 1546.

45. Sternberg, A., McKee, D.L., Naujokat, C. (2020). Novel drugs targeting the SARS-CoV-2/COVID-19 machinery. *Curr. Topics Med. Chem.* 20, 1423–1433.

46. Doi, K., Ikeda, M., Hayase, N., et al. (2020). COVID-UTH Study Group, Nafamostat mesylate treatment in combination with favipiravir for patients critically ill with COVID-19: A case series. *Crit. Care* 24, 392.

47. Jang, S., Rhee, J.-Y. (2020). Three cases of treatment with nafamostat in elderly patients with COVID-19 pneumonia who need oxygen therapy. *Int. J. Infect. Dis.* 96, 500–502.

48. Theoharides, T.C., Conti, P. (2020). Dexamethasone for COVID-19? Not so fast. *J. Biol. Regul. Homeostas. Agents* 34, 1241–1243.

49. Horby, P., Lim, W.S., Emberson, J.R., et al. (2021). Dexamethasone in hospitalized patients with COVID-19. *N. Engl. J. Med.* 384, 693–704.

50. Tomazini, B.M., Maia, I.S., Cavalcanti, A.B., et al. (2020). Efffect of dexamethasone on days alive and ventilator-free in patients with moderate to severe acute respiratory distress syndrome and COVID-19: The CoDEX randomized clinical trial. *JAMA* 324, 1307–1316.

51. Han, Y.J., Ren, Z.G., Li, X.X., et al. (2020). Advances and challenges in the prevention and treatment of COVID-19. *Int. J. Med. Sci.* 17, 1803–1810.

52. Muller, M.P., Dresser, L., Raboud, J., et al. (2007). Adverse events associated with high-dose Ribavirin: Evidence from the Toronto outbreak of severe acute respiratory syndrome. *Pharmacotherapy* 27, 494–503.

53. Totura, A.L., Bavari, S. (2019). Broad-spectrum coronavirus antiviral drug discovery. *Expert Opin. Drug Discov.* 14, 397–412.

54. Thilakarathna, S.H., Vasantha Rupasinghe, H.P. (2013). Flavonoid bioavailability and attempts for bioavailability enhancement. *Nutrients* 5, 3367–3387.

55. Zhang, H., Cui, W., Qu, X., et al. (2019). Photothermal-responsive nanosized hybrid polymersome as versatile therapeutics codelivery nanovehicle for effective tumor suppression. *Proc. Natl. Acad. Sci. USA* 116, 7744–7749.

56. Rubin, D., Chan-Tack, K., Farley, J., et al. (2020). FDA approval of Remdesivir: A step in the right direction. *N. Engl. J. Med.* 383, 2598–2600.

57. Gérard, A.O., Laurain, A., Fresse, A., et al. (2021). Remdesivir and acute renal failure: A potential safety signal from disproportionality analysis of the WHO safety database. *Pharmacol. Ther.* 109, 1021–1024.

58. Joshi, S., Parkar, J., Ansari, A., et al. (2021). Role of favipiravir in the treatment of COVID-19. *Int. J. Infect. Dis.* 102, 501–508.

59. Fathi, M., Vakili, K., Sayehmiri, F., et al. (2021). The prognostic value of comorbidity for the

severity of COVID-19: A systematic review and meta-analysis study. *PLoS One* 16, e0246190.

60. Thakur, B., Dubey, P., Benitez, J., et al. (2021). A systematic review and meta-analysis of geographic differences in comorbidities and associated severity and mortality among individuals with COVID-19. *Sci. Rep.* 11, 8562.

61. Ng, W.H., Tipih, T., Makoah, N.A., et al. (2021). Comorbidities in SARS-CoV-2 patients: A systematic review and meta-analysis. *mBio* 12, e03647–20.

62. Zhang, Y., Qin, L., Zhao, Y., et al. (2020). Interferon-induced transmembrane protein 3 genetic variant rs12252-C associated with disease severity in coronavirus disease 2019. *J. Infect. Dis.* 222, 34–37.

63. Fricke-Galindo, I., Falfán-Valencia, R. (2021). Genetics insight for COVID-19 susceptibility and severity: A review. *Front. Immunol.* 12, 622176.

64. Zhao, J., Yang, Y., Huang, H., et al. (2020). Relationship between the ABO blood group and COVID-19 susceptibility. *Clin. Infect. Dis.* Aug 4:ciaa1150. doi:10.1093/cid/ciaa1150.

65. Bastard, P., Rosen, L.B., Zhang, Q., et al. (2020). Autoantibodies against type I IFNs in patients with life-threatening COVID-19. *Science* 370, eabd4585. doi:10.1126/science.abd4585.

66. The COVID-19 Host Genetics Initiative. (2020). The COVID-19 Host Genetics Initiative, a global initiative to elucidate the role of host genetic factors in susceptibility and severity of the SARS-CoV-2 virus pandemic. *Eur. J. Hum. Genetics* 28, 715.

67. Barh, D., Aljabali, A.A.A., Tambuwala, M.M., et al. (2021). Predicting COVID-19—Comorbidity pathway crosstalk-based targets and drugs: Towards personalized COVID-19 management. *Biomedicines* 9, 556.

68. Kates, O.S., Haydel, B.M., Florman, S.S., et al. (2020). COVID-19 in solid organ transplant: A multi-center cohort study. *Clin. Infect. Dis.* 2020 August 7, ciaa1097.

69. Malinis, M., Cohen, E., Azar, M.M. (2021). Effectiveness of SARS-CoV-2 vaccination in fully-vaccinated solid organ transplant recipients. *Am. J. Transpl.* doi:10.1111/ajt.16713. Online ahead of print.

70. Kincaid, E. (2021). One year into the pandemic, more than 3000 healthcare workers have died of COVID-19. *MedScape* 8, www.medscape.com/viewarticle/947304.

71. Wiersinga, W.J., Rhodes, A., Cheng, A.C., et al. (2020). Pathophysiology, transmission, diagnosis, and treatment of coronavirus disease 2019 (COVID-19): A review. *JAMA* 324, 782–793.

72. Kumar Mishra, S., Tripathi, T. (2021). One year update on the COVID-19 pandemic: Where are we now? *Acta Trop.* 214, 105778.

73. Li, T., Lu, H., Zhang, W. (2020). Clinical observation and management of COVID-19 patients. *Emerg. Microb. Infect.* 9, 687–690.

74. Tobaiqy, M., Qashqary, M., Al-Dahery, S., et al. (2020). Therapeutic management of patients with COVID-19: A systematic review. *Infect. Prev. Pract.* 2, 100061.

75. Fernandez-Quintela, A., Milton-Laskibar, I., Trepiana, J., et al. (2020). Key aspects in nutritional management of COVID-19 patients. *J. Clin. Med.* 9, 2589.

76. Perrin, R., Riste, L., Hann, M., et al. (2020). Into the looking glass: Post-viral syndrome post COVID-19. *Med Hypotheses* 144, 110055.

77. Moldofsky, H., Patcai, J. (2011). Chronic widespread musculoskeletal pain, fatigue, depression and disordered sleep in chronic post-SARS syndrome: A case-controlled study. *BMC Neurol.* 11, 37.

78. Davido, B., Seang, S., Tubiana, R., et al. (2020). Post-COVID-19 chronic symptoms: A postinfectious entity? *Clin. Microbiol. Infect.* 26, 1448–1449.

79. Dani, M., Dirksen, A., Taraborelli, P., et al. (2021). Autonomic dysfunctions in "long COVID": Rationale, physiology and management strategies. *Clin. Med.* 21, e63–e67.

80. Wang, T., Du, Z., Zhu, F., et al. (2020). Comorbidities and multi-organ injuries in the treatment of COVID-19. *Lancet* 395, e52.

81. Zaim, S., Chong, J.H., Sankaranarayanan, V., et al. (2020). COVID-19 and multiorgan response. *Curr. Probl. Cardiol.* 45, 100618.

Chapter 4   Prevention and Control Strategies for the COVID-19 Pandemic

Isfendiyar Darbaz, Gizem Morris, and Şükrü Tüzmen

4.1 INTRODUCTION

Both physical and mental health have been severely impacted by the COVID-19 pandemic. COVID-19 has been shown to cause extrapulmonary manifestations in the cardiovascular, gastrointestinal, urinary, and nervous systems, as well as serious respiratory pathology. Mental health problems related to the pandemic include depression, anxiety, fatigue, and post-traumatic stress disorder The development of specific, efficient, and safe COVID-19 prevention and therapeutics, such as vaccines, antiviral agents, and passive immunotherapy, is extremely beneficial. Several problems, however, remain unresolved, and systemic and effective prevention and care may prove difficult to achieve in the immediate future [1].

School and business closure on a wide scale and over a long period of time results in a drastic decline in daily activities and lifestyle behaviors. People who are affected by economic downturns, quarantines, and curfews are more likely to indulge in unhealthy activities such as overeating, smoking, and drinking. Psychological distress caused by COVID-19 has been linked to increased energy intake and decreased physical activity, resulting in weight gain and higher rates of overweight and obesity [1].

At this time, avoiding virus exposure by physical isolation, face masks, hand washing and eye protection is unquestionably the most effective way of reducing COVID-19 transmission and preventing associated chronic complications. Changes in lifestyle factors such as diet, exercise, smoking, alcohol intake, screen time, and sleep can also help to shift the COVID-19 risk distribution. These factors are also important in the treatment of mental disorders, which are common in pandemics like this one [1].

In addition to mass vaccination, the best solution for controlling the pandemic would be to use preventive strategies, responsive diagnostic techniques, and currently available medications at the same time. This segment contains the most up-to-date details on COVID-19 transmission, prevention, and control.

4.2 PANDEMICS ARE EXPECTED TO INCREASE IN FREQUENCY

4.2.1 Macro Environmental Analyses

The outbreak of COVID-19 has put a greater social, economic, and psychological strain on society than ever before. The battle between response – advanced technology and immediate medical research – is still a long way from being able to respond effectively to the assault of new virus variants under time pressure. Researchers warn that "pandemics are expected to become more common" [2]. As a result, the unexpected effect of COVID-19 increases the burden on the medical and social capacities of global health systems, which have become increasingly reliant on global collaboration and are being harmed by current insufficient systems [3]. Moreover, outbreaks and the transmission of new viruses are expected to rise. This poses serious problems for human populations that lack antibody defense, and it is unclear how their immune systems can cope [4].

4.2.2 Pre-Disposal Factors at Community Level – Outbreak and Transmission

Economic and psychological effects on pastoral populations that are underserved as a result of a shortage of health personnel, fewer accessible health facilities, lack of diagnostic testing kits and protective equipment, and an overall inadequate healthcare delivery system. Low- and middle-income countries are vulnerable and underserved, posing significant challenges to monitoring the spread of the disease. These populations are overcrowded, with little opportunity for physical separation. Similarly, farming communities are more susceptible to zoonotic diseases. Recent research suggests that intensive animal husbandry and unregulated animal-derived food intake may be a major factor in the spread of COVID-19. Furthermore, the pastoral community's close interaction with these animal husbandries, such as camels, is considered a significant exposure and risk factor for viral transmission to humans [5].

In comparison to the rest of the world, Africa has a higher proportion of people with health problems. Consequently, higher rates of malnutrition, anemia, malaria, HIV/AIDS, and tuberculosis in many African countries could be linked to, and exacerbated by, ongoing COVID-19 pandemic prevention and control efforts [3].

Pastoral communities are also found to be uneducated, or less likely to follow public health recommendations for infection prevention and

DOI: 10.1201/9781003190394-4

control. Furthermore, cultural and traditional barriers associated with controversial health theories and low health-seeking habits remain a concern in these trying times [5].

The ramifications on social and economic levels are also concerning. The COVID-19 pandemic in Africa has dramatically increased unemployment rates, according to a World Bank survey, and the African economy will be severely impacted [3]. Economic conditions are expected to worsen because of current fragile healthcare and public health systems, insufficient healthcare facilities, lack of access to clean water, sanitation, food protection, and political unrest, as well as restrictions on primary commodity exports and imports [6].

4.3 COVID-19 POSING DIFFERENT THREATS AND CHALLENGES FOR CONTROL MECHANISMS

4.3.1 Unique Viral Characteristics of the SARS-CoV-2

Severe acute respiratory syndrome-coronavirus 2 (SARS-CoV-2) is a single-stranded RNA virus [7]. The word "corona" is derived from the Latin word for "crown", which refers to the crown-like spikes on the surface of the virus. Coronaviruses are zoonotic, which means that they can spread from animals to humans. Since zoonotic diseases have an animal reservoir, eradication is extremely difficult. For example, avian influenza virus can be eradicated in farmed animals, turkeys, and ducks, but it returns every year because of its presence in wild birds. Avian influenza virus does not spread from person to person, but outbreaks in poultry farms happen every year all over the world [7]. Coronaviruses have been associated with other outbreaks in humans, including Severe Acute Respiratory Syndrome (SARS) caused by SARS-CoV, and Middle East Respiratory Syndrome (MERS) caused by MERS-CoV [8].

Both direct and indirect contact (droplet and human-to-human transmission) will spread SARS-CoV-2 (contaminated objects and airborne contagion). SARS-CoV-2 is believed to spread mainly through respiratory droplets, which are produced when a patient coughs, sneezes, or even speaks or sings. Droplets will spread only a few feet and remain in the air for a few seconds. SARS-CoV-2, on the other hand, can remain stable and infectious in droplets for up to three hours after being suspended in the air. As a result, airborne isolation, good room ventilation, and proper disinfectant application (especially in restrooms, bathrooms) can all help to keep the virus from spreading [9].

SARS-CoV-2 can be transmitted from asymptomatic individuals (or individuals during the incubation period). For this reason, faster and more responsive diagnostic methods for detecting infected people are needed to address a variety of problems for prevention and control measures [9]. The SARS-CoV-2 spread may be more complicated than in previous outbreaks. The importance of a home quarantine requiring full society lockdown is highlighted by the relatively long incubation period, the prevalence of asymptomatic patients, and the persistence of viral shedding after recovery [9]. The following section will concentrate on non-vaccination-based prevention steps, as vaccination alone cannot and will not stop the COVID-19 pandemic. As a result, low-cost, evidence-based, integrated control methods will be required [10].

4.3.2 Aerosol Exposure Risk and Mitigation Strategies

The COVID-19 pandemic has completely changed people's views on otorhinolaryngologic treatments and procedures. Respiratory disease can be caused by contact (touching a contaminated surface followed by self-inoculation of the eyes, nose, or mouth), droplets (inhalation in the nasal/upper airway or direct inoculation of the eyes, nose, or mouth), or aerosol transmission (inhalation into upper or lower airways) (Figure 4.1) [11].

Four factors affect the likelihood of indoor viral respiratory transmission: (1) the properties of aerosols and droplets; (2) indoor airflow; (3) virus-specific factors; and (4) host-specific factors The transmission of a respiratory viral pathogen requires both exposure to, and successful inoculation with, an infectious titer of virus. Protective goggles and face shields are not currently differentiated in face safety guidelines; however, we recommend using face shields because they provide additional protection beyond just covering the eyes. Face shields prevent early exposure to cough or sneeze-generated aerosols by intercepting droplets and high-velocity airborne particles before they enter a face mask or respirator. Since aerosol particles will "slip" around the face shield as particle transport associated with bulk airflow takes over, face-shield effectiveness decreases with time. At this stage, wearing a good face mask or respirator is needed. While current clinical evidence on the effectiveness of N95 masks versus surgical masks in preventing disease transmission is inconclusive, a recent study indicated that N95 masks may be more effective than surgical masks in reducing coronavirus-associated disease transmission [11].

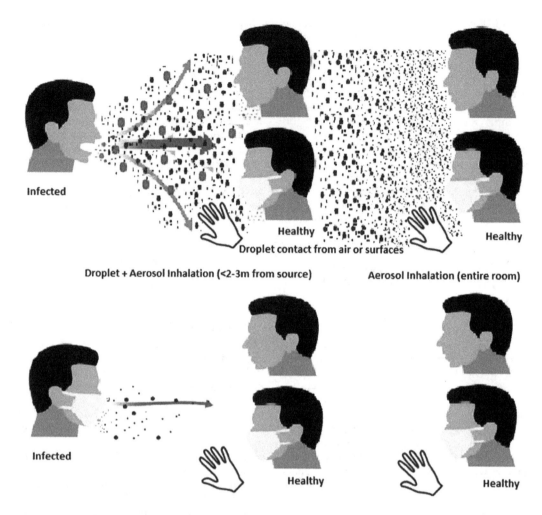

Droplet + Aerosol Inhalation (<2-3m from source)   Aerosol Inhalation (entire room)

Figure 4.1 There are three potential pathways for the transmission of respiratory pathogens. Self-inoculation after contact with droplets that settle on surfaces, direct deposition/ inspiration of infectious droplets in the mouth or nose, and deposition on the skin, as well as airborne transmission through inhalation of aerosols, are all possible modes of transmission. Aerosol transmission over short distances (2 to 3 meters) can be difficult to distinguish from droplet transmission. Long-range transmission of viral respiratory pathogens such as influenza and coronaviruses is still debatable.

Infectious aerosols can be reduced by the rate of building ventilation (dilution) and using higher-efficiency filtration. According to the American Society for Heating, Refrigeration, and Air-Conditioning Engineers (ASHRAE), the key technique for building protection during the pandemic reopening process is to reduce aerosol exposure. Most heating, ventilation, and air-conditioning (HVAC) systems in homes use intentional particle filtration, which decreases aerosol concentrations even more. The most powerful filter (MERV 16) can remove >95% of particles when properly built [11].

4.4 STRATEGIES FOR SHORT-TERM IMMEDIATE ACTIONS REQUIRED FOR PREVENTION AND CONTROL

In the current situation, infection prevention measures are critical for disease management. To minimize the risk of SARS-CoV-2 infection and transmission, several preventive measures have been recommended for general public health, including hand and respiratory hygiene, as well as good food practices (in relation to raw animal products) [12]. In the meantime, there is a pressing need to recommend successful preventive measures that could reduce the risk of COVID-19 infection [13]. Education, separation, prevention, transmission control, and treatment of infected people, according to the WHO, are crucial measures in controlling infectious diseases like COVID-19. Having the following guidelines will help to limit the spread of infection [9].

Shielding entails remaining at home (home quarantine) and avoiding direct contact with someone who is either a potentially asymptomatic or symptomatic COVID-19 patient, avoiding congested public places, excessive travel, and keeping a distance of at least two meters between people, particularly if they are coughing or sneezing; hand shaking should be avoided, hands should be washed for at least 20 seconds with soap and water, or a hand sanitizer containing at least 75% alcohol should be used on a regular basis, particularly after touching common surfaces in public spaces. Touching eyes, nose, and mouth should be avoided and surfaces should be wiped with disinfectant sprays. Use of medical masks (especially N95, 12–16-layer cotton or surgical masks) or a respirator may be necessary because of the long incubation period and the presence of asymptomatic patients (especially FFP3). Furthermore, medical shields or protective suits are recommended, particularly for healthcare workers. Since gloves may easily become infected, wearing gloves in public does not provide adequate protection against COVID-19 [9, 14]

Effective preventative measures and health responses from governments, physicians, and the general public are expected to prevent the spread of COVID-19 infection. The transmission of a virus from person to person is important, and super-spreading events can occur in public gatherings. The following are some of the critical measures that must be taken to prevent COVID-19 from spreading across the population:

(a) Isolation of affected individuals or potential carriers as well as individuals traveling from affected countries. COVID-19 is transmitted by asymptomatic carriers, according to some reports.
(b) Prevention of transmission by ensuring a high degree of hygiene at home and in public spaces and public transport.
(c) Avoidance of social gatherings because they present high risk events for virus spread.
(d) Increase in public education and perception.
(e) Everyone, especially infected, elderly people, and immunocompromised individuals should wear masks and protective clothing to prevent infection and protect themselves from COVID-19.
(f) Maintenance of good immunity by eating a nutrient-dense diet, and the intake of vitamins, especially C and E, along with physical exercise, to aid in the fight against COVID-19.
(g) Maintenance of social isolation is strongly recommended because of the spread of SARS-CoV-2 from person to person [15].

4.4.1 Physical Avoidance

The goal of social distancing is to flatten the curve of new infections, preventing an increase in demand on healthcare services. [16, 17].

Masks and face shields cannot fully eliminate pathogen exposure, but they do minimize the amount of exposure. Even if it fails to avoid infection, wearing a mask will minimize the amount of pathogen exposure, resulting in a relatively mild disease. As a result, wearing masks in the general population will reduce at least a significant portion of COVID-19 infections [18–20].

Handwashing and wearing a mask are critical for slowing the spread of SARS-CoV-2. However, washing hands in the correct manner is often difficult, and existing medical masks, also known as surgical masks, are in short supply in many countries. People in some countries have been encouraged to make their own SARS-CoV-2 masks at home, but it is unclear if these are successful at blocking the virus [21].

4.4.2 Lifestyles and Behavior

Appropriate nutrition is essential for a healthy immune system, and both malnutrition and overnutrition can have negative effects on immune responses. Malnourishment and malnutrition can cause nutritional deficiencies in energy, protein, and micronutrients, which can weaken the immune system and make it more susceptible to infections. Specific nutrients can influence immune function by affecting gut microbiota composition, cell activation, gene expression, and signaling pathway activity [1].

Plants have been used as traditional medicines in almost all of the cultures around the world for centuries to treat a variety of chronic illnesses, including viral diseases. Scientists have attempted to validate scientifically the health-improving ability of functional and nutraceutical foods in recent decades. Different parts and extracts from medicinal plants have demonstrated similar medicinal properties as synthesized pharmaceuticals [1]. Various groups of compounds, such as alkaloids, flavonoids, terpenoids, and polysaccharides, exhibit immunomodulatory properties with fewer side effects than allopathic medications, prompting a surge in interest in using medicinal plants to modulate the human immune system. We believe that functional food plants can assist people in overcoming infection by: (1) modulating the immune system, (2) producing antiviral activity against the infection, and (3) reducing other respiratory issues. The potential immunomodulatory activity of plants is a relatively new idea in the field of phytomedicine. Immunomodulators not only boost humoral and cell-mediated immunity, but they also stimulate non-specific immune responses including natural killer (NK) cells, macrophages, granulocytes, and complement systems, all of which boost infection resistance in a non-specific way. Table 4.1 lists 20 popular and easily accessible functional food plants with immunomodulatory and antiviral properties that can modulate the immune system and are biologically active against a variety of medical indications caused by respiratory tract infections. These plants have been shown to stimulate the immune system in a variety of ways. However, their efficacy in humans may be limited. When used in large quantities, they can be poisonous. As a result, caution should be exercised in their applications [1].

Probiotics are live microorganisms with potential health benefits when ingested, primarily by enhancing or restoring gut flora. Probiotics have been shown to stimulate multiple immune pathways, influence host immunological networks, improve immune responses, and reduce the frequency and length of viral respiratory tract infections by a small amount. Microbial dysbiosis has been found in some COVID-19 patients, with a decrease in Lactobacillus and Bifidobacterium, and probiotics have been suggested in COVID-19 management guidelines. However, it is unknown whether conventional probiotics are effective in the prevention or treatment of COVID-19 [1].

Obesity appears to have a significant negative impact on pathogen protection and immunity, and a correlation between obesity and various infectious diseases has been established. Low-grade chronic inflammation is a symptom of obesity, and it can weaken innate and adaptive immune responses, making the immune system more susceptible to infections. Obesity has been shown to negatively impact host immunity, infection resistance, post-infection complications, and mortality from serious infections. COVID-19 has a high chance of causing serious or fatal outcomes in overweight and obese individuals. These individuals need special care, with a focus on infection prevention and weight loss [1].

While home confinement can help to prevent the spread of SARS-CoV-2, it also alters exercise habits and decreases physical activity. In reality, the COVID-19 pandemic is exacerbating an already-existing physical inactivity epidemic. Restricted exercise lowers energy consumption and raises the risk of gaining weight. Increased eating as a result of boredom, depression, or anxiety may also lead to a rise in body weight. During the pandemic, exercise is critical for avoiding the health hazards associated with inactivity, as well as for improving wellbeing and immunity, and reducing stress and anxiety [1].

Individuals with elevated anxiety and those dealing with anxiety disorders have demonstrated that aerobic exercise is successful in treating behavioral illnesses, with high-intensity exercise becoming more effective than lower-intensity activities [22]. A physically active lifestyle is also important for mental and physical health during confinement. During the COVID-19 pandemic, regular physical activity can help with infection prevention, mental health issues such as anxiety and depression, body weight maintenance, and chronic disease prevention and management. Given the negative effects of the COVID-19 pandemic on the mobility and playing habits of children, motivating children to engage in physical activity deserves special consideration [1].

Long periods of confinement at home can cause boredom, stress, and mental issues, which can contribute to increased alcohol consumption. Alcohol is considered to have little benefit on one's health, and is a significant risk factor for chronic illness and injury. However, according to GBD 2016 Alcohol Collaborators (2018), moderate consumption of alcohol may provide some benefits [23].

With increasing levels of alcohol consumption, the risk of all-cause mortality increases, and only total abstinence reduces the risk of damage to health. Chronic alcohol use, in particular, has been shown to impair the ability to fight infections such as tuberculosis and pneumonia by disrupting the innate and adaptive immune systems. Alcohol affects a variety of pathways that impair immunity, and it is likely to be harmful in the case of infection with the SARS-CoV-2. Acute respiratory distress syndrome (ARDS), one of the most serious COVID-19 complications, has been shown to be substantially increased by high chronic alcohol intake [1].

Various mechanisms can increase the risk of respiratory tract infections in smokers. Smoking impairs immune function and has been shown to nearly double the risk of tuberculosis infection, increase the risk 3–5-fold of several types of pneumonia infection, and enhance the risk by approximately 5-fold for influenza virus infection [24, 25]. In terms of COVID-19–related dangers, electronic cigarettes and other alternative devices are unlikely to be a safer choice. They can cause the

Table 4.1 Immunomodulatory and antiviral functional plant food

Plant Name	Plant Parts Used (Preparation Methods)	Chemical Content	Healing Benefits
Onion (*Allium cepa* L.)	Bulb (Crushed, mixed with honey)	Quercetin, thiosulfinates, anthocyanins	Quercitin has been shown to lower cholesterol, prevent heart disease, thin the blood and ward off blood clots, good for asthma, chronic bronchitis, diabetes, and infections. It has even been linked to prohibiting some forms of cancer.
Garlic (*Allium sativum* L.)	Bulb (Crushed, mixed with honey)	Diallyl disulphide, alliin, polyphenols, proteins	Garlic has been used to treat bronchitis, hypertension, TB (tuberculosis), liver disorders, dysentery, flatulence, colic, intestinal worms, rheumatism, diabetes, and fevers.
Barberry (*Berberis vulgaris* L.)	Fruit, stem and root (Boiled extract, poultice)	Berbamine, berberine	Studies showed that barberries have numerous health benefits, including anti-inflammatory ones. Moreover, it can be used as a medicinal herb to treat a variety of disorders, such as diabetes, liver disease, gallbladder pain, digestive, urinary tract diseases, and gallstones.
Tea Plant (*Camellia sinensis* (L.) Kuntze)	Leaf (Boiled, beverage)	Catechins, quercetin, gallic acid, theaflavin-3,3'-digallate	The tea plant is a herb used in cancer (prevention), cognitive improvement, Crohn's disease, diuresis, genital warts, headaches, heart disease (prevention), Parkinson's disease (prevention), stomach disorders, weight loss (combination products), and hypercholesterolemia.
Papaya (*Carica papaya* L.)	Fruit and leaves (Leaves, ground to prepare juice; fruit can be eaten directly)	Caricaxanthin, violaxanthin, zeaxanthin, carpaine, dehydrocarpaine I, II and cardenolide	Papaya is used for preventing and treating gastrointestinal tract disorders, intestinal parasite infections, and as a sedative and diuretic. It is also used for nerve pains (neuralgia) and elephantoid growths.
Bitter orange (*Citrus aurantium* L.)	Fruit, peel (Dried peel or fruit juice)	Polysaccharides, polyphenolic compounds	Bitter orange and its extracts are used in Traditional Chinese Medicine (TCM) to treat indigestion, diarrhea, dysentery, and constipation. In other regions, the fruit is used to treat anxiety and epilepsy.
Turmeric (*Curcuma longa* L.)	Rhizome (Pounded, tincture, powder)	Curcumin	Taken orally, turmeric is used as treatment for indigestion (dyspepsia), abdominal pain, hemorrhage, diarrhea, flatulence, abdominal bloating, loss of appetite, jaundice, hepatitis, and liver disease, gallbladder complaints, headaches, bronchitis, colds, respiratory infections, fibromyalgia, leprosy, fever.
Fig (*Ficus carica* L.)	Fruit, leaves (Decoction with honey)	Terpenoids, anthocyanins, steroids	Fig leaves are used for diabetes, high cholesterol, and skin conditions such as eczema, psoriasis, and vitiligo. Some people apply the milky sap (Latex) from the tree directly to the skin to treat skin tumors and warts.
Soybean (*Glycine max* (L.) Merr.)	Seeds (Cooked, roasted)	Isoflavones, flavonoids, phytosterols, organic acid, saponins	Long-term use of soybean (*Glycine max*) may prevent the progression of breast cancer.
Liquorice (*Glycyrrhiza glabra* L.)	Root (Dried roots extracted. The extract is vacuum dried to a dark paste, then dried to a powder)	Glycyrrhizin	Efficient hepatoprotective medication in patients with chronic hepatitis C and more broadly to protect from a variety of hepatic diseases such as chronic viral hepatitis, drug- or chemical-induced liver injury, nonalcoholic fatty liver disease, autoimmune hepatitis, and hepatocellular

(Continued)

Table 4.1 (Continued) Immunomodulatory and antiviral functional plant food

Plant Name	Plant Parts Used (Preparation Methods)	Chemical Content	Healing Benefits
Wolfberry (*Lycium barbarum* L.)	Fruit (Fresh fruit eaten directly)	Polysaccharide-protein complexes, phenolic compounds	Nourishing the eyes, kidney, lungs, and liver.
Mango (*Mangifera indica* L.)	Bark, leaves, roots, fruits, flowers (Boiling, powdering of bark, leaves, root and flowers; fruit can be directly eaten)	Flavonoids, xanthones (Mangiferin), phenolic acids, triterpenes	Used as a dentrifrice, antiseptic, astringent, diaphoretic, stomachic, vermifuge, tonic, laxative and diuretic and to treat diarrhea, dysentery, anemia, asthma, bronchitis, cough, hypertension, insomnia, rheumatism, toothache, leucorrhoea, haemorrhage and piles.
Mulberry (*Morus alba* L.)	Fruit leaf, root (Fruit juice, leaves, root bark decoction or tea)	Carotene, vitamin B1, folic acid, folinic acid, vitamin D, polyhydroxylated alkaloids, glycoprotein, Anthocyanins, benzofurans, stilbenes	In folk remedies, have been traditionally used for the treatment of fever, cough, hyperlipidaemia, hypertension, and hyperglycaemia.
Black Cumin (*Nigella sativa* L.)	Seeds (Roasted)	Quinones, alkaloids, saponins	The medicinal use of black cumin seeds in various traditional herbal systems is known for a wide range of ailments which include different airway disorders, for pain such as chronic headache and back pain, diabetes, paralysis, infection, inflammation, hypertension, and administered in digestive tract related problems.
Long pepper (*Piper longum* L.)	Fruit, root (Decoction)	Piperine	Long pepper is used to improve appetite and digestion, as well as treat stomach ache, heartburn, indigestion, intestinal gas, diarrhea, and cholera. It is also used for lung problems including asthma, bronchitis, and cough
Black pepper (*Piper nigrum* L.)	Fruit (Dried, used as spice)	Piperine	Oral use for arthritis, asthma, upset stomach, bronchitis, cholera, colic, depression, diarrhea, gas, headache, sex drive, menstrual pain, stuffy nose, sinus infection, dizziness, discolored skin (vitiligo), weight loss, and cancer.
Plum (*Prunus domestica* L.)	Fruit (Eaten fresh)	Anthocyanins, protocatechuic acid	Used for the treatment of leukorrhea, irregular menstruation, and debility following miscarriage
Guava (*Psidium guajava* L.)	Fruit, shoots, leaves (Fruit can be eaten directly. Decoction and poultice of leaves, shoots)	Phenolic, flavonoid, carotenoid, terpenoid, triterpenes	Compounds in guava leaf extract may have a positive effect on a range of illnesses and symptoms, including menstrual cramps, diarrhea, the flu, type 2 diabetes, and cancer.
Pomegranate (*Punica granatum* L.)	Fruit, seeds, bark (Fruit juice, decoction of seeds, dried bark)	Anthocyanins, fatty acids, alkaloids, vitamins	Used as an antiparasitic agent and to treat diarrhea, ulcers, diabetes and cardiovascular disease.
Ginger (*Zingiber officinale* Roscoe)	Root (Dried, roasted, eaten with honey)	Essential oil, crude fiber proteins, fatty oils, carbohydrates	Ginger extract reduces inflammation in rheumatoid arthritis, inflammatory gut disease, asthma, and certain cancers

Notes: (1) The immunomodulatory properties of these plants are for the overall immune system of the body, not for any specific disease, illness, or organ. (2) Antiviral properties are often used against viruses that infect the respiratory tract.

contagious lung damage seen with conventional cigarettes because they also use tobacco and emit smoke or vapor [1, 26].

In the context of homeschooling, teleworking or home-offices, and online socializing, prevention and lockdown initiatives implemented in several countries resulted in a growing dependence on screens. Sleep and immunity are intertwined, and sleep deprivation and irregular sleeping patterns can increase susceptibility to SARS-CoV-2 infection [27]. Sleep quality may be compromised during the pandemic as a result of COVID-19–related anxiety and stress, and it can be damaged even more by repetitive screen-related behaviors such as watching television, using computers and mobile devices, and playing electronic games. A controlled management of screen time, adequate sleep quality and quantity, and regular daily sleep cycles should be encouraged, to provide the best possible function of the immune system to reduce SARS-CoV-2 infections [1].

4.4.3 Medical Supplements

Micronutrients, such as vitamins and trace elements, are known to play important roles in both innate and adaptive immune responses, and maintaining micronutrient homeostasis is critical for immune system health. Micronutrient deficiencies can lower immunity to disease, but supplementation has been shown to boost immunity against viral infections. Vitamin D deficiency, for example, tends to be linked to weakened immune responses and an increased risk of systemic infections. Vitamin D supplementation can help to prevent respiratory infections by reducing the development of proinflammatory cytokines and thus the risk of pneumonia caused by cytokine storm [1, 28, 29].

N-acetyl-L-cysteine (NAC) is a common health supplement that has been proposed as a nutraceutical that can help in the control of RNA viruses such as influenza and coronaviruses [30]. Based on a systematic literature search, a possible function of NAC and copper in combination with antiviral drugs, such as remdesivir has been hypothesized for treatment of COVID-19 [30].

SARS-CoV-2 is a deadly virus that has spread around the world. This virus, on the other hand, is vulnerable to increased body heat, which boosts the immune system. According to researchers, repeated treatments of heat accompanied by cold are the most successful first-line treatment for mild SARS-CoV-2infections. They suggest using the most available form of hydrothermotherapy treatments for all stages of COVID-19 [31]. However, studies involving larger-scale populations are needed in order to obtaining more representative results.

4.5 STRATEGIES FOR LONG-TERM PREPAREDNESS AND READINESS IN RESPONSE TO ONE HEALTH AND WORLD HEALTH SYSTEMS (WHO)

In practice, preventative approaches seek to enhance communicable and zoonotic disease monitoring and response by coordinating multisectoral and inter-disciplinary health prevention and intervention efforts. The One Health initiative is a movement to form all-inclusive, co-equal alliances between physicians, osteopathic doctors, veterinarians, dentists, nurses, and other scientific-health and environmental disciplines. To determine the feasibility of multisectoral interventions, other relevant fields must be included in discussions of methodologies, the definition of benchmarks, and the actual implementation of multicenter pilot studies. Since each region, such as countries and continents, is unique, potential synergies with COVID-19 public health strategies and other sector goals will need to be evaluated and adapted to each social-ecological background. Future potential strategies will need to reconsider the determinants of health in neglected tropical diseases (NTDs) in order to galvanize efforts and develop comprehensive, well-defined programs that will lay the groundwork for a multi-sectorial approach. These multi-sectorial approaches may involve medical developmental sectors, environmental sectors, agricultural sectors, education, economy, communications, bilateral agribusiness, and public–private partnerships [32].

4.6 CONCLUSION

To summarize, SARS-CoV-2 is a new and highly contagious virus, and while vaccines for prevention of COVID-19 disease have now been developed, there is no perfectly successful treatment. Sporadic social distancing will most likely continue until 2022 if no substantial action is taken. As a result, before the world at large has been vaccinated and successful medications are discovered, it is advisable to continue using preventive methods and public health programs. COVID-19 will ultimately be defeated by a combination of therapies that include all of the above drugs or supplements, as well as a proper immunomodulatory diet, adequate mental support, and adherence to standards [9].

REFERENCES

1. Lange, K.W., Nakamura, Y. (2020). Lifestyle factors in the prevention of COVID-19. *Global Health J.* 4, 146–152.

2. Kucharski, A.J., Russel, T.W., Diamond, C., Liu, Y., Edmunds, J., Funk, S. (2020). Early dynamics of

transmission and control of COVID-19: A mathematical modelling study. *Lancet Infect. Dis.* 20(5), 553–558.

3. Rutayisire, E., Nkundimana, G., Mitonga, H.K., Boye, A., Nikwigize, S. (2020). What works and what does not work in response to COVID-19 prevention and control in Africa. *Int. J. Infect. Dis.* 97, 267–269.

4. El-Sayed, A., Kamel, M. (2020). Climatic changes and their role in emergence and re-emergence of diseases. *Environ Sci. Pollut. Res. Int.* 27, 22336–22352. doi:10.1007/s11356-020-08896-w.

5. One Health. (2020). Editorial commentary: Prevention and control of COVID-19 in pastoral community through One Health approach. *One Health* 11, 100181.

6. El-Sadr, W.M., Justman, J. (2020). Africa in the path of COVID-19. *N. Engl. J. Med.*, 383, e11 doi:10.1056/NEJMp2008193.

7. Heymann, D., Shindo, N. (2020). COVID-19: What is next for public health? *Lancet* 395(10224), 542–545.

8. Baloch, S., Baloch, M.A., Zheng, T., Pei, X. (2020). The coronavirus disease 2019 (COVID-19) pandemic. *Tohoku J. Exp. Med.* 250, 271–278.

9. Lotfi, M., Hamblin, M.R., Rezaei, N. (2020). COVID-19: Transmission, prevention, and potential therapeutic opportunities. *Clin. Chim. Acta* 508, 254–266.

10. Aziz, A.B., Raqib, R., Khan, W.A., Rahman, M., Haque, R., Alam, M., Zaman, K., Ross, A.G. (2020). Integrated control of COVID-19 in resource-poor countries. *Int. J. Infect. Dis.* 101, 98–101.

11. Kohanski, M.A., Lo, L.J., Waring, M.S. (2020). Review of indoor aerosol generation, transport and control in the context of COVID. *Int. Forum Allergy Rhinol.* doi:10.1002/alr.22661.

12. Goldust, M., Abdelmaksoud, A., Navarini, A.A. (2020). Hand disinfection in the combat against COVID-19. *J. Eur. Acad. Dermatol. Venereol.* 34, e454–e455.

13. Fan, Y., Zhang, Y., Tariq, A., Jiang, X., Ahamd, Z., Zhihao, Z., Idrees, M., Azizullah, A., Adnan, M., Bussmann, R.W. (2020). Food as medicine: A possible preventive measure against coronavirus disease (COVID-19). *Phytother Res.* doi:10.1002/ptr.6770.

14. Chu, D.K., Akl, E.A., Duda, S., Solo, K., Yaacoub, S., Schünemann, H.J. (2020). Physical distancing, face masks, and eye protection to prevent person-to-person transmission of SARS-CoV-2 and COVID-19: A systematic review and meta-analysis. *Lancet* 395(10242), 1973–1987.

15. Srivastava, N., Saxena, S.K. (2020). Chapter 11; Prevention and control strategies for SARS-CoV-2 infection. *Coronavirus Disease 2019 (COVID-19)*, pp. 127–140. S.K. Saxena (ed.), Medical Virology: From Pathogenesis to Disease Control, doi:10.1007/978-981-15-4814-7_11.

16. Ling, L., Wong, W.T., Wan, W.T.P., Choi, G., Joynt, G.M. (2020). Infection control in non-clinical areas during the COVID-19 pandemic. *Anaesthesia.* doi:10.1111/anae.15075.

17. Jessop, Z.M., Dobbs, T.D., Ali, S.R., Combellack, E., Clancy, R., Ibrahim, N., Jovic, T.H., Kaur, A.J., Nijran, A., O'Neill, T.B., Whitaker, I.S. (2020). Personal protective equipment (PPE) for surgeons during COVID-19 pandemic: A systematic review of availability, usage, and rationing. *Br. J. Surg.* doi:10.1002/bjs.11750.

18. Han, G., Zhou, Y.H. (2020). Possibly critical role of wearing masks in general population in controlling COVID-19. *J. Med. Virol.* 92(10), 1779–1781.

19. Mitze, T., Kosfeld, R., Rode, J., Wälde, K. (2020). Face masks considerably reduce COVID-19 cases in Germany. *Proc. Natl. Acad. Sci. USA.* 117 (51), 32293–32301.

20. Ha, J.F. (2020). The COVID-19 pandemic and face shields. *Br. J. Surg.* 107, e398.

21. Ma, Q.X., Shan, H., Zhang, H.L., Li, G.M., Yang, R.M., Chen, J.M. (2020). Potential utilities of mask wearing and instant hand hygiene for fighting SARS-CoV-2. *J. Med. Virol.* 1–5.

22. De Flora, S., Balansky, R., La Maestra, S. (2020). Rationale for the use of N-acetylcysteine in both prevention and adjuvant therapy of COVID-19. *FASEB J.* 34(10), 13185–13193. doi:10.1096/fj.202001807.

23. GBD 2016 Alcohol Collaborators. (2018). Alcohol use and burden for 195 countries and territories, 1990–2016: A systematic analysis for the Global Burden of Disease Study 2016. *Lancet* 392, 1015–1035.

24. Cheng, J., Qiong, C., Mingxuan, X. (2020). Smoking increases the risk of infectious disease: A narrative review. *Tob Induc. Dis.* 18, 60. doi:10.18332/tid/123845.

25. Huttunen, R., Heikkinen, T., Syrjanen, J. (2011). Smoking and the outcome of infection. *J. Intern. Med.* 269(3), 258–269. doi:10.1111/j.1365-2796.2010.02332.x.

26. Marco T.D., Silva, A., de Carvalho Guerreiro, R., Da-Silva, F.R., Esteves, A.M., Poyares, D., Piovezan, R., Treptow, E., Starling, M., Rosa, D.S., Pires, G.N. (2020). Sleep and COVID-19: Considerations about immunity, pathophysiology, and treatment. *Sleep Sci.* 13(3), 199–209. doi:10.5935/1984-0063.20200062.

27. Cao, Y., Chen, M., Dong, D., Xie, S., Liu, M. (2020). Environmental pollutants damage airway epithelial cell cilia: Implications for the prevention of obstructive lung diseases. *Thorac Cancer* 11(3), 505–510. doi:10.1111/1759-7714.13323.

28. Ferder, L., Giménez, V.M.M., Inserra, F., Tajer, C., Antonietti, L., Mariani, J., Manucha, W. (2020). Vitamin D supplementation as a rational pharmacological approach in the COVID-19 pandemic. *Am. J. Physiol. Lung Cell Mol. Physiol.* 319(6), L941–L948.

29. Panfili, F.M., Roversi, M., D'Argenio, P., Rossi, P., Cappa, M., Fintini, D. (2020). Possible role of vitamin D in COVID-19 infection in pediatric population. *J. Endocrinol. Invest.* 15, 1–9.

30. Sultana, J., Mazzaglia, G., Luxi, N., Cancellieri, A., Capuano, A., Ferrajolo, C., De Waure, C., Ferlazzo, G., Trifirò, G. (2020). Potential effects of vaccinations on the prevention of COVID-19: Rationale, clinical evidence, risks, and public health considerations. *Expert Rev. Vac.* 19(10), 919–936.

31. Ramirez, F.E., Sanchez, A., Pirskanen, A.T. (2021). Hydrothermotherapy in prevention and treatment of mild to moderate cases of COVID-19. *Med. Hypotheses* 146, 110363.

32. Ehrenberg, J.P., Zhou, X.N., Fontes, G., Rocha, E.M.M., Tanner, M., Utzinger, J. (2020). Strategies supporting the prevention and control of neglected tropical diseases during and beyond the COVID-19 pandemic. *Infect Dis. Poverty* 9, 86. doi:10.1186/s40249-020-00701-7.

Chapter 5   Global Focus and Interdisciplinary Approaches in COVID-19 Research and Their Outcomes

Hülya Şenol and Şükrü Tüzmen

5.1 INTRODUCTION

5.1.1 Challenges and Strategies Taken by Different Countries to Combat the Effects of the COVID-19 Pandemic

The deadly Severe Acute Respiratory Syndrome-Coronavirus 2 (SARS-CoV-2), which triggered the current COVID-19 pandemic, belongs to the family of coronaviruses (CoVs) and is the third human zoonotic coronavirus to have caused an outbreak [1]. In late December 2019, the first COVID-19 patients were registered in Wuhan, China. The majority were market workers, stall owners, or tourists to the city's Huanan Wholesale Seafood Market. However, later research revealed that many of the first human cases had no prior contact with the Huanan Wholesale Seafood Market and began experiencing symptoms on December 1, 2019. As a result, they contracted the SARS-CoV-2 virus in November after coming in contact with previously undetected cases. The SARS-CoV-2 virus has most likely not been manipulated or engineered, according to investigations, but it has an ecological reservoir in bats. The World Health Organization (WHO) declared on January 30, 2020, that the COVID-19 outbreak was an international public health emergency, and on March 11, 2020, it was declared as a pandemic disease. COVID-19 has spread to 221 countries and territories, with 140,322,903 confirmed cases and 3,003,794 deaths registered by the World Health Organization (WHO) on April 18, 2021 [2]. At the

time of writing, the number of cases and deaths continues to rise on a daily basis as a result of rapid human-to-human transmission (Figure 5.1), there are critical issues that must be addressed immediately in many parts of the world.

In this chapter, we present the challenges and strategies used by various countries to tackle the issues of COVID-19 in order to assist other states in adjusting and improving their preparedness policies for the pandemic.

5.1.1.1 China, Thailand, and Korea

China, Thailand, and Korea showed a lower total number of COVID-19 cases on April 13, 2021 than 86 countries on the WHO list. During the pandemic, China has responded rapidly, conducting an epidemiological inquiry on December 29, 2019, shutting the seafood market in Wuhan, South China, on January 1, 2020, and putting the city on lockdown on January 23, 2020. Using digital media, the pandemic crisis was tracked and publicized in real time, and government-planned epidemic prevention strategies were implemented, with people actively cooperating throughout the country. By February 19, 2020, China's national emergency response had slowed the spread of COVID-19 and averted numerous cases [3]. Thailand was the first country outside China to report a new case of COVID-19, on January 13, 2020. In the first week of April 2020, national lockdown was declared, and all international airports were

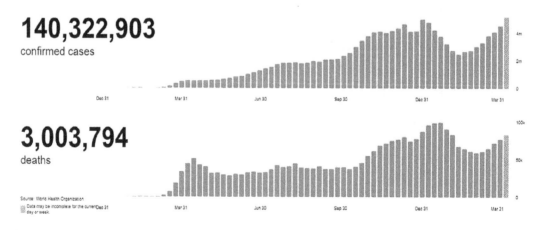

140,322,903
confirmed cases

3,003,794
deaths

Source: World Health Organization
Data may be incomplete for the current day or week

Figure 5.1   Global situation on April 18, 2021.
Source: WHO, 2021. https://covid19.who.int/

    DOI: 10.1201/9781003190394-5

Table 5.1 Strategies used by China, Thailand, and Korea

China [3]	Thailand [4]	Korea [5]
– Monitoring of wildlife sources	– National lockdown	– Aggressive screening and immediate testing
– International cooperation	– Collection of data from all domestic airports	– Testing of employees at hospitals and in-patients
– Lockdown of communities/cities at the national level, travel restrictions	– Use of applications such as Facebook, Line, Tik Tok, and Twitter to inform the public about outbreaks, to provide accurate information and preventive measures	– Contact tracing of patients
– Speedy mobilization of healthcare personnel		– Fast treatment and quarantining of patients
– Development of guidelines		– Conversion of private hospitals into COVID-19 dedicated hospitals
– Use of cloud computing and big data	– Use of the Chiang Mai Hospital information system (CMC-19)	– Creation of group chatroom for the control team experts
– Minimizing of social contacts, aggressive quarantine, mask wearing, regular disinfection, and efficient hand washing	– Use of Self-Screening application (SSA) provided in Thai, Chinese, and English	– Implementation of walk-in and drive-in testing centers
– Early testing, reporting, isolation and treatment	– Use of Self-Health Check (SHC) application by the public	– Implementation of mobile screening centers
– Nucleic acid testing and CT examination for diagnosis		– Providing care to self-quarantined patients by video calls
– Use of public facilities as flexible temporary hospitals		– Management of residential treatment centers by each local government independently
– Admittance of patients with mild/moderate disease to mobile, temporary, or field facilities, and admittance of patients with severe disease to COVID-19 dedicated hospitals		– Use of the self-quarantine protection app and mandatory use of self-diagnosis app
– Critical care medicine, multi-disciplinary, multi-organ treatment, supplementation with oxygen, and mechanical ventilation for patients having severe/critical disease		– Dashboard developed to send patient data (self-assessed body temperature, blood pressure, pulse) to healthcare providers
– Treatment with traditional Chinese medicine (TCM) and Western medicine		– Collection and release of relevant information on COVID-19 patients in real time
– Acceleration of development of vaccines		

ordered to shut down [4]. Korea had previously struggled to manage the Middle East Respiratory Syndrome (MERS) outbreak, so the Korean government managed to respond to COVID-19 on February 23, 2020, at the highest level. To respond to pandemic emergencies, the Central Disaster and Safety Countermeasure Headquarters collaborated with the KCDC (Korea Center for Disease Control and Prevention). China, Thailand, and Korea increased the quality of their public health and medical staff through effective strategies [5] (Table 5.1).

Finland, Mongolia, Norway, Iceland, Vietnam and New Zealand have implemented multiple effective measures and restrictions, managed the pandemic very well and have been very successful in restraining the pandemic (Tables 5.2–5.4). Several lessons can be learned from their COVID-19 management, and these lessons could be useful to other countries who are struggling with the pandemic.

5.1.1.2 Australia

The first positive case was confirmed in Australia on January 25, 2020, but the rates of COVID-19–related cases and deaths were substantially lower than in Italy, the United Kingdom, the United States, and China [2]. This disparity may be a result of successful measures taken in Australia that have resulted in a lower infection rate. For example, decisive and rapid lockdown procedures that enabled Australians to leave the house for only five reasons (shopping only for essential supplies; work or study that cannot be done remotely; visiting friends or family with a limited number of people; exercise; and medical or care needs). Individuals who violated these restrictions were fined AUD$1,000, and all travelers were quarantined for 14 days. The federal government invested AUD$1 billion in telehealth, a suicide prevention telephone service, and crisis support, as well as AUD$10 million in training volunteers to communicate with elderly people

Table 5.2 Strategies used by Vietnam and Iceland

Vietnam [6]

- Formation of the Taskforce Group for prevention and control
- Suspension of flights from epidemic areas
- Health check and 14 days of quarantine for people returning from abroad
- Closure of schools and introduction of online education
- Financial support to individuals affected by COVID-19
- Aggressive testing, tracing and treatment
- Coverage of testing and treatment by health insurance
- Reduction of the scale of festivals and gatherings
- Mandatory mask wearing in public places
- Limited travel in spring 2020
- Clear leadership
- Activation of the Emergency Public Health Operations Center
- Application of measures to suspend visa exemption and restriction of entry
- Daily broadcasting of COVID-19–related information by all national media, MOH's website, newspapers, governmental website
- Public installment of NCOVI health notification software to report on health status daily
- Implementation of social isolation measures from April 1 to April 15, 2020
- Issuing clinical guidelines on diagnosis and treatment of COVID-19 patients in February 2020 and adjusting it according to upgraded global scientific reports
- Provision of health education about preventive measures to all people
- Mobilizing provision of medical equipment and protective measures for health facility workers
- Hand washing
- Promotion of social distancing, at least 2 m apart in public places and avoiding gathering in large numbers
- Creation of an official account on social media (Zalo), providing SMS to all citizens
- Changing waiting ringtones/music to a voice message to remind of COVID-19 measures
- Applying research to active treatment and improvement of survival rates

Iceland [7]

- Purchase of substantial amounts of medical supplies, increase in intensive care unit (ICU) beds and ventilators, creation of special COVID-19 wards in two large hospitals
- Suspension of outpatient clinics and elective surgery, establishment of a contact tracing unit and case management teams
- Travel vouchers given to all citizens to increase national tourism
- Quarantine of 14 days for arriving passengers and COVID-19 testing at borders
- Reduced schedule at airports during first wave
- Reduced freight at ports during first wave
- Restrictions in the number of people allowed at gatherings
- Adherence to personal hygiene
- Social distancing (2 m from May to August 2020: 1 m from September 7, 2020)
- Closure of universities and high schools
- Preschool, elementary schools remained open during first wave; on August 14, 2020, all schools opened
- Closing of non-essential retail during first wave
- No mask recommendation during first wave, but mandatory on public transport, in high schools and universities between May and September 2020
- May 4, 2020: maximum 4 individuals doing sport together, September 7, 2020: 75% capacity of sport complexes
- Religious venues and services to remain open with social distancing and restricted number of people between May and September 2020
- Setting up swab hubs, conducting a high daily appointment-based swab rate, undergoing two border COVID-19 swab tests five days apart for visitors who did not opt for a 14-day quarantine
- Providing swab test results within a 24-hour period while individuals remained in quarantine

Table 5.3 Strategies used by Mongolia and Finland

Mongolia [8]	Finland [9]
– Initiation of precautionary measures before the WHO declaration of pandemic – Governmental meeting for emergency preparedness – One-window policy - all announcements at a set time through all media and channels – Text message alerts sent nationwide to the public's mobile phones – Closure of educational institutions at all levels – Restriction of travel to China – Chinese border restrictions with ban on import of foods – Isolation of incoming travelers from countries with COVID-19 cases – Restriction of Tsagaan Sar lunar New Year celebrations – Increased health system preparedness – Setting up isolation camps and isolation of travelers at high risk for 2 weeks in these camps – Widespread public face mask wearing – Banning domestic travel between provinces and inter-cities until March 3, 2020 – Providing disinfection protocols for trains and trucks – Preparation of risk assessment for all provinces – Banning of all religious gatherings – Cancellation of international flights, land travel and rail travel – Establishment of emergency call service with a 4-digit number – Contact tracing – Closing of public businesses (except grocery stores) – Seven measures to protect public health and income – Preparation of a 300-bed emergency hospital – Hospitalization of all confirmed, suspected cases and their primary contacts by the National Centre for Communicable Diseases – Introduction of legislation with sanctions and criminal charges for intentionally falsifying health conditions and misreporting – Testing of incoming travelers in quarantine – Random community testing and walk-in testing sites – Coverage of most of healthcare and emergency expenses of children, pregnant women, patients with tuberculosis, and cancer, by government – Provision of COVID-19 related healthcare, isolation and quarantine services free of charge	– Support of government to all municipalities – Funding of all measures by municipalities – Selection of five university hospitals to plan and coordinate care and all hospital districts for epidemic preparedness and management – Production of materials for use by public health officials – Provision of guidance for healthcare and social providers – Provision of guidelines for COVID-19 prevention in workplaces – Implementation of early lockdown – Physical distancing interventions – General advice on hygiene, respiratory etiquette, physical distancing by the Finnish Institute for Health and Welfare (THL, Terveyden ja Hyvinvoinnin Laitos) – Issuing guidance on testing patients with severe respiratory tract infection symptoms, social and healthcare personnel and elderly individuals – Effective testing, contact tracing, isolation, and treatment – Effective testing at airports, land borders and harbors – Drive-in testing by hospitals and the public sector – Mandatory mask wearing – Isolation of patients at their homes or in hospitals – Healthcare resource prioritization – Two-week quarantine for all exposed people, four economic packages (one for emergency measures, three as strong economic stimulus packages) – Stay-home advice to people developing respiratory symptoms – Information of public and media on THL website – Nationwide use of the digital self-assessment tool "Omaolo" available in Finnish, Swedish and English – Contacting of patients using this tool by physicians and nurses – Medical helpline (116117) – Sharing information between municipalities by an open access Innokylä website moderated by THL – Use of the app "Koronavilkku" to alert people who have come into contact with COVID-19 cases – Quarantine-like conditions for persons over 70 years – Self-quarantine for 14 days after traveling abroad – Instructing private-sector employees to work from home – Closing sports centers, libraries, youth centers, clubs, rehabilitative work facilities, museums, swimming pools, daycare services for the elderly, restaurants (except takeaway), and workshops – Ban public events – Prohibition of visiting people in high-risk groups – Closure of all educational institutions – Severe punishable measures

over the phone and online. However, the federal government took a long time to provide housing for the homeless and to support mental health services for individuals under 16 years of age [12]. Government subsidies promoted and supported diabetes services via telehealth and included diabetes educators in sponsored telehealth support. Australian health professionals collaborated with consumer groups to develop guidelines and educational resources for COVID-19 [13].

5.1.1.3 *United Kingdom*
On June 18, 2020, the Health Secretary announced a COVID-19 outbreak in Leicester, England, but

only a quarter of all COVID-19 patients were confirmed between June 1 and June 15, 2020. The majority of the new cases were Asian, black, minority ethnic, and South Asian residents in 10 wards in Leicester's east end. Testing of patients admitted to hospital by National Health Service hospital laboratories (Pillar 1 testing) and community-based swab testing by remote lighthouse laboratories (Pillar 2 testing) were the subject of the national plan for COVID-19 management. The major issue revealed during the second peak was the inadequacy of information exchange regarding Pillar 2 data to local authority and local health organizations, which did not

Table 5.4 Strategies used by New Zealand and Norway

New Zealand [10]	Norway [11]
– Rapid and science-based risk assessment	– Nationwide lockdown
– Early decisive government action	– Isolation of cases and close contacts
– Emphatic leadership of Prime Minister	– High-trust of society in government (Trustworthy Leadership)
– Border control by keeping international incoming travelers in government-managed quarantine or isolation for 14 days	– Contact tracing, widespread testing, and surveillance
– Limitations on mass social gathering	– Social distancing (in public places, 1 m apart and indoors 2 m)
– Encouraging physical distancing (on March 21, 2020)	– Self-isolation following travel
– Implementing countrywide lockdown on March 26 for a total of 7 weeks	– Restrictions of mass gatherings (no more than five people in a group)
– Closing all schools	– Closure of childcare centers, primary schools, lower secondary schools, upper secondary schools, universities and colleges, and other educational institutions with the exception of childcare for children of parents working in healthcare services
– Closing non-essential workplaces	– Ban on cultural and sports events
– Severe movement and travel restrictions on March 25, 2020	– Closing restaurants, bars, pubs, and nightclubs, with the exception of restaurants where food is served; applying social distancing of at least 1 m between guests
– High case and contact follow-up	– Closure of hairdressing, skin care, massage, tattooing, piercing and similar services
– Rapid contact tracing and quarantine of contacts	– Closure of gyms, swimming pools, water parks, etc.
– Widespread testing, rapid case detection and isolation	– Early border closure
– Intensive handwashing	– Continuation of domestic transport, avoidance of unnecessary leisure travel and journeys
– Cough etiquette	– Mandatory 14-day quarantine for everyone entering Norway from other countries
– Provision of hand hygiene facilities for the public	– Ban on healthcare professionals traveling abroad
– Intensive physical distancing	– Border control of the international Schengen borders
– Well-coordinated communication with the public	– Rejection at the borders of foreign nationals who do not live or work in Norway
– Use of mobile phone technology to speed up contact tracing and quarantine	– Continuation of public transport for people with critical functions in society
– Enhancing infection control measures at hospitals	– Ban on using public transport
– Outsourcing of staff and equipment to hospitals	– Public should work from home
– Expansion of intensive care unit (ICU) and ventilator spaces for patients	– Ban on visiting vulnerable groups (elderly people, psychiatric institutions, prisons)
– Governmental spending program to support businesses and employees, who lost their jobs or whose jobs were threatened	– Ban on visitors entering health institutions
	– Safeguarding of infection control for all patients
	– Daily government press conferences to inform the public

provide demographic information such as ethnicity, age, address, or place of work. Increase in Pillar 2 testing capacity including mobile testing was ineffective so that lockdown measures were reintroduced on June 30, 2020. Local authorities, clinicians, and public health teams should have been empowered to implement area-specific and context-specific approaches in existing programs. Tests, and track-and-trace systems should also have been done in a culturally sensitive manner, allowing ethnic minority communities to readily access these resources [14].

5.1.1.4 Spain

COVID-19 first emerged in Barcelona, Spain, on February 25, 2020, and healthcare professionals were unable to protect themselves during visits of many patients who did not meet the epidemiologic requirements of Primary Healthcare Centers (PHCs), resulting in over 40,000 healthcare professionals being contaminated and many dying by May 21, 2020 [15]. General Practitioners and nurses avoided physical contact with the patients and used telemedicine as one of the recommendations of the European Centre for Disease Prevention and Control. Separate areas were built for patients with respiratory problems. In periods when safety equipment was scarce, nurses and General Practitioners wore self-made facemasks. The number of patients visiting centers decreased as a result of a high number of virtual consultations via phone or e-mail. PHCs opened at weekends, and patients were visited at their homes by healthcare professionals. A chest X-ray was ordered for patients who had serious symptoms. Primary Healthcare professionals (PCs) called their COVID-19 patients every 24, 48, or 72 hours, depending on their clinical status. Patients and their families were taught to take hygienic precautions, isolate themselves, control their symptoms, and contact PHCs if their condition worsened. PHC professionals looked after the elderly in 200 nursing homes, while PCs provided emotional support to the patients and their families. Patients with social issues, as well as disabled people with multi-morbidity or other conditions, were put in specially designed hotels.

5.1.1.5 *Africa*

Egypt's Minister of Health and Population announced the first case of SARS-CoV-2 in Africa on February 14, 2020. Because of their close ties with China, 13 countries, including Kenya, the Democratic Republic of the Congo, Nigeria, and South Africa were designated as high-risk priority zones. Because of lessons learned from the 2014–2016 Ebola outbreak and other previous outbreaks, as well as significant investments in monitoring and preparedness, Africa was better prepared than ever before. Personal protective equipment, diagnostic kits, and positive controls were sent by the WHO, while reagents were shipped by Charité–Universitätsmedizin Berlin Institute of Virology, a PANDORA-ID-NET partner in Germany. The African Union and the Africa Centres for Disease Control and Prevention convened on February 22, 2020, in an emergency ministerial conference. The WHO Strategic Preparedness and Response Plan was developed to assist Africa's most vulnerable countries, and the WHO trained African health workers via free online courses on COVID-19 [1]. Several SARS-CoV-2 variants have been reported globally. One of them is B.1.351, known as 20H/501Y.V2. This variant was first reported in Nelson Mandela Bay, South Africa and surrounding areas in October 2020. The B.1.351 variant has multiple mutations in the spike protein such as K417N, E484K, and N501Y. Computer models showed that the B.1.351 variant is 50% more transmissible and 20% better at evading the immune response than previous variants. Early reports found no evidence to prove that this variant impacts disease severity. This variant is responsible for all current COVID-19 cases in South Africa and has spread to the UK and the USA. The rise in the number of cases because of the B.1.351 variant has increased the burden on the healthcare system in South Africa.

5.1.1.6 *United States*

COVID-19, which was announced on January 20, 2020 in the United States, demonstrated the inequities in the healthcare system. The fatality rate was 3.6% on April 10, 2020. Delay in testing increased the spread of COVID-19, healthcare demand, and fatality rates. Obesity and diabetes are serious, common chronic diseases in the USA, increasing the risk of having severe symptoms from COVID-19 and tripling the risk of hospitalization because of COVID-19 infections. In addition, obesity is linked to impaired immune function, decreases lung capacity making breathing more difficult. Recently, the Centers for Disease Control and Prevention reported that 30.2% of hospitalizations were attributed to obesity in the USA. Hispanic and non-Hispanic black adults are more likely to suffer severely from COVID-19 because of a higher prevalence of obesity. The American Diabetes Association also reported that while there is not enough data to prove that people with diabetes are more likely to get COVID-19, people at any age with multi-morbidities including type 2 diabetes, are at increased risk of having serious symptoms and complications from COVID-19. The increase in the fatality rate may be because of the lack of hospital resources in some US states. In many US states such as in New York, Illinois, and Louisiana, documented prison-related outbreaks occurred because 17% of prisons across the US operate at or above 100% capacity. There are disparities in access to employment, education, housing, and healthcare in the United States historically, and COVID-19 has reinforced health disparities. African Americans, Native Americans, and Latino people have higher exposures to COVID-19 and higher mortality rates because of limited access to preventive services and an inability to obey physical distancing recommendations. There are hundreds of thousands of immigrants, refugees and asylum seekers in the USA, and viral transmission among these communities was heightened by overcrowding, unsafe and unsanitary living conditions, and medical neglect. In the USA, one in four adults has a mobility, cognitive or independent living disability and most of them are African Americans. The death rate caused by COVID-19 among people with disabilities was very high in late April because these people are unable to socially distance, they are unemployed, and poor, so that they cannot afford or access essential medical equipment, specialty care, and prescription medications. In addition, COVID-19 epidemic posed an increased threat to the lives of millions of unsafely housed and homeless people in the USA. Many of them died because of their unsafe and unsanitary living conditions, and by not obeying critical measures such as social distancing. The slow implementation of plans such as emergency housing reinforced the risks of transmission of COVID-19 among these people. States should take measures to provide homes, adequate cleaning supplies and care for prisoners, people with disabilities, and homeless people to protect human rights and public health [16].

5.1.1.7 India, Brazil, and Sweden

Several countries, such as Brazil could not implement effective interventions to reduce transmission of the virus during early waves and have confirmed cumulative total cases are still increasing. India and Brazil have the second and third highest numbers of COVID-19 cases in the world. The huge population (1.3 billion) and population density in India are big barriers in fighting the pandemic. However, India has quickly overcome the pandemic through the CoWiN tracking and surveillance platform, providing free food for months to 800 million citizens during lockdown, converting stadiums and train coaches to COVID specialty hospitals with millions of beds and emergency medical facilities, adopting holistic preventive approaches through Ayurveda and other Indian traditional medicines along with yoga, installing oxygen plants even in remote hospitals, rapid testing, developing and mass production of indigenous vaccines like Covaxin

and vaccinating 100 million people per day. On April 15, 2021, Sweden, one of the most developed countries and highly rated for its medical awareness in the world, has been reported to have one of the highest COVID-19 infection rates in Western Europe. The number of cases and deaths are still rising. Many critical voices have addressed the lack of government-led legal interventions such as reinforcing lockdown and quarantine. The challenges faced by these countries are presented in Table 5.5.

5.1.1.8 Iran

COVID-19 was discovered in Iran on February 20, 2020, prompting the President to create the Corona National Headquarters. After that, several steps were taken to respond gradually to and control the disease, including the establishment of 16- and 24-hour health centers for face-to-face and telephone contacts with patients, enlisting external help from

Table 5.5 Challenges of India, Brazil, and Sweden during the initial phase of the COVID-19 pandemic

India [17–20]	Brazil [21–23]	Sweden
– Sudden shortage of healthcare services due to high infection rate – Inappropriate ratio of patients to medical professionals – Shortage of hospital beds and medical equipment (ventilators) due to high volume of patients – Low testing rate – Burden of high population density and COVID-19 transmission Difficulty to adhere to social distancing before national lockdown – High urban living density complicates social distancing – Absence of cough hygiene – Political and religious events Shortage of personal protective equipment	– No cohesive political leadership at national and local levels (president, governors, and mayors) – Lack of efficient prevention and control measures – Limited testing capacity – Limited contact tracing – High urban density – High number of urban slums with poor sanitation and limited healthcare access – large household sizes and crowding in urban slums – Poor social distancing in areas where the poorest populations live – Poor hygiene measures in areas where the poorest populations live – High number of homeless people living in insecure, unhealthy conditions – Overcrowded and precarious housing conditions – Clean water not available to all people – Patients turned away by oversaturated healthcare systems – Inability to self-isolate – Relaxation of social distancing measures from April 13 onwards – Untested large number of samples – Failing of municipalities to take into consideration the surveillance and monitoring indicators of the pandemic – Large prison population with limited social distancing	– Allowing uncontrolled community transmission – No mandatory measures in crowded places until March 29, 2020 – Limited and inadequate source identification, testing, contact tracing, and reporting – Insufficient recognition of face mask use, aerosol transmission, presymptomatic and asymptomatic transmission by the national strategy – Start of the use of facemasks in healthcare facilities and care homes only on November 11, 2020, in Stockholm and on public transport at certain times from January 7, 2021 – Unresolved structural factors related to the organization of the care of older people – Government did not put the translation of the WHO's hygiene recommendations into practice until December 18, 2020 – Failures in the legal frameworks and governance of social services and health, problems in sharing responsibilities, and transparency problem in policy-making and decision-making processes – Insufficient participation and engagement of key stakeholders (informed scientists, change in behavior, communications expertise, civil society)

the Medical System Organization, the Armed Forces, donors and nongovernmental organizations, the Red Crescent Society and the Social Security Organization, forming an epidemiology committee, and implementing a "4030" response system for responding to and counseling the general public, forming a scientific committee to establish recommendations in collaboration with the Ministry of Health and Medical Education (MOHME) and universities. Activities included holding scientific webinars and video conferences with the media, establishment of a committee for documentation, expansion of laboratory networks, enhancement of the electronic data registration system, and provision of emergency professionals with instructions [24].

5.1.1.9 Turkey

The first COVID-19 patients in Turkey were reported on March 10, 2020. Within 30 days of the outbreak, the number of patients increased dramatically, and Turkey was listed in the top ten countries with community transmission. Turkey had the opportunity to benefit from the experience of Europe and China, and had 280 hospitals with intensive care unit beds, equivalent to 40 beds per 100,000 people. Public measures taken to mitigate COVID-19 included a meeting of the National Scientific Board for risk assessment; the preparation of National COVID-19 Guidelines; the suspension of all flights to and from countries with high COVID-19 incidences, including China, Iran, Spain, Iraq, and Italy; the use of thermal cameras on all international arrivals at airports; the closure of the land border with Iran; and adherence to the 14 Rules, which included social distancing, restriction on access to recreational areas, public places, and shopping malls; and advice to stay at home for people aged 20 and below, and 65 and above; school closures and starting distance-education at universities; a travel ban between 31 cities and total lockdown in 31 cities. However, there was a need to expand management strategies including sharing available data, timely analyses, and conducting and analyzing data obtained from epidemiologic field research in Turkey [25]. Recently, weekend lockdowns and Ramadan restrictions were reinstated, following the confirmation of an increasingly high number of new cases. Turkey recorded 22,388 new cases, 4,977,982 confirmed cases, and 42,187 confirmed deaths on May 7, 2021, the highest numbers in the country since the beginning of the pandemic [2]. The Turkish Health Minister stated that the increase in the number of cases was because of a new, more transmissible, strain of SARS-CoV-2. In addition, there have been other reasons that led to an increase in confirmed cases and deaths. The hidden asymptomatic cases in the population, easing of restrictions, violation of social distancing and hygiene rules, exemption of travel restrictions for short tourist trips to Turkey, gatherings in crowded places and organization of indoor political party congresses across the country has added to the increase of cases.

5.1.1.10 North Cyprus

A female German tourist was the first COVID-19 case in North Cyprus, on March 10, 2020. People who had come into contact with the patient, including any passengers on the same plane, were quarantined on March 10 in three separate hotels (TRNC Ministry of Health). Foreign nationals have been prohibited from entering North Cyprus since March 11, 2020 with the exception of those with valid Alien Resident Certificates, diplomatic credentials, or other official documents or special permits.

All international flights to North Cyprus, as well as cross-border trips from the island's southern sections, were prohibited. On March 12, the country's second case was registered, this time the spouse of the German tourist who was diagnosed with COVID-19. To avoid the spread of the SARS-CoV-2, the Turkish Republic of Northern Cyprus government closed schools and outlawed mass gatherings on March 12, 2020.

On-site teaching was suspended at all educational levels, from nursery to university level. The digital online system was implemented in primary schools, middle schools, high schools and universities. North Cyprus has over 20 higher education institutions. There are 18 universities in total, with about 100,000 foreign students. For the international university students, restrictions have since been eased by allowing them to enter the country and stay in quarantine hotels for 15 days.

The Ministry of Health confirmed on March 13, 2020 that five people had tested positive for the SARS-CoV-2. Due to the outbreak, the 2020 Northern Cypriot presidential election was postponed for six months on March 17. After being quarantined for 14 days at the expense of the Northern Cyprus Ministry of Health, over 840 German tourists were sent back to Germany on March 24, 2020. On March 28, 2020, the first COVID-19–related death in the country was registered. There were no COVID-19 cases after 76 days of curfew and countrywide quarantine, but the cases rose dramatically after the ports were reopened to foreign arrivals.

Northern Cyprus had 5,410 confirmed cases, 4,593 recoveries, 28 deaths, and a death rate of 87 per million people as of April 16, 2021, one of the lowest rates in the world (Coronavirus [COVID-19] deaths worldwide per one million population as of April 12, 2021, by region, Statista; "Mortality Analyses", Johns Hopkins University, 2021). The ensuing surge of infections has not yet threatened to overwhelm the North Cyprus healthcare system.

5.2 FOCUSED AREAS OF RESEARCH

The use of technologies including artificial intelligence (AI), 5G technology, telemedicine, Internet of Medical Things (IoMT), geospatial technology, big data, blockchain, smart applications, and robotics are vital for the diagnosis of COVID-19, screening, monitoring, tracking, mapping, and for the creation of awareness [26].

The COVID-19 pandemic has resulted in an increase in the number of people suffering from post-traumatic stress disorder (PTSD) [27], traumatization, psychological distress, suicide [28], depressive symptoms, and extreme anxiety [29], all of which have negative psychological consequences because of the fear of contracting the virus, lack of sufficient knowledge about COVID-19, and long quarantine periods [30].

Many environmental studies analyzed and reported the effects of lockdown measures on the quality of air and water. Many researchers observed a decrease in air pollutants and other gaseous pollutants in India [31], nitrogen dioxide, and nitrogen oxides in Ontario, Canada, and fine particulate matter ($PM_{2.5}$ and NO_2 in New York [32]. Also, an increase in ozone concentrations (O_3) was reported in Brazil [33] and in China [34]. Decrease in levels of suspended particulates in Vembanad Lake, Kerala, in India [35]. Reduced levels of As, Se, Pb, and Fe metals and in NO_3, and fecal coliforms and total coliforms in 22 groundwater samples collected from Tuticorin city in Southern India [36] were also observed during the COVID-19 lockdown. Recovery around existing policy frameworks such as climate change conventions and agreements, Sendai Framework for Disaster Risk Reduction, and United Nations Sustainable Development Goals, investing in preparedness and multi-sector pandemic planning, strengthening international communication, collaboration and cooperation are also essential. In addition, there is a need to determine the inequalities in the disaster risk management cycle, design information, risk communication systems, and data sharing systems accepted by the community [37].

5.2.1 Research Challenges and Recommendations

The literature on COVID-19 research supports the need for developing and maintaining quality health systems for effective control and mitigation of the COVID-19 pandemic. In this part of the chapter we review the experiences and recommendations of several authors from different disciplines.

5.2.1.1 Geriatric Care

Geriatric care is a serious concern globally because older people are very fragile, vulnerable to infections, and the fatality rate of older people is higher compared to other age groups. All countries need a country-level geriatric policy and effective urgent measures to address all challenges related to healthcare of the geriatric population, such as providing financial security, increasing the capacity of domiciliary health workers, and the establishment of an integrated multi-sectoral network [38].

These essential strategies were addressed to battle the challenges of geriatric care in Hong Kong [39]:

- Long-term care services were expanded and provided at a nominal fee for all residents under the control of Hong Kong government.

- "The money follows the older person" project was initiated. Funds were given to older people in the form of vouchers, which could be used by signing a contract with care providers.

- Hong Kong's Social Welfare Department provided financial support and prepared guidelines for nonprofit nongovernmental care organizations, and announced many measures such as keeping daycare centers open for elderly people who do not have any help with providing home-delivered meals, the administration of medicine, nursing care, and having an escort to medical appointments.

- All face-to-face visits were terminated and remote meetings organized between patients and their visitors.

- Very strict hygiene practices, such as wearing masks, washing hands, and checking body temperatures were observed in all care services. Most of the time residents stayed and ate their meals in their rooms [39].

In Japan, more than a quarter of the population is elderly and they follow strict hygiene rules and stay at home, but they may lose their muscle strength, flexibility, and aerobic capacity because of reduced physical activity. A home-version video including 10-minute exercises each day for a week has been introduced to elderly people to promote antiviral immunity and prevent functional decline [40].

In the USA, COVID-19 revealed the importance and need for strengthening the workforce of caretakers for the elderly. Their socio-economic conditions and skills can be improved by increasing Medicaid and other healthcare support programs, and revamping training and regulation for the caretakers [41].

5.2.1.2 Medicine, Health Equity, and Management

COVID-19 has caused severe disruption and inequalities in healthcare delivery services globally. Recommendations to enhance the quality and equity of healthcare delivery will be critical. Some of these recommendations are as follows:

- Serving people in their own neighborhood through mini-clinics and increasing the role of school-based clinics [41]

- Enhancement and support of telemedicine capability, use of communication platforms based on tiered urgency, the speedy enabling of novel electronic workflows, and suspension of noncritical administrative functions [42]

- Creation of well-equipped and well-funded scientific and medical research centers, discontinuing or reducing import and export of foods to reduce the spread of COVID-19 via foodstuffs, providing homes for homeless people who are at high risk of being infected, and locking down non-essential industrial activities to reduce potential airborne infections [43]

- Ensuring displaced populations and refugees access to testing and treatment, effective communication, public trust, transparency, and community partnership for COVID-19 control, the thoughtful application of isolation and safe quarantine by respecting rights and specific circumstances, and ensuring quarantined individuals have continued access to basic needs [44]

- Strengthening integrated health care systems, the rapid reorganization of service delivery, enhancing technology use, engagement of talented management and employees, community involvement, development of effective housing and labor regulations, and a need for agile leadership [45]

- Suspension of new treatments, non-urgent diagnostic procedures, and elective surgeries, cancellation of embryo transfers, increasing the utilization of telehealth, minimizing in-person interactions [46]

- Understanding and resolution of barriers to recognize the role of nurse leaders in infection prevention and control [47]

5.2.1.3 Psychiatry and Psychology

COVID-19 has caused loss of social connectedness, personal autonomy and impacted mental health and wellbeing of individuals resulting from unemployment, loss of income, and the fear of falling victim to COVID-19 in many countries. In a study, many Australians reported depression and mild-level anxiety, of which 30% reported moderate to high depression and anxiety levels during the pandemic. In addition, negative mental health effects have increased in disabled, homeless, elderly, unemployed people, teachers, and frontline medical workers. Easily accessible and coordinated online mental health services, training the workforce in providing support, online interventions, and research to determine factors that predict psychological distress are needed [12].

As Spain had the second-highest number of COVID-19 deaths recorded on April 2, 2020 the following effective measures were taken to control the pandemic:

- The number of intensive care units were increased, and new beds were set up in recovery rooms, operating theatres, libraries, and rehabilitation gyms of hospitals

- Only patients with serious conditions were admitted to hospitals, and COVID-19 positive patients were sent to nearby hotels or homes converted for patient treatment

- Rehabilitation units, day hospitals, and vocational units were closed for psychiatric patients, and COVID-19 patients occupied most of the beds. There were three programs (the first related to the mental health of staff, the second related to relatives of patients and setting up video conference call systems for them, and the third for arrangements related to persons who had passed away) available 24/7 in the Psychiatric Liaison Department

Appointments were handled by telephone or videoconference, and nurses provided health services to patients at their homes.

Psychiatric in-patients diagnosed with COVID-19 should be separated from COVID-19 negative patients, with their own staff and space. Replacement staff need to be trained ahead of time [48]. People infected by SARS-CoV-2 may present diverse psychiatric conditions. In a study based on experiences of Early Career Psychiatrists from 10 countries, the importance of worldwide preparedness regarding mental health during pandemics was pointed out, and it was suggested that good mental health services such as telepsychiatry, enhanced community services, and proactive consultation–liaison units can be adopted by all countries, and new guidelines should be developed to manage psychiatric conditions during pandemics [49].

5.3 CONCLUSIONS

The COVID-19 pandemic has had catastrophic effects on many facets of life, and it will most likely be a long-term global threat. COVID-19 has exposed fundamental inequities, shortcomings, and flaws in global healthcare systems. Countries have been increasingly implementing a variety of policies to combat the disease. Some countries were able to react effectively to COVID-19 pandemics by implementing efficient policies, but the majority were unable. Examining global COVID-19 interventions is important for adapting effective policies, improving healthcare services, and developing national preparedness plans for future crises. We discovered that using facemasks, physical distancing, social distancing, hygiene procedures, lockout steps, screening individuals, and quarantine are all effective ways to reduce the risk of COVID-19 transmission from person to person. Pandemic management and control necessitate the participation of many stakeholders, including the government, the general public, accountability and access to accurate data, risk evaluation and communication, and healthcare staff training. To mitigate and stop the spread of COVID-19, the successful implementation of application technologies (telehealth, self-screening application) in multiple languages are needed to handle an enormous amount of data. A significant number of studies has been carried out over a brief period of time to reveal the detailed structure of SARS-CoV-2 and its effects on human health. Many vaccines and drugs have been developed in a single year. Mass vaccinations are in progress in many parts of the world. However, recommendations and actions described in this chapter are still important to minimize the effect of the pandemic and to save lives.

REFERENCES

1. Kapata, N., Ihekweazu, C., Ntoumi, F., Raji, T., Chanda-Kapata, P., Mwaba, P., Mukonka, V., Bates, M., Tembo, J., Corman, V., Mfinanga, S., Asogun, D., Elton, L., Arruda, L.B., Thomason, M.J., Mboera, L., Yavlinsky, A., Haider, N., Simons, D., Hollmann, L., Lule, S.A., Veas, F., Abdel Hamid, M.M., Dar, O., Edwards, S., Vairo, F., McHugh, T.D., Drosten, C., Kock, R., Ippolito, G., Zumla, A. (2020). Is Africa prepared for tackling the COVID-19 (SARS-CoV-2) epidemic? Lessons from past outbreaks, ongoing pan-African public health efforts, and implications for the future. *Int. J. Infect. Dis.* 93:233–236. doi:10.1016/j.ijid.2020.02.049. Epub 2020 February 28. PMID: 32119980; PMCID: PMC7129026.

2. WHO. (2021). WHO coronavirus (COVID-19) dashboard. Retrieved from https://covid19.who.int/

3. Liu, Q., Xu, K., Wang, X., Wang, W. (2020). From SARS to COVID-19: What lessons have we learned? *J. Infect. Public Health* 13(11):1611–1618. doi:10.1016/j.jiph.2020.08.001. Epub 2020 August 21. PMID: 32888871; PMCID: PMC7442131.

4. Intawong, K., Olson, D., Chariyalertsak, S. (2021). Application technology to fight the COVID-19 pandemic: Lessons learned in Thailand. *Biochem. Biophys. Res. Commun.* 538:231–237. doi:10.1016/j.bbrc.2021.01.093. Epub 2021 February 12. PMID: 33589143; PMCID: PMC7880622.

5. Lee, S.M., Lee, D. (2020). Lessons learned from battling COVID-19: The Korean experience. *Int. J. Environ. Res. Public Health* 17(20):7548. doi:10.3390/ijerph17207548.

6. Ha, B.T.T., Ngoc, Q.L., Mirzoev, T., Tai, N.T., Thai, P.Q., Dinh, P.C. (2020). Combating the COVID-19 epidemic: Experiences from Vietnam. *Int. J. Environ. Res. Public Health* 17(9):3125. doi:10.3390/ijerph17093125.

7. Cuschieri, S., Pallari, E., Hatziyianni, A., Sigurvinsdottir, R., Sigfusdottir, I.D., Sigurðardóttir, Á.K. (2020). Withdrawn: Dealing with COVID-19 in small European island states: Cyprus, Iceland and Malta. *Early Hum. Dev.* 105261. Advance online publication. doi:10.1016/j.earlhumdev.2020.105261.

8. Ryenchindorj, E., Emma, D., Darmaa, B., Indermohan, N., David, W., Graham, N.T., Chimedsuren, O., Semira, M.H. (2020). Early policy actions and emergency response to the COVID-19 pandemic in Mongolia: Experiences and challenges. *Lancet Global Health* 89:e1234–e1241. doi:10.1016/S2214-109X(20)30295-3.

9. Tiirinki, H., Tynkkynen, L.K., Sovala, M., Atkins, S., Koivusalo, M., Rautiainen, P., Keskimäki, I. (2020). COVID-19 pandemic in Finland: Preliminary analysis on health system response and economic consequences. *Health Policy Technol.* 440. doi:10.1016/j.hlpt.2020.08.005.

10. Michael, G.B., Nick, W., Andrew, A. (2020). Successful elimination of COVID-19 transmission in New Zealand. *N. Engl. J. Med.* 383:e56. doi:10.1056/NEJMc2025203.

11. Sigrun, M.M., Ella, M.S. (2021). "Everybody needs to do their part, so we can get this under control." Reactions to the Norwegian Government meta-narratives on COVID-19 measures. *Political Psychol.* 00. doi:10.1111/pops.12727.

12. Berger, E., Reupert, A. (2020, July). The COVID-19 pandemic in Australia: Lessons learnt. *Psychol. Trauma* 12(5):494–496. doi:10.1037/tra0000722. Epub 2020 June 11. PMID: 32525385.

13. Andrikopoulos, S., Johnson, G. (2020). The Australian response to the COVID-19 pandemic and diabetes: Lessons learned. *Diabetes*

Res. Clin. Pract. 165:108246. doi:10.1016/j. diabres.2020.108246. Epub 2020 June 2. PMID: 32502693; PMCID: PMC7266597.

14. Joshua, N., Jatinder, S.M., David, R.J.A., Kamlesh, K., Pranab, H., Manish, P. (2020). Early lessons from a second COVID-19 lockdown in Leicester UK. *Lancet* 396. doi:10.1016/S0140-6736(20)31490-2.

15. Muñoz, M.A., López-Grau, M. (2020). Lessons learned from the approach to the COVID-19 pandemic in urban primary health care centres in Barcelona, Spain. *Eur. J. Gen. Pract.* 26(1):106–107. doi:10.1080/13814788.2020.1796962. PMID: 32715802; PMCID: PMC7470118.

16. Okonkwo, N.E., Aguwa, U.T., Jang, M., Barré, I.A., Page, K.R., Sullivan, P.S., Beyrer, C., Baral, S. (2020). COVID-19 and the US response: Accelerating health inequities. *BMJ Evid. Based Med.*. doi:10.1136/bmjebm-2020-111426. Epub ahead of print.

17. Bhadra, A., Mukherjee, A., Sarkar, K. (2021). Impact of population density on COVID-19 infected and mortality rate in India. *Model Earth Syst. Environ.* 7:623–629. doi:10.1007/s40808-020-00984-7.

18. Mele, M., Magazzino, C. (2021). Pollution, economic growth, and COVID-19 deaths in India: A machine learning evidence. *Environ. Sci. Pollut. Res.* 28:2669–2677. doi:10.1007/s11356-020-10689-0.

19. Anat, K.K., Rajasekharan, N., Shaffi, F.K. (2020, November). COVID-19: Challenges and its consequences for rural health care in India. *Public Health Pract.* 1: 100009. doi:10.1016/j.puhip.2020.100009.

20. Kamath, S., Kamath, R., Salins, P. 2020 COVID-19 pandemic in India: Challenges and silver linings. *Postgrad. Med. J.* 96:422–423. doi:10.1136/postgradmedj-2020-137780.

21. Estela, M.L., Aquino, I., Henrique, S., et al. (2020). Social distancing measures to control the COVID-19 pandemic: Potential impacts and challenges in Brazil. *Ciênc saúde coletiva* 25 (suppl 1). doi:10.1590/1413-81232020256.1.10502020.

22. de Monteiro, O.M., Fuller, T.L., Brasil, P., Gabaglia, C.R., Nielsen-Saines, K. (2020). Controlling the COVID-19 pandemic in Brazil: A challenge of continental proportions. *Nat. Med.* 26:1505–1506. doi:10.1038/s41591-020-1071-5.

23. Freitas, C.M., Silva, I.V.M., Cidade, N.C. (2020). COVID-19 as a global disaster: Challenges to risk governance and social vulnerability in Brazil. *Ambiente Sociedade São Paulo* 23:1–12.

24. Maziar, P., Razavi, S., Hosseini Ghavamabad, L. (2020). Letter to editor: COVID-19 and dealing with it - lessons learned in Iran. *Med. J. Islamic Repub. Iran* 34:110. doi:10.34171/mjiri.34.110.

25. Cakir, B. (2020). COVID-19 in Turkey: Lessons learned. *J. Epidemiol. Global Health* 10(2):115–117.

doi:10.2991/jegh.k.200520.001. PMID: 32538025; PMCID: PMC7310785.

26. Mbunge, E., Akinnuwesi, B., Fashoto, S.G., Metfula, A.S., Mashwama, P. (2021). A critical review of emerging technologies for tackling COVID-19 pandemic. *Hum. Behav. Emerg. Technol.* 3(1):25–39. doi:10.1002/hbe2.237.

27. Dutheil, F., Mondillon, L., Navel, V. (2020). PTSD as the second tsunami of the SARS-Cov-2 pandemic. *Psychol. Med.* 24:1–2. doi:10.1017/S0033291720001336. Epub ahead of print. PMID: 32326997; PMCID: PMC7198460.

28. Reger, M.A., Stanley, I.H., Joiner, T.E. (2020). Suicide mortality and coronavirus disease 2019: A perfect storm? *JAMA Psychiatry* doi:10.1001/jamapsychiatry.2020.1060. Epub ahead of print. PMID: 32275300.

29. Wang, C., Pan, R., Wan, X., Tan, Y., Xu, L., Ho, C.S., Ho, R.C. (2020). Immediate psychological responses and associated factors during the initial stage of the 2019 coronavirus disease (COVID-19) epidemic among the general population in China. *Int. J. Environ. Res. Public Health* 17(5):1729. doi:10.3390/ijerph17051729.

30. Brooks, S.K., Webster, R.K., Smith, L.E., Woodland, L., Wessely, S., Greenberg, N., Rubin, G.J. (2020). The psychological impact of quarantine and how to reduce it: Rapid review of the evidence. *Lancet* 395:10227. doi:10.1016/S0140-6736(20)30460-8.

31. Karuppasamy, M.B., Seshachalam, S., Natesan, U. et al. (2020). Air pollution improvement and mortality rate during COVID-19 pandemic in India: Global intersectional study. *Air Qual. Atmos. Health* 13:1375–1384. doi:10.1007/s11869-020-00892-w.

32. Zangari, S., Hill, D.T., Charette, A.T., Mirowsky, J.E. (2020). Air quality changes in New York City during the COVID-19 pandemic. *Sci. Total Environ.* 742:140496. doi:10.1016/j.scitotenv.2020.140496. Epub 2020 June 25. PMID: 32640401; PMCID: PMC7314691.

33. Siciliano, B., Dantas, G., da Silva, C.M., Arbilla, G. (2020). Increased ozone levels during the COVID-19 lockdown: Analysis for the city of Rio de Janeiro, Brazil. *Sci. Total Environ.* 737:139765. doi:10.1016/j.scitotenv.2020.139765. Epub 2020 May 28. PMID: 32480061; PMCID: PMC7263276.

34. Zhao, Y., Zhang, K., Xu, X., Shen, H., Zhu, X., Zhang, Y., Hu, Y., Shen, G. (2020). Substantial changes in Nitrate Oxide and Ozone after excluding meteorological impacts during the COVID-19 outbreak in Mainland China. *Environ. Sci. Technol. Lett.*, acs. Est lett. 0c00304. doi:10.1021/acs.estlett.0c00304.

35. Yunus, A.P., Masago, Y., Hijioka, Y. (2020). COVID-19 and surface water quality: Improved lake water quality during the lockdown. *Sci. Total Environ.* 731:139012. doi:10.1016/j.scitotenv.2020.139012. Epub 2020 April 27. PMID: 32388159; PMCID: PMC7185006.

36. Selvam, S., Jesuraja, K., Venkatramanan, S., Chung, S.Y., Roy, P.D., Muthukumar, P., Kumar, M. (2020). Imprints of pandemic lockdown on subsurface water quality in the coastal industrial city of Tuticorin, South India: A revival perspective. *Sci. Total Environ.* 738:139848. doi:10.1016/j.scitotenv.2020.139848. Epub 2020 May 31. PMID: 32574914; PMCID: PMC7832982.

37. Fakhruddin, B., Blanchard, K., Ragupathy, D. (2020). Are we there yet? The transition from response to recovery for the COVID-19 pandemic. *Progress Disaster Sci.* 7:100102. doi:10.1016/j.pdisas.2020.100102.

38. Mazumder, H., Hossain, M.M., Das, A. (2020). Geriatric care during public health emergencies: Lessons learned from novel corona virus disease (COVID-19) pandemic. *J. Gerontol. Soc. Work* 63(4):257–258. doi:10.1080/01634372.2020.1746723. Epub 2020 March 26. PMID: 32216550.

39. Lum, T., Shi, C., Wong, G., Wong, K. (2020, July–October). COVID-19 and long-term care policy for older people in Hong Kong. *J. Aging Soc. Policy* 32(4–5):373–379. doi:10.1080/08959420.2020.1773192. Epub 2020 May 31. PMID: 32476597.

40. Aung, M.N., Yuasa, M., Koyanagi, Y., Aung, T.N.N., Moolphate, S., Matsumoto, H., Yoshioka, T. (2020, April 30). Sustainable health promotion for the seniors during COVID-19 outbreak: A lesson from Tokyo. *J. Infect. Dev. Ctries* 14(4):328–331. doi:10.3855/jidc.12684. PMID: 32379708.

41. Butler, S.M. (2020). Four COVID-19 lessons for achieving health equity. *JAMA* 324(22):2245–2246. doi:10.1001/jama.2020.23553. PMID: 33289815.

42. Hsu, H., Greenwald, P.W., Laghezza, M.R., Steel, P., Trepp, R., Sharma, R. (2021, March 18). Clinical informatics during the COVID-19 pandemic: Lessons learned and implications for emergency department and inpatient operations. *J. Am. Med. Inform. Assoc.* 28(4):879–889. doi:10.1093/jamia/ocaa311. PMID: 33247720; PMCID: PMC7799016.

43. Moustafa, K. (2020). Lessons to Learn from COVID-19. *Oman Med. J.* 35(4):e159. doi:10.5001/omj.2020.81. PMID: 32802418; PMCID: PMC7420288.

44. Lau, L.S., Samari, G., Moresky, R.T., Casey, S.E., Kachur, S.P., Roberts, L.F., Zard, M. (2020). COVID-19 in humanitarian settings and lessons learned from past epidemics. *Nat. Med.* 26(5): 647–648. doi:10.1038/s41591-020-0851-2. PMID: 32269357.

45. Al Fannah, J., Al Harthy, H., Al Salmi, Q. (2020, September 7). COVID-19 Pandemic: Learning lessons and a vision for a better health system. *Oman Med. J.* 35(5):e169. doi:10.5001/omj.2020.111. PMID: 32953143; PMCID: PMC7477518.

46. Antonio La, M., Craig, N., Antonio, P., Scott, M. (2020). COVID-19: Lessons from the Italian reproductive medical experience. *Fertil. Steril.* 113(5). doi:10.1016/j.fertnstert.2020.03.021.

47. Cruickshank, M., Shaban, R. Z. (2020). COVID-19: Lessons to be learnt from a once-in-a-century global pandemic. *J. Clin. Nurs.* 29(21–22):3901–3904. doi:10.1111/jocn.15365. Epub 2020 June 22. PMID: 32498115; PMCID: PMC7301028.

48. Arango, C. (2020). Lessons learned from the coronavirus health crisis in Madrid, Spain: How COVID-19 has changed our lives in the last 2 weeks. *Biol. Psychiatry* 88(7):e33–e34. doi:10.1016/j.biopsych.2020.04.003.

49. Ojeahere, M.I., de Filippis, R., Ransing, R., et al. (2020). Management of psychiatric conditions and delirium during the COVID-19 pandemic across continents: Lessons learned and recommendations. *Brain Behav. Immun. Health* 9:100147. doi:10.1016/j.bbih.2020.100147.

Chapter 6   The Evolution of COVID-19 Diagnostics

Praveen Rai, Ballamoole Krishna Kumar, Deekshit Vijaya Kumar, Prashant Kumar,
Anoop Kumar, Shashi Kumar Shetty, and Biswajit Maiti

6.1 INTRODUCTION

Coronaviruses are a family of single-stranded RNA (ssRNA) viruses capable of causing mild to lethal infections in mammals and birds. The first case of human coronavirus was reported in the 1960s, and since then, seven coronaviruses have emerged with the potential of causing mild to severe diseases in humans. Since the year 2000, three highly pathogenic coronaviruses (CoV), namely, Severe Acute Respiratory Syndrome-Coronavirus (SARS-CoV), Middle East Respiratory Syndrome-Coronavirus (MERS-CoV), and SARS-CoV-2 have emerged. The SARS-CoV first appeared in 2003 in Guangdong, China; the MERS-CoV emerged in 2012 in Saudi Arabia; and the SARS-CoV-2 emerged in 2019 in the Wuhan province of China. While SARS-CoV and MERS-CoV did not cause pandemics, they had a very high mortality rate of 9.7% and 34%, respectively, which is in fact much higher compared to the mortality rate observed in the ongoing COVID-19 pandemic caused by SARS-CoV-2 [1]. The diseases caused by the three CoVs range from the mild common cold to severe diseases such as Severe Acute Respiratory Syndrome (SARS), Middle East Respiratory Syndrome (MERS), and COVID-19.

6.2 CORONAVIRUS DISEASE 2019 (COVID-19)

SARS-CoV-2, initially named as 2019-nCoV, quickly spread across international borders, infecting people in a number of countries, and prompting the World Health Organization (WHO) to declare SARS-CoV-2 infection as "a very high-risk global pandemic" [2]. As of May 21, 2021, 166,492,036 cases, including 3,458,041 deaths caused by COVID-19 have been registered worldwide, with a case fatality rate of 2.05%. Transmission of SARS-CoV-2 occurs primarily via respiratory droplets or aerosols (<5 μm) exhaled by an infected individual [3]. The virus can also be transmitted to a healthy individual via fomites carrying the virus, or by direct contact between an infected and a healthy individual. The incubation period for SARS-CoV-2 ranges from two to fourteen days with a median incubation period of 5–6 days, but an infected individual starts shedding the virus before the onset of symptoms or even if he or she is asymptomatic. Individuals infected with SARS-CoV-2 may be an asymptomatic carrier or may exhibit mild, moderate or severe acute respiratory syndrome distress (ARDS). The patients usually show symptoms such as a high fever above 39°C (102°F), headache, dry cough, sore throat, chest congestion, chest pain, shortness of breath, loose motions, runny nose, redness in eyes, pneumonia etc. In severe cases, the patients may show a respiratory rate above 30/min, oxygen saturation in blood below 95% and in this critical stage, severe pneumonia, septic shock, respiratory failure, cardiac arrest and multiple organ failures, leading to the death of the individual [4]. Health complications have also been observed in cases of asymptomatic infections, where the patients show relatively normal lung function without dyspnea, but with low blood oxygen saturation level, a condition referred to as 'silent hypoxia' and indicates severe respiratory failure, which may lead to the sudden death of the patient [5].

6.3 EMERGENCE AND STRUCTURAL FEATURES OF SARS-CoV-2

SARS-CoV-2 is a new member of the genus Betacoronavirus in the Coronaviridae family of the order Nidovirales [6]. SARS-CoV-2 and other two human CoVs, SARS- CoV and MERS-CoV, have most likely originated from bats and have been transmitted to humans through intermediates, with pangolin being the potential intermediate for SARS-CoV-2. Whole-genome analysis reveals that SARS-CoV-2 is 79% similar to SARS-CoV and 50% similar to MERS-CoV. It is 96.2% similar to the RaTG13 bat coronavirus, which indicates that RaTG13 could be the origin of SARS-CoV-2 [7]. SARS-CoV-2 like other CoVs has a crown-shaped appearance through the uniform distribution of spike proteins on the virion surface as observed by electron microscopy (Figure 6.1). SARS-CoV-2 is an enveloped virus with a non-segmented positive-sense ssRNA genome of 29,891 bases encoding 9,860 amino acids. The genome encodes four structural proteins, namely the spike protein (S), the Envelope protein (E), the Nucleoprotein (N) and the Membrane protein (M), in addition to six accessory and sixteen non-structural proteins. The trimeric S glycoprotein is responsible for host cell tropism and entry into the target cells via the angiotensin-converting enzyme 2

DOI: 10.1201/9781003190394-6

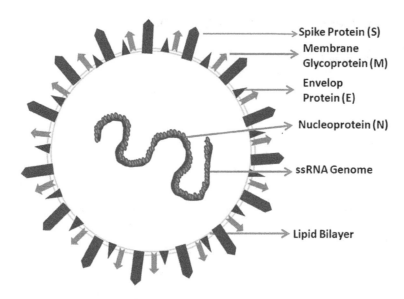

Figure 6.1 Schematic representation of SARS-CoV-2. The spike protein (S), Membrane glycoprotein (M) and Envelope protein (E). The nucleoprotein (N) wraps the positive sense single stranded RNA genome in the viral core and constitutes the ribonucleoprotein (RNAP) complex.

(ACE2) receptor. The S glycoprotein consists of two subunits (S1and S2) and shows a structural difference from the S protein of other similar CoVs by having a furin cleavage site (S1/S2) rich in basic amino acid residues (SPRRARSVAS), which favors efficient viral entry into host cells [3]. There are six crucial amino acid residues in the Receptor-Binding Domain (RBD) of the S protein, responsible for viral attachment to the ACE2 receptor on the host cells. Five of them are different between SARS-CoV and SARS-CoV-2, while all six are identical for SARS-CoV-2 and Pangolin CoV, which suggest that pangolin is the intermediate host [8]. Other structural proteins, such as the N and E proteins, are relatively more conserved between SARS-CoV and SARS-CoV-2, with a sequence identity of 89.6% and 96%, respectively [7].

6.4 LABORATORY DIAGNOSIS OF COVID-19

Molecular and serological assays are available for the diagnosis of COVID-19. Though the specimens required for these tests depend on the clinical presentations in affected individuals, respiratory specimens are the most common for the diagnosis of SARS-CoV-2 infection. The nucleic acid amplification test (NAAT) is the most accurate test available for the diagnosis of COVID-19. It involves procedures such as sample collection, sample processing, RNA extraction, and real-time Reverse Transcriptase-Quantitative Polymerase Chain

Reaction (RT-qPCR) and its analysis. As far as possible, the patients suspecting SARS-CoV-2 infection should be diagnosed based on RT-qPCR. Amplification of more than one target on the SARS-CoV-2 genome is needed for an accurate diagnosis of viral infection. The commonly used RT-qPCR targets in SARS-CoV-2 include the E, N, RNA dependent RNA Polymerase (RdRP) and S genes (Table 6.1). Because of the enhanced rate of mutation in the viral genome, at least three of the mentioned targets must be included in the diagnosis to avoid any false-negative results [9]. Recently, a fully automated NAAT system has been developed that integrates the stages of sample processing, RNA extraction, amplification, and reporting. This automated system can be installed in remote resource-limited areas with limited numbers of high-performance trained staff.

Additionally, other amplification methods for the detection of SARS-CoV-2 are under development or undergoing the process of commercialization. These methods involve technologies such as Reverse Transcription Loop-Mediated Isothermal Amplification (RT-LAMP), Clustered Regularly Interspersed Short Palindromic Repeats (CRISPR), and molecular microarray assays. An overview of the nuclei acid–based diagnostic assays available for the diagnosis of COVID-19 infection is presented in Figure 6.2. The serological assays include the detection of viral protein in respiratory tract specimens. These are rapid tests that are based on Lateral

Table 6.1 Comparison of nucleic acid amplification tests for the detection of SARS-CoV-2

Method	LOD (Limit of Detection)	Clinical Sensitivity	Specificity	Target Regions	Advantages	Limitations	References
RT-PCR	0.15–100 copies/μL	90–100	100	RdRp, N, E, S and ORF1b or ORF8	High throughput; highly sensitive and specific; detects active cases; useful in clinical decision-making	Labor intensive; requires numerous reagents; specialized equipment; costly; less accurate after ~5 days since symptom onset	[20]
TMA	5.5×10^3 copies/mL	98–100	100	N1 and N2	Provides an effective, highly sensitive means of detection of SARS-CoV-2 in nasopharyngeal specimens	None	[28]
RT-LAMP	80 copies/mL	90–100	100	N, S and orf1 ab	Rapid, simple and sensitive method for large screening in public domain and at hospitals	Requires multiple detection primers	[23]
RT-NEAR	0.13 copies/μl	95–100	100	RdRp	Compact, integrated hands-on technique	Formation of nonspecific products that limits the sensitivity and thereby increases the threshold of detection methods	[30]
RT-HDA	1.16×10^4 copies/mL	95–100	100	Pp1ab	Simple cost-efficient method	Negative results do not preclude infection with SARS-CoV-2 and should not be the sole basis of a patient treatment decision.	https://www.quidel.com/molecular-diagnostics/helicase-dependent-amplification-tests
CRISPR	0.9 copies/μL	90–100	100	N	Simple and efficient; low cost; low turnaround time; improved specificity; visual readout	Risk of contamination	[35]
ddPCR	1.8 copies/reaction	83–99	100	ORF1ab	Highly sensitive and accurate method	Expensive	[37]
RT-RPA	20 copies/μL 1 copy/μL	95–100	100	RdRp N	One tube rapid detection method, can be used for high-throughput clinical testing or combined with lateral flow strips for individual testing	None	[39]
SDA	10 copies/reaction	95–100	100	N	Alternative method for rapid diagnosis while maintaining the advantages of aligner-mediated cleavage and isothermal amplification in terms of simplicity, convenience, and affordability	Requires standardization	[43]

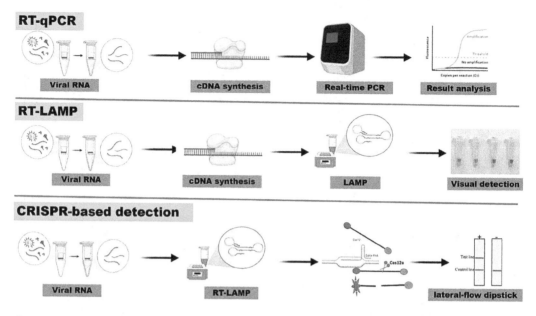

Figure 6.2 Overview of the nucleic acid–based diagnostic assays available for diagnosis of COVID-19 infection.

Flow Immunoassays (LFI) and can be completed within 30 minutes. However, the sensitivity of LFI-based rapid tests is lower than for NAAT [9]. Moreover, false-positive results can also exist for the rapid tests if the antibodies on the test strip cross-react with the antigen of other viruses than SARS-CoV-2.

6.4.1 Computed Tomography (CT) Scans

Chest computed tomography (CT) scans are presently one of the first live imaging techniques to detect pneumonia-related illnesses in the lung. It was found to be more sensitive than X-rays in detecting lung defects in SARS and MERS [10]. Recently the technique has also been used for the diagnosis and management of COVID-19. However, this technique has its own set of limitations. Though the RT-qPCR assay is considered to be the gold standard for the detection of SARS-CoV-2, recently several studies have shown the importance of chest CT scans in COVID-19 patients with false-negative RT-qPCR results and showed a sensitivity of 98% [11]. In addition, chest CT scans can be used in complicated cases of COVID-19.

Chest CT scans play an essential role in promptly detecting lung abnormalities in COVID-19 pneumonia. CT scan features include bilateral, peripheral, and basal predominant ground-glass opacities (GGOs) with or without consolidation in nearly 85% of patients, with superimposed irregular lines and interfaces or mixed pattern evolve with crazy-paving,

architectural distortion and perilobular abnormalities superimposed on GGOs with slow resolution [12]. In addition, thickening of the bronchial wall, mucoid impactions, and centrilobular nodules are common during infection, whereas lymphadenopathy and pleural effusion are uncommon [13]. It is important to note that the results of chest CT scanning are dependent on the patient's stage of infection. Figure 6.3 shows the lung abnormalities in COVID-19 pneumonia and other lung diseases.

In a recent meta-analysis, the effectiveness of RT-PCR and chest CT scan in the diagnosis of COVID-19 was evaluated [14]. For chest CT scans, the pooled sensitivity was 94% (95 % CI: 91%, 96%; I 2 = 95%) and for RT-PCR, it was 89% (95% CI: 81%, 94%; I 2 = 90%), but the pooled specificity for chest CT scans was low 35% (95% CI: 26%, 50%; I 2 = 95%). The positive predictive value (PPV) of chest CT scans ranged from 1.5% to 30.7%, while the negative predictive value (NPV) was 95.4% to 99.8%. The PPV ranged from 47.3% to 96.4% for RT-PCR, while the NPV was 96.8% to 99.9%. Considering the huge difference in PPV between chest CT scans and RT-PCR, as well as the low specificity of CT scans, the use of chest CT scans can result in a high percentage of false-positive results, demanding additional diagnostic investigations, higher medical costs, hospital load, and patient anxiety [14].

Another meta-analysis study compared chest CT scans to RT-PCR. The overall sensitivity, specificity, PPV, and NPV were 87% (95% CI 85–90%),

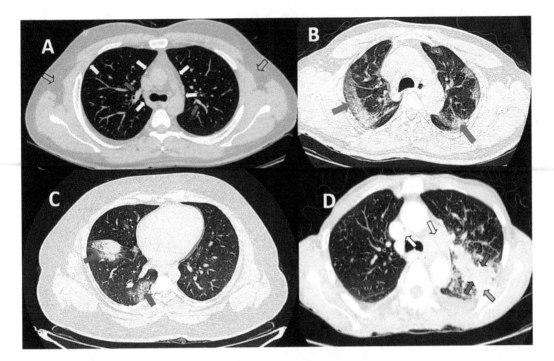

Figure 6.3   Chest CT scan images. (A) Normal cross-sectional image shows both lung fields, which are normally aerated and applied to the chest wall on all sides. There is no sign of pleural thickening (yellow arrow) and no fluid collection. The pulmonary structure is normal (red arrows) and shows normal vascular markings. No intrapulmonary nodules or patchy opacities are present. The mediastinum is centered and of normal width (white arrows). The hilar region on each side and the main broncho remain normal. The thoracic skeleton and soft tissues show no abnormalities (green arrows). (B) Patient with COVID-19 pneumonia shows patchy subpleural ground-glass opacities (red arrow) and consolidation in both lungs predominantly involving peripheral and suggestive of infectious etiology (CORAD 6 – moderate disease [17/25]). (C) Patient with COVID-19 pneumonia shows patchy ground-glass opacities involving right lung (red arrows), predominantly in the periphery and a patch of consolidation in the right lower lobe and suggestive of infectious etiology (CORAD 6 – mild disease [06/25]). (D) Patient with malignant etiology shows heterogeneously enhancing lesion (red arrows) of left lung upper lobe involving pleura (green arrow), perihilar structures with multiple enlarged mediastinal lymph nodes (yellow arrows).

46% (95% CI 29–63%), 69% (95% CI 56–72%), and 89% (95% CI 82–96%), respectively [15]. It was also concluded that, mainly in negative samples, it is critical to rely on three rounds of RT-qPCR to achieve 99% accuracy. Bollineni et al. [16] found that chest CT imaging shows high sensitivity and NPV for diagnosis of COVID-19 and can be used as an alternative primary screening tool in epidemic areas. Furthermore, despite a negative RT-qPCR examination, positive CT scan findings can still indicate COVID-19 infection [16]. In a retrospective study of 64 patients conducted in Hong Kong, chest radiography had a sensitivity of 69% compared to 91% for RT-qPCR. On a chest radiograph, 20% of the RT-qPCR positive

cases showed no lung anomalies [17]. In another study, 75% of RT-qPCR negative cases had chest CT scan findings, with 48% of those likely to be COVID-19 positive cases [18].

Even though the chest CT scan can have a role in the diagnosis of COVID-19 where initial RT-qPCR testing has been inconclusive, there are a few major challenges associated with CT scans for COVID-19, as listed below:

■ Possible danger of radiation exposure.

■ The risk of infection from surface contamination and aerosolization during the process of a CT scan of a COVID-19 patient, and exposure to healthcare workers.

- Challenges in the interpretation of CT scan data and possible false-positive results as the pathology can overlap with other infections such as SARS, influenza, MERS and bacterial pneumonia.

- Lower sensitivity of CT scans for COVID-19 diagnosis in children.

6.4.2 Molecular Diagnosis

6.4.2.1 Reverse Transcription Real-Time Quantitative Polymerase Chain Reaction (RT-qPCR)

As per the WHO recommendation, the most widely used nucleic acid–based test for the detection of SARS-CoV-2 is RT-qPCR [19]. Several RT-qPCR assays targeting different genes of the SARS-CoV-2 genome, such as RdRp, N, E, and S genes, and ORF1b or ORF8 regions, have been used for the detection of SARS-CoV-2 from clinical samples. However, the WHO recommends an RT-qPCR-based assay targeting the E gene for screening the RdRp gene to confirm SARS-CoV-2. While the US Centers for Disease Control and Prevention (CDC) recommends an RT-qPCR assay based on two nucleocapsid protein genes (N1, N2) [19], to minimize the chances of false-positive results, CDC has developed a new RT-qPCR diagnostic panel including No Template Control (NTC) and Human Specimen Control (HSC). The method has also undergone tremendous modifications to improve the sensitivity, specificity, and feasibility of the technique. A multiplex RT-qPCR has been developed recently, targeting different regions of SARS-CoV-2 and seasonal influenza virus simultaneously with a limited quantification range between 5 and 10 copies per reaction for influenza and SARS-CoV-2, respectively [20]. Furthermore, a significant improvement has been made in the technique to achieve the results with greater accuracy in a short period of time at a low cost to detect SARS-CoV-2 RNA directly from samples without involving an extraction procedure [21]. The HID-RT-PCR (Heat Inactivated Direct-RT-PCR) developed in this study had an accuracy, sensitivity and specificity of 98.8%, with a limit of detection of 0.009 TCID50/ml for the ORF1 and 0.003 TCID50/ml for E genes.

6.4.2.2 Reverse Transcription Loop-Mediated Isothermal Amplification (RT-LAMP)

LAMP is a rapid DNA amplification technique that has been widely used to detect pathogens such as viruses, bacteria, and protozoan malarial parasites. The technique works by the principle of using four different primers specifically designed to bind six different regions of the target DNA [22]. The method is widely used for the detection of SARS-CoV-2 viral RNA by incorporating the reverse transcriptase enzyme in the LAMP reaction and can be completed within 20 minutes with a detection limit of 80 copies of viral RNA per ml of the sample [23]. Since then, several modifications to this assay have been introduced to achieve a greater level of specificity and sensitivity. For example, an RT-LAMP assay was developed, wherein swabs are dipped into synthetic nasal fluid spiked with the virus, moved to a viral transport medium, and then a volume of sample is used to perform the RT-LAMP without the RNA extraction step. The assay showed a detection limit of around 50 copies of viral RNA per µl of the sample within 30 minutes. Similarly, an RT-LAMP was developed for the detection of ORF8 and N genes of SARS-CoV-2 directly from the nasopharyngeal swabs with a sensitivity of detection of about 100 copies/µl [24]. An RT-LAMP was developed that targets the NSP3 region of the virus. The technique could detect 100 copies/reaction of SARS-CoV-2 RNA [25]. A commercially available RT-LAMP (Loopamp® 2019-SARS-CoV-2 Detection Reagent Kit [http://loopamp.eiken.co.jp/]) showed high sensitivity with a detection limit of 1.0×10^1 copies/µl within 35 minutes. More recently, the RT-LAMP technique was developed to detect SARS-CoV-2 on heat-inactivated samples using non-commercial RT-LAMP reagents [26]. Though the study showed low sensitivity, it aimed mainly at detecting samples with high to medium SARS-CoV-2 content in a global setting to curb the spread of infection. Similarly, a field-deployable High-Performance Loop-Mediated Isothermal Amplification (HP-LAMP) technique was developed to detect SARS-CoV-2 rapidly from saliva [27]. The technique has a limit of detection of 1.38 copies/ml of saliva. This simple one-step protocol may allow samples to be analyzed at home with pooling strategies (involves mixing several samples together).

6.4.2.3 Transcription Mediated Amplification (TMA)

TMA refers to the isothermal amplification of RNA by the process of reverse transcription and generation of multiple transcripts by RNA polymerase. Following amplification, these transcripts are hybridized with oligonucleotide probes with a chemiluminescent tag for detection. This technique has a capacity to produce 100–1,000 copies/cycle with a 10-billion-fold increase within 15–30 minutes of reaction. The technique has been used widely in food and water safety laboratories to detect pathogens such as Listeria, Salmonella, and

Campylobacter. However, more recently, the method has also been used efficiently for the detection of SARS-CoV-2. Recently, a highly sensitive transcription-mediated amplification method, Hologic Panther, was developed for the detection of SARS-CoV-2 [28]. It showed high analytical sensitivity of 98.1%, and less inconclusive results when compared to real-time PCR. In addition, the assay was found to process and generate results for >1,000 samples within a day, thereby enabling healthcare sectors to process a large volume of samples for the detection of SARS-CoV-2 RNA [29].

6.4.2.4 *Nicking Endonuclease Amplification Reaction (NEAR)*

NEAR is an isothermal method used for the amplification of short ON (Base modified oligonucleotides) sequences. The technique mainly utilizes the combination of both strand displacement DNA polymerase (*Bst*) and a nicking endonuclease, which is based on the primer extension of the longer primer in the presence of a template, cleavage of the extended primer by nicking endonuclease, and release of the resulting short oligonucleotides caused by insufficiently stable duplexes below the elevated reaction temperature (55°C). The primer is then regenerated and undergoes another round of extension and nicking, and so on, resulting in linear amplification of the short oligonucleotides. The technique was found to be highly efficient with the analytical sensitivity of 0.13 copies/µl, specificity of 100% for the detection of SARS-CoV-2 at an operating temperature range of 55–59°C in less than 15 minutes. However, the major limitation of this technique is the formation of non-specific products that limits the sensitivity and thereby increases the threshold of detection methods [30].

6.4.2.5 *Helicase-Dependent Amplification (HDA)*

The helicase dependent isothermal DNA amplification technique uses DNA helicase to separate double-stranded DNA and to generate a single-stranded template for hybridization of a primer with subsequent primer extension by a DNA polymerase, resulting in an exponential amplification of a selected DNA target [31]. This method helps to maintain a constant temperature from the beginning to the end of the reaction by eliminating the initial PCR denaturation step [32]. Quidel has developed an isothermal helicase dependent amplification with fluorescence detection of SARS-CoV-2 (https://www.quidel.com/molecular-diagnostics/helicase-dependent-amplification-tests). The technique operates in individual tubes at one temperature

reducing the time required to 25 minutes. It also avoids the need for specialized training in molecular techniques.

6.4.2.6 *Clustered Regularly Interspaced Short Palindromic Repeats (CRISPR)*

CRISPR is short palindromic repeat DNA sequences usually found in prokaryotes as a part of their defense mechanism. CRISPR requires a small RNA fragment called the guide RNA (gRNA), which binds to the complementary target sequence, and a nuclease enzyme cleaves at the precise site. In the case of viral nucleic acid detection, the gRNA in turn binds to the target segment of the viral gene. Several CRISPR associated Cas proteins (cas9, cas12 or cas13) have been shown to exert nonspecific endonuclease activity to cleave DNA or RNA. More recently, it was reported that the CRISPR-Cas12a protein could detect nucleic acids of exogenous viruses, like the human papillomavirus from cervical cancer patients in raw plasma, without the need for RNA extraction [33]. Recently, a CRISPR-based technology DETECTR was used to detect SARS-CoV-2 in RNA extracted clinical specimens [32]. Subsequently, a combination of CRISPR-Cas13a with a reader device based on a mobile phone was developed for detection of SARS-CoV-2 RNA extracted from nasal swabs [34]. Furthermore, SHERLOCK (Specific High sensitivity Enzymatic Reporter unlocking) a CRISPR-Cas12b-based test for detecting SARS-CoV-2, was developed [35]. In addition, Ding et al. developed the All-In-One Dual CRISPR-Cas12a (AIOD-CRISPR) assay for SHERLOCK Testing in One-Pot (STOP) and visual detection of SARS-CoV-2 [32]. However, the majority of these methods involve isolation of SARS-CoV-2 RNA from the specimens that might further increase the risk of cross-contamination and virus transmission. To avoid such complications, a CRISPR-Cas12a-based point of care SARS-CoV-2 test was developed recently, where CRISPR Cas-12a was combined with RT-RPA to directly analyze lysed samples without the need for any RNA extraction. The test showed a sensitivity of 0.1 copies /µl for the detection of SARS-CoV-2 from clinical specimens in 60 minutes [36].

6.4.2.7 *Digital Droplet PCR (ddPCR)*

The ddPCR is a third-generation polymerase chain reaction technique based on the principles of limited dilution, endpoint PCR, and Poisson statistics with absolute quantification. In the technique, the sample is divided into discrete partitions of thousands of droplets. Some droplets might contain no template and others one or more templates. This will allow the technique to detect even very low (1.8 copies/reaction) amount of viral nucleic acid from the sample. The partitioned droplets are amplified by PCR and counted by a droplet reader to determine the number of positive droplets, and then estimated by modelling as a Poisson distribution. The feasibility of ddPCR was mainly assessed to improve the diagnostic accuracy of SARS-CoV-2 nucleic acid in specimens with low viral load [37]. The technique was found to be effective in detecting low viral load during the convalescent stage of the disease, where RT-PCR would otherwise fail to detect the virus.

6.4.2.8 Reverse Transcription – Recombinase Polymerase Amplification (RT-RPA)

RT-RPA is a technique developed using proteins involved in DNA synthesis, repair and recombination. In this technique, a recombinase protein uvsX from T4-like bacteriophages was used to bind to primers in the presence of ATP and a crowding agent (polyethylene glycol), forming a recombinase-primer complex. The complex is then allowed to interact with the double-stranded DNA with a homologous sequence that in turn promotes strand invasion by the primer. The proteins in the complex will stabilize the displaced DNA strand. Finally, the recombinase enzyme disassembles, and a strand displacing DNA polymerase binds to the 3' end of the primer to elongate it in the presence of dNTPs. The process is then repeated in several cycles to achieve exponential amplification [38]. The technique has been widely used in combination with reverse transcription for the detection of SARS-CoV-2 on an OR-DETECTR platform that combines RPA and CRISPR/Cas12 technologies for two transcripts, the RdRp and N genes. The limit of detection for RdRp was found to be 20 copies/µl and 1 copy/µl of the N gene. A similar one-tube method based on RT-RPA and SHERLOCK (OR-SHERLOCK) combines RT-RPA and CRISPR/Cas13a detection with the same level of sensitivity and specificity as that of OR-DETECTR [39]. A microfluidic-integrated lateral flow recombinase polymerase amplification (MI-IF-RPA) assay was developed for rapid detection of SARS-CoV-2. The technique combines RT-RPA and a universal lateral flow (LF) dipstick detection system into a single microfluidic chip. The RT-RPA reaction components are mixed with running buffer and then delivered to the LF detection strips for biotin- and FAM-labeled amplified analyte sequences, which can provide easily interpreted positive or negative results. The technique showed the limit of detection of 1 copy/µl or 30 copies per sample with 97% to 100% specificity [40].

6.4.2.9 Strand Displacement Amplification (SDA)

SDA is another isothermal amplification method, where a nicking endonuclease is used to generate a nick in one strand of the double-stranded DNA followed by an extension of sequence from the nicking site catalyzed by strand displacement polymerase [41]. In this method, two pairs of primers that recognize the target regions are designed. The first is a bumper primer, and the second an SDA primer that binds next to the bumper primer at the target sequences. The two enzymes, HincII and Exo Klenow, are added to cleave at the recognition site of the phosphorothioate of the DNA probe, and to initiate the replication of the sequence, respectively. Subsequently, the exponential reaction begins with the repeated cycle of nicking, extension, and strand displacement. This amplification is enhanced by additional primers flanking the inner region of the target sequence. The final product can be amplified 10^7-fold within 2 hours [42]. This principle of SDA has been used in combination with other nucleic acid–based methods as a hybrid amplification technique to improve the detection of SARS-CoV-2 nucleic acid. For example, a PCDR (polymerase chain displacement reaction) is a modified SDA method developed for the detection of SARS-CoV-2, where PCR and isothermal amplification was carried out in one assay. The method showed tenfold increased sensitivity compared to RT-qPCR with the detection limit of 5 copies/reaction. Another modified SDA method is aligner mediated cleavage-SDA (AMC-SDA), wherein specific recognition sequences will be created in the template nucleic acid for nicking endonucleases by using aligner primers [43]. The method can detect 10 copies/reaction of SARS-CoV-2 nucleic acid under isothermal amplification through a real-time fluorescence detection system within 25 minutes.

6.5 SEROLOGICAL ASSAYS

While RT-qPCR is the gold standard technique used to detect SARS-CoV-2 active cases, it comes with its own set of challenges when used in resource-constrained settings and sero-epidemiological studies. The test protocol for the laboratory diagnosis of COVID-19 is complex and expensive, placing high demands on experimental instruments, testing reagents, and the skills of research personnel [44]. The assay typically takes 4–6 hours to complete, but the logistical requirement to ship clinical samples leads to a turnaround time of more than 24 hours, which delays the reporting [9]. Further, false-negative results because of low viral load in the upper respiratory tract region may occur using RT-PCR analysis [45]. Hence several intergovernmental organizations have encouraged researchers and clinicians to develop and investigate the use of serology tests in community settings [46, 47]. The development of serological assays continues apace internationally; to date, over 400 assays have been commercialized for the rapid diagnosis of COVID-19 (https://www.finddx.org/). The fundamental principle behind serological assays is the detection of antibodies developed in response to viral infection (IgG and IgM) and/or viral antigen through means of immunodiagnostic techniques [47]. Studies have shown that antigen-specific antibodies could be detected in a COVID-19 patient after 3–6 days, and IgG could be detected at the later stages of infection [48, 49]. Though positive IgM and IgG ELISA results have been seen as early as the fourth day after symptom onset, serological tests with high sensitivity are seen in the second and third weeks of illness [50, 51]. The presence of IgM antibodies indicates recent exposure to viral infection, whereas IgG antibodies indicate earlier exposure to SARS-CoV-2 viral infection [47]. Because of the simplicity of the testing protocol, serological assays can be ramped up to analyze thousands of samples at labs with resource-limited settings [46, 52]. Besides, serological assays are becoming an increasingly valuable method for determining the degree of COVID-19 infection in the community, and identifying individuals who are immune and potentially "protected" from infection. Given the incredible demand for rapid tests for the diagnosis of COVID-19 infections, R&D companies around the world have launched many rapid diagnostics technologies with varying degrees of sensitivity. Comparative data on the analytical and clinical performances of the immunoassays is essential to evaluate the utility of the diagnostic test in diagnosing COVID-19 infection with the lowest possible error rate. Padoan et al. [53] have conducted a study to evaluate the analytical and clinical performances of five commercially available serological assays for the detection of SARS-CoV-2 antibodies [53]. Their findings indicated that all immunoassays had excellent specificity, while sensitivity differed between immunoassays and was highly dependent on the time between the onset of symptoms and the sample selection. An overview of the serological diagnostics assays available for the diagnosis of COVID-19 infection is depicted in Figure 6.4.

6.5.1 Enzyme-Linked Immunosorbent Assay (ELISA)

There are several ELISA-based methods available, with high levels of reproducibility and enduring sensitivity, which makes the test an excellent tool for the diagnosis of various infectious diseases. ELISA-based IgM and IgG antibody tests have proved to have more than 95% specificity in the diagnosis of COVID-19. To detect SARS-CoV2 specific antibodies in patient serum, a known capture antigen is immobilized on the ELISA microtiter plate. On the addition of a patient serum sample, virus-specific antibodies bind to the immobilized capture antigen. Subsequently, the addition of enzyme-labelled detection antibody specific to antibody isotypes (i.e., IgG, IgM, etc.) forms a complex with the patient antibodies. Next, the interaction of the enzyme and its substrate causes a colorimetric change that can be quantified and correlated to the presence and/or concentration of the antibody. This assay can be qualitative or quantitative, with a turnaround time of 2–5 hours. The analytical specificity and clinical performances of the various commercially available ELISA have been reviewed by several researchers [9, 19, 53]. In India, the National Institute of Virology, Pune, in collaboration with Zydus Diagnostics, has developed an indigenous IgG-based ELISA (COVID KAVACH ELISA) for the detection of antibodies in COVID-19 infection. Preliminary validation of the COVID KAVACH ELISA has shown to have high sensitivity and specificity in detecting SARS-CoV-2 infections. The systematic review and meta-analysis of the diagnostic accuracy of ELISA for the detection of COVID-19 showed that ELISA had a pooled sensitivity of 84.3% in measuring the SARS-COV-2 specific IgM and IgG [54].

6.5.2 Point-of-Care Serological Assays

Point-of-care (POC) serological assays are simple and rapid tests based on lateral flow immunoassay (LFIA) technology. The primary advantage of these assays is their simplicity, with a time-to-result anywhere between 10 and 30 minutes. A typical lateral flow test strip is made of overlapping membranes mounted on a backing card. When a sample is added to the lateral flow, it migrates through the conjugate pad, which includes antibodies unique to the target analyte that has been conjugated to colored or fluorescent particles. The analyte-bound conjugated antibody then flows through the immobilized antibody in a test and control line of the nitrocellulose membrane. The read-out, represented by the lines appearing with different intensities, can be assessed by eye or by using a dedicated reader. The utility of low-cost, rapid, and accurate POC tests prompted the development and marketing of several lateral flow immunoassays for the diagnosis of COVID-19. However, the study by Bastos et al. [54] raised

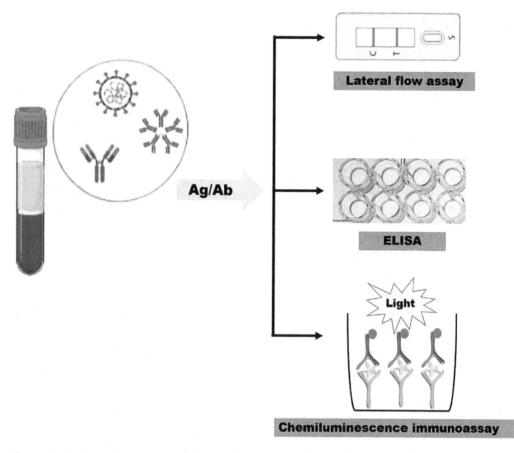

Figure 6.4 Overview of the serological diagnostics assays available for diagnosis of COVID-19 infection.

concerns about detection sensitivity of the commercially available lateral immunoassays as they demonstrated the pooled sensitivity of 66% in detecting COVID-19 cases [54].

6.5.3 Chemiluminescence Immunoassay

Over the past few years, chemiluminescence immunoassays (CLIAs) have gained increasing attention as a rapid and sensitive PoC test in different fields, including clinical diagnosis. The detection of the analyte is based on the reaction wherein enzymes used for the immunochemical reaction converts the chemiluminescence substrate to a reaction product, which emits a photon of light instead of color development [55]. Based on this principle, few CLIAs are available for the detection of serum immunoglobulin IgG and IgM against SARS-CoV-2 [56–58]. The performance of four different chemiluminescence immunoassay systems for the detection of COVID-19 showed varying degrees of diagnostic accuracy, thereby suggesting the

necessity of evaluation of the performance of diagnostic tests before actual use [58].

6.6 CHALLENGES WITH EXISTING TECHNOLOGIES

To date, RT-qPCR is considered the gold standard for the detection of SARS-CoV-2 globally. This is primarily because it offers a high level of sensitivity with a very low limit of detection and specificity. Additionally, several other assays based on an array of technologies have either been developed or are in the process of development. Many of these have also been commercialized and approved for emergency use by the respective authorities. Existing methods available for the diagnosis of COVID-19 may comprise (a) NAAT including RT-qPCR and isothermal amplification-based assays, (b) immunoassays including antibody tests (serology) and antigen tests, or (c) imaging-based diagnosis including CT scans. However, all these methods have their own limitations and challenges (Table 6.2).

Table 6.2 Key challenges with existing technologies for the detection of SARS-CoV-2

Name of the Detection Technology	Key Challenges
RT-qPCR	• Do not qualify as a PoC or for bedside testing in resource-limited setting • Technical complexity, high testing costs, and requirement of skilled research personnel • It may require up to one full day or beyond to provide a final result report
Isothermal Amplification-Based Assays	• Not able to generate accurate quantitative results data • If not optimized well, it can generate a false-positive result
Antibody Tests	• Do not offer high specificity • Less sensitive compared to other technologies
Antigen Tests	• Relatively less specific and can cross-react with other RNA viruses • Less sensitive compared to NAAT assays
CT Scan Examination	• Limited availability in diagnostic centers and hospitals • It cannot be used for field-level or bedside diagnosis of COVID-19 disease

6.6.1 Challenges with RT-qPCR

RT-qPCR is considered to be the best method for detection of SARS-CoV-2. In addition to the sensitivity and specificity, the assay can be used for quantitative estimation of viral load. However, the method has several limitations, which include:

■ It cannot be deployed as a PoC or for bedside testing in resource-limited settings.

■ Technical complexity and high costs place a high demand on experimental instruments, testing reagents, and the skill of research personnel.

■ Tests typically take 4–6 hours to complete, but the logistical requirement to ship clinical samples leads to a turnaround time of more than 24 hours that delays the reporting.

6.6.2 Challenges with Isothermal Amplification-Based Assays

Isothermal amplification-based assays such as the LAMP assay are another NAAT-based emerging method that can be considered a good alternative for the detection of SARS-CoV-2 [59].

The US Food and Drug Administration (US-FDA) has recently approved this assay for commercial use (https://www.fda.gov/media/138248/download). Despite having several advantages, it also has a few limitations, such as:

■ The assays usually provide only qualitative results.

■ Can be susceptible to contaminations and chances of generating false-positive results.

■ The sensitivity of the assays can be slightly on the low side compared to the gold standard RT-qPCR.

6.6.3 Challenges of Antibody Tests

Serological tests for COVID-19 have also been recommended by the CDC as an indirect method of detecting SARS-CoV-2, as it detects the presence of antibodies in patients' blood [60]. Though this is a rapid testing method, there can be limitations, such as:

■ Cross-reactivity to other coronaviruses can be challenging.

■ Less sensitive than other methods.

■ Test results are sometimes difficult to correlate with the patient's condition.

6.6.4 Challenges of Antigen Tests

Immunoassays such as antigen tests are rapid and can detect the presence of the SARS-CoV-2. While the assays can be a good alternative to NAAT assays, they have a few disadvantages, such as:

■ The assays are less specific and can cross-react with other coronaviruses, which can be challenging.

■ Less sensitive compared to other NAAT assays.

■ Negative results may require further confirmation by NAAT.

6.6.5 Challenges of CT Examination

CT examination has also been considered by various clinicians for the diagnosis of COVID-19 through the early screening and to assess the disease's severity. This type of examination is very useful to deal with the disease and to detect lung lesions. However, there are major limitations of this technology, such as:

■ The CT examination can be used for the specific detection of SARS-CoV-2 but only performed in few diagnostic centers and hospitals.

- Another shortcoming of the technology is that it cannot be used for field level or bedside diagnosis of COVID-19 disease. This is primary because of the requirement for sophisticated instruments and well-trained personnel to carry out the examination.

6.7 CONCLUSIONS AND FUTURE PERSPECTIVES

As the ongoing COVID-19 pandemic has profoundly impacted human life, the use of accurate, quality diagnostics is paramount in the development and implementation of strategies for the treatment and control of COVID-19. Several nucleic acid–based and antigen/antibody-based diagnostic methods for COVID-19 identification have been approved by health authorities around the world in order to meet the need for rapid testing in a variety of healthcare settings, and the selection of appropriate methods should be based on patients' medical history or the purpose of investigation, type of sample to be analyzed, and turnaround time of the test. It is essential to perform the correct test at the correct time in the right biological sample to fight COVID-19. Even though RT-qPCR remains the frontline and gold standard technique for the detection of SARS-CoV-2 infections, considering its limited capacity for laboratory-based molecular testing and high turnaround time, several alternative detection modalities for screening for SARS-CoV-2 infections have been established, and more are in the pipeline. By integrating different disciplines, it is possible to formulate an "ASSURED" (Affordable, Sensitive, Specific, User-friendly, Rapid and robust, Equipment-free, and Deliverable to end-users) COVID-19 diagnostics to manage the pandemic effectively. All of the recent breakthroughs in COVID-19 research, whether in diagnostics or vaccines, offer a ray of hope and will be a giant leap forward for combating the current COVID-19 pandemic.

ACKNOWLEDGEMENTS

This study was supported by the Science and Engineering Research Board (SERB), DST-Government of India, through the COVID-19 project (CVD/2020/000150).

REFERENCES

1. Petersen, E., Koopmans, M., Go, U., Hamer, D.H., Petrosillo, N., Castelli, F., Storgaard, M., Khalili, S.A., Simonsen, L. (2020). Comparing SARS-CoV-2 with SARS-CoV and influenza pandemics. *Lancet Infect. Dis.* 20, e238–e244. doi:10.1016/S1473-3099(20)30484-9.

2. Muralidar, S., Ambi, S.V., Sekaran, S., Krishnan, U.M. (2020). The emergence of COVID-19 as a global pandemic: Understanding the epidemiology, immune response and potential therapeutic targets of SARS-CoV-2. *Biochimie* 179, 85–100. doi:10.1016/j.biochi.2020.09.018.

3. Malik, Y.S., Kumar, N., Sircar, S., Kaushik, R., Bhat, S., Dhama, K., Gupta, P., Goyal, K., Singh, M.P., Ghoshal, U., El Zowalaty, M.E., VinodhKumar, O.R., Yatoo, M.I., Tiwari, R., Pathak, M., Patel, S.K., Sah, R., Rodriguez-Morales, A.J., Ganesh, B., Kumar, P., Singh, R.K. (2020). Coronavirus disease pandemic (COVID-19): Challenges and a global perspective. *Pathogens* 9(7), 519. doi:10.3390/pathogens9070519.

4. Huang, C., Wang, Y., Li, X., Ren, L., Zhao, J., Hu, Y., Zhang, L., Fan, G., Xu, J., Gu, X., Cheng, Z., Yu, T., Xia, J., Wei, Y., Wu, W., Xie, X., Yin, W., Li, H., Liu, M., Xiao, Y., Gao, H., Guo, L., Xie, J., Wang, G., Jiang, R., Gao, Z., Jin, Q., Wang, J., Cao, B. (2020). Clinical features of patients infected with 2019 novel coronavirus in Wuhan, China. *Lancet* 395, 497–506. doi:10.1016/S0140-6736(20)30183-5.

5. Wilkerson, R.G., Adler, J.D., Shah, N.G., Brown, R. (2020). Silent hypoxia: A harbinger of clinical deterioration in patients with COVID-19. *Am. J. Emerg. Med.* 38(10), 2243.e5–2243.e6. doi:10.1016/j.ajem.2020.05.044.

6. Grifoni, A., Sidney, J., Zhang, Y., Scheuermann, R.H., Peters, B., Sette, A. (2020). Candidate targets for immune responses to 2019-Novel Coronavirus (nCoV): Sequence homology and bioinformatic-based predictions. *SSRN* doi:10.2139/ssrn.3541361. PMID: 32714104; PMCID: PMC7366807. [Preprint]

7. Zhou, P., Yang, X.L., Wang, X.G., Hu, B., Zhang, L., Zhang, W., Si, H.R., Zhu, Y., Li, B., Huang, C.L., Chen, H.D. (2020). A pneumonia outbreak associated with a new coronavirus of probable bat origin. *Nature* 579(7798), 270–273. doi:10.1038/s41586-020-2012-7.

8. Tang, X., Wu, C., Li, X., Song, Y., Yao, X., Wu, X., Duan, Y., Zhang, H., Wang, Y., Qian, Z., Cui, J., Lu, J. (2020). On the origin and continuing evolution of SARS-CoV-2. *Natl. Sci. Rev.* 7(6), 1012–1023. doi:10.1093/nsr/nwaa036.

9. Kubina, R., Dziedzic, A. (2020). Molecular and serological tests for COVID-19. A comparative review of SARS-CoV-2 coronavirus laboratory and point-of-care diagnostics. *Diagnostics* 10(6), 434. doi:10.3390/diagnostics10060434.

10. Memish, Z.A., Al-Tawfiq, J.A., Assiri, A., AlRabiah, F.A., Al Hajjar, S., Albarrak, A., Flemban, H., Alhakeem, R.F., Makhdoom, H.Q., Alsubaie, S., Al-Rabeeah, A.A. (2014). Middle East respiratory syndrome coronavirus disease in children. *Pediatr. Infect. Dis. J.* 33(9), 904–906 doi:10.1097/INF.0000000000000325.

11. Xie, X., Zhong, Z., Zhao, W., Zheng, C., Wang, F., Liu, J. (2020). Chest CT for typical coronavirus

disease 2019 (COVID-19) pneumonia: Relationship to negative RT-PCR testing. *Radiology* 296(2), E41–E45. doi:10.1148/radiol.2020200343.

12. Wang, Y., Dong, C., Hu, Y., Li, C., Ren, Q., Zhang, X., Shi, H., Zhou, M. (2020). Temporal changes of CT findings in 90 patients with COVID-19 pneumonia: A longitudinal study. *Radiology* 296, E55–E64. doi:10.1148/radiol.2020200843.

13. Chung, M., Bernheim, A., Mei, X., Zhang, N., Huang, M., Zeng, X., Cui, J., Xu, W., Yang, Y., Fayad, Z.A., Jacobi, A. (2020). CT imaging features of 2019 novel coronavirus (2019-nCoV). *Radiology* 295(1), 202–207. doi:10.1148/radiol.2020200230.

14. Kim, H., Hong, H., Yoon, S.H. (2020). Diagnostic performance of CT and reverse transcriptase polymerase chain reaction for coronavirus disease 2019: A meta-analysis. *Radiology* 296(3), E145–E155. doi:10.1148/radiol.2020201343.

15. Khatami, F., Saatchi, M., Zadeh, S.S., Aghamir, Z.S., Shabestari, A.N., Reis, L.O., Aghamir, S.M. (2020). A meta-analysis of accuracy and sensitivity of chest CT and RT-PCR in COVID-19 diagnosis. *Sci. Rep.* 10(1), 1–2. doi:10.1038/s41598-020-80061-2.

16. Bollineni, V., Nieboer, K.H., Döring, S., Buls, N., de Mey, J. (2021). The role of CT imaging for management of COVID-19 in epidemic area: Early experience from a University Hospital. *Insights Imaging* 12(1), 1–5. doi:10.1186/s13244-020-00957-5.

17. Wong, H.Y., Lam, H.Y., Fong, A.H., Leung, S.T., Chin, T.W., Lo, C.S., Lui, M.M., Lee, J.C., Chiu, K.W., Chung, T., Lee, E.Y. (2020). Frequency and distribution of chest radiographic findings in COVID-19 positive patients. *Radiology* 296, 201160. doi:10.1148/radiol.2020201160.

18. Ai, T., Yang, Z., Hou, H., Zhan, C., Chen, C., Lv, W., Tao, Q., Sun, Z., Xia, L. (2020). Correlation of chest CT and RT-PCR testing in coronavirus disease 2019 (COVID19) in China: A report of 1014 cases. *Radiology* doi:10.1148/radiol.2020200642.

19. Rai, P., Kumar, B.K., Deekshit, V.K., Karunasagar, I., Karunasagar, I. (2021). Detection technologies and recent developments in the diagnosis of COVID-19 infection. *Appl. Microbiol. Biotechnol.* 1–5. doi:10.1007/s00253-020-11061-5.

20. Mancini, F., Barbanti, F., Scaturro, M., Fontana, S., Di Martino, A., Marsili, G., Puzelli, S., Calzoletti, L., Facchini, M., Di Mario, G., Fabiani, C. (2021). Multiplex real-time reverse-transcription polymerase chain reaction assays for diagnostic testing of severe acute respiratory Syndrome coronavirus 2 and seasonal influenza viruses: A challenge of the phase 3 pandemic setting. *J. Infect. Dis.* 223(5), 765–774. doi:10.1093/infdis/jiaa658.

21. Smyrlaki, I., Ekman, M., Lentini, A., de Sousa, N.R., Papanicolaou, N., Vondracek, M., Aarum, J., Safari, H., Muradrasoli, S., Rothfuchs, A.G., Albert, J. (2020). Massive and rapid COVID-19 testing is feasible by extraction-free SARS-CoV-2

RT-PCR. *Nat. Commun.* 11(1), 1–2. doi:10.1038/s41467-020-18611-5.

22. Tomita, N., Mori, Y., Kanda, H., Notomi, T. (2008). Loop-mediated isothermal amplification (LAMP) of gene sequences and simple visual detection of products. *Nat. Protoc.* 3, 877–882. doi:10.1038/nprot.2008.57.

23. Huang, W.E., Lim, B., Hsu, C.C., Xiong, D., Wu, W., Yu, Y., Jia, H., Wang, Y., Zeng, Y., Ji, M., Chang, H. (2020). RT-LAMP for rapid diagnosis of coronavirus SARS-CoV-2. *Microb. Biotechnol.* 13(4), 950–961. doi:10.1111/1751-7915.13586.

24. Mautner, L., Baillie, C.K., Herold, H.M., Volkwein, W., Guertler, P., Eberle, U., Ackermann, N., Sing, A., Pavlovic, M., Goerlich, O., Busch, U. (2020). Rapid point-of-care detection of SARS-CoV-2 using reverse transcription loop-mediated isothermal amplification (RT-LAMP). *Virol. J.* 17(1), 1–4. doi:10.1186/s12985-020-01435-6.

25. Park, G.S., Ku, K., Baek, S.H., Kim, S.J., Kim, S.I., Kim, B.T., Maeng, J.S. (2020). Development of reverse transcription loop-mediated isothermal amplification assays targeting severe acute respiratory syndrome coronavirus 2 (SARS-CoV-2). *J. Mol. Diagn.* 22(6), 729–735 doi:10.1016/j.jmoldx.2020.03.006.

26. Alekseenko, A., Barrett, D., Pareja-Sanchez, Y., Howard, R.J., Strandback, E., Ampah-Korsah, H., Rovšnik, U., Zuniga-Veliz, S., Klenov, A., Malloo, J., Ye, S. (2021). Direct detection of SARS-CoV-2 using non-commercial RT-LAMP reagents on heat-inactivated samples. *Sci. Rep.* 11(1), 1–10. doi:10.1038/s41598-020-80352-8.

27. Wei, S., Suryawanshi, H., Djandji, A., Kohl, E., Morgan, S., Hod, E.A., Whittier, S., Roth, K., Yeh, R., Alejaldre, J.C., Fleck, E. (2021). Field-deployable, rapid diagnostic testing of saliva for SARS-CoV-2. *Sci. Rep.* 11(1), 1–9. doi:10.1101/2020.06.13.20129841.

28. Gorzalski, A.J., Tian, H., Laverdure, C., Morzunov, S., Verma, S.C., VanHooser, S., Pandori, M.W. (2020). High-throughput transcription-mediated amplification on the Hologic Panther is a highly sensitive method of detection for SARS-CoV-2. *J. Clin. Virol.* 129, 104501. doi:10.1016/j.jcv.2020.104501.

29. Pham, J., Meyer, S., Nguyen, C., Williams, A., Hunsicker, M., McHardy, I., Gendlina, I., Goldstein, D.Y., Fox, A.S., Hudson, A., Darby, P. (2020). Performance characteristics of a high-throughput automated transcription-mediated amplification test for SARS-CoV-2 detection. *J. Clin. Microbiol.* 58(10). doi:10.1128/JCM.01669-20.

30. Kilic, T., Weissleder, R., Lee, H. (2020). Molecular and immunological diagnostic tests of COVID-19–current status and challenges. *iScience* 101406. doi:10.1016/j.isci.2020.101406.

31. Zanoli, L.M., Spoto, G. (2013). Isothermal amplification methods for the detection of nucleic acids

in microfluidic devices. *Biosensors* 3(1), 18–43. doi:10.3390/bios3010018.

32. Qin, Z., Peng, R., Baravik, I.K., Liu, X. (2020). Fighting COVID-19: Integrated micro- and nanosystems for viral infection diagnostics. *Matter* doi:10.1016/j.matt.2020.06.015.

33. Tsou, J.H., Leng, Q., Jiang, F. (2019). A CRISPR test for detection of circulating nuclei acids. *Transl. Oncol.* 12, 1566–1573. doi:10.1016/j.tranon.2019.08.011.

34. Fozouni, P., Son, S., de León Derby, M.D., Knott, G.J., Gray, C.N., D'Ambrosio, M.V., Zhao, C., Switz, N.A., Kumar, G.R., Stephens, S.I., Boehm, D. (2021). Amplification-free detection of SARS-CoV-2 with CRISPR-Cas13a and mobile phone microscopy. *Cell.* 184(2), 323–333. doi:10.1016/j.cell.2020.12.001.

35. Joung, J., Ladha, A., Saito, M., Kim, N.G., Woolley, A.E., Segel, M., Barretto, R.P.J., Ranu, A., Macrae, R.K., Faure, G., Ioannidi, E.I. (2020). Detection of SARS-CoV-2 with SHERLOCK One-Pot Testing. *N. Engl. J. Med.* 383, 1492–1494. doi:10.1056/NEJMc2026172.

36. Tsou, J.H., Liu, H., Stass, S.A., Jiang, F. (2021). Rapid and sensitive detection of SARS-CoV-2 using clustered regularly interspaced short palindromic repeats. *Biomedicines* 9(3), 239. doi:10.3390/biomedicines9030239.

37. Suo, T., Liu, X., Feng, J., Guo, M., Hu, W., Guo, D., Ullah, H., Yang, Y., Zhang, Q., Wang, X., Sajid, M. (2020). ddPCR: A more accurate tool for SARS-CoV-2 detection in low viral load specimens. *Emerg. Microb. Infect.* 9(1), 1259–1268. doi:10.1080/22221751.2020.1772678.

38. Lobato, I.M., O'Sullivan, C.K. (2018). Recombinase polymerase amplification: Basics, applications and recent advances. *Trac Trends Anal. Chem.* 98, 19–35. doi:10.1016/j.trac.2017.10.015.

39. Sun, Y., Yu, L., Liu, C., Ye, S., Chen, W., Li, D., Huang, W. (2021). One-tube SARS-CoV-2 detection platform based on RT-RPA and CRISPR/Cas12a. *J. Transl. Med.* 19(1), 1–10. doi:10.1186/s12967-021-02741-5.

40. Liu, D., Shen, H., Zhang, Y., Shen, D., Zhu, M., Song, Y., Zhu, Z., Yang, C. (2021). A microfluidic-integrated lateral flow recombinase polymerase amplification (MI-IF-RPA) assay for rapid COVID-19 detection. *Lab Chip* doi:10.1039/d0lc01222j.

41. Walker, G.T., Fraiser, M.S., Schram, J.L., Little, M.C., Nadeau, J.G., Malinowski, D.P. (1992). Strand displacement amplification: An isothermal, in vitro DNA amplification technique. *Nucleic Acids Res.* 20(7), 1691–1696. doi:10.1093/nar/20.7.1691.

42. Walker, G.T., Nadeau, J.G., Spears, P.A., Schram, J.L., Nycz, C.M., Shank, D.D. (1994). Multiplex strand displacement amplification (SDA) and detection of DNA sequences from Mycobacterium tuberculosis and other mycobacteria. *Nucleic Acids Res.* 22(13), 2670–2677. doi:10.1093/nar/22.13.2670.

43. Zhang, C., Zheng, T., Fan H., Zhang, T., Han, D. (2021). Aligner-mediated cleavage-based isothermal amplification for SARS-CoV-2 RNA detection. *ACS Appl. Bio Mater.* doi:10.1021/acsabm.0c01674.

44. Shen, Y., Anwar, T.B., Mulchandani, A. (2021). Current status, advances, challenges and perspectives on biosensors for COVID-19 diagnosis in resource-limited settings. *Sens. Actuat. Rep.* 100025. doi:10.1016/j.snr.2021.100025.

45. Arevalo-Rodriguez, I., Buitrago-Garcia, D., Simancas-Racines, D., Zambrano-Achig, P., Del Campo, R., Ciapponi, A., Sued, O., Martinez-Garcia, L., Rutjes, A.W., Low, N., Bossuyt, P.M. (2020). False-negative results of initial RT-PCR assays for COVID-19: A systematic review. *PLoS One* 15(12), e0242958. doi:10.1371/journal.pone.0242958.

46. Vandenberg, O., Martiny, D., Rochas, O., van Belkum, A., Kozlakidis, Z. (2020). Considerations for diagnostic COVID-19 tests. *Nat. Rev. Microbiol.* 1–3. doi:10.1038/s41579-020-00461-z.

47. Peeling, R.W., Wedderburn, C.J., Garcia, P.J., Boeras, D., Fongwen, N., Nkengasong, J., Sall, A., Tanuri, A., Heymann, D.L. (2020). Serology testing in the COVID-19 pandemic response. *Lancet Infect. Dis.* 20, e245–e249. doi:10.1016/S1473-3099(20)30517-X.

48. Young, B.E., Ong, S.W., Ng, L.F., Anderson, D.E., Chia, W.N., Chia, P.Y., Ang, L.W., Mak, T.M., Kalimuddin, S., Chai, L.Y., Pada, S. (2020). Viral dynamics and immune correlates of coronavirus disease 2019 (COVID-19) severity. *Clin. Infect. Dis.* doi:10.1093/cid/ciaa1280.

49. Zhao, J., Yuan, Q., Wang, H., Liu, W., Liao, X., Su, Y., Wang, X., Yuan, J., Li, T., Li, J., Qian, S. (2020). Antibody responses to SARS-CoV-2 in patients with novel coronavirus disease 2019. *Clin. Infect. Dis.* 71(16), 2027–2034. doi:10.1093/cid/ciaa344.

50. Long, Q.X., Liu, B.Z., Deng, H.J., Wu, G.C., Deng, K., Chen, Y.K., Liao, P., Qiu, J.F., Lin, Y., Cai, X.F., Wang, D.Q. (2020). Antibody responses to SARS-CoV-2 in patients with COVID-19. *Nat. Med.* 26(6), 845–848. doi:10.1038/s41591-020-0897-1.

51. Hou, H., Wang, T., Zhang, B., Luo, Y., Mao, L., Wang, F., Wu, S., Sun, Z. (2020). Detection of IgM and IgG antibodies in patients with coronavirus disease 2019. *Clin. Transl. Immunol.* 9(5), e1136. doi:10.1002/cti2.1136.

52. Sidiq, Z., Hanif, M., KumarDwivedi, K., Chopra, K.K. (2020). Benefits and limitations of serological assays in COVID-19 infection. *Ind. J. Tuberc.* 67, S163–S166. doi:10.1016/j.ijtb.2020.07.034.

53. Padoan, A., Bonfante, F., Pagliari, M., Bortolami, A., Negrini, D., Zuin, S., Bozzato, D., Cosma, C., Sciacovelli, L., Plebani, M. (2020). Analytical and

clinical performances of five immunoassays for the detection of SARS-CoV-2 antibodies in comparison with neutralization activity. *EBioMedicine* 62, 103101. doi:10.1016/j.ebiom.2020.103101.

54. Bastos, M.L., Tavaziva, G., Abidi, S.K., Campbell, J.R., Haraoui, L.P., Johnston, J.C., Lan, Z., Law, S., MacLean, E., Trajman, A., Menzies, D. (2020). Diagnostic accuracy of serological tests for COVID-19: Systematic review and meta-analysis. *BMJ* 370. doi:10.1136/bmj.m2516.

55. Chen, Y., Spiering, A.J., Karthikeyan, S., Peters, G.W., Meijer, E.W. (2012). Sijbesma RP mechanically induced chemiluminescence from polymers incorporating a 1,2-dioxetane unit in the main chain. *Nat. Chem.* 4(7), 559–562. doi:10.1038/nchem.1358.

56. Cai, X.F., Chen, J., li Hu, J., Long, Q.X., Deng, H.J., Liu, P., Fan, K., Liao, P., Liu, B.Z., Wu, G.C., Chen, Y.K. (2020). A peptide-based magnetic chemiluminescence enzyme immunoassay for serological diagnosis of coronavirus disease 2019. *J. Infect. Dis.* 222(2), 189–193. doi:10.1093/infdis/jiaa243.

57. Infantino, M., Grossi, V., Lari, B., Bambi, R., Perri, A., Manneschi, M., Terenzi, G., Liotti, I., Ciotta, G., Taddei, C., Benucci, M. (2020). Diagnostic accuracy of an automated chemiluminescent immunoassay for anti-SARS-CoV-2 IgM and IgG antibodies: An Italian experience. *J. Med. Virol.* 92(9), 1671–1675. doi:10.1002/jmv.25932

58. Wan, Y., Shang, J., Graham, R., Baric, R.S., Li, F. (2020). Receptor recognition by the novel coronavirus from Wuhan: An analysis based on decade-long structural studies of SARS coronavirus. *J. Virol.* 94(7). doi:10.1128/JVI.00127-20.

59. Maiti, B., Anupama, K.P., Rai, P., Karunasagar, I., Karunasagar, I. Isothermal amplification-based assays for rapid and sensitive detection of SARS-CoV-2: Opportunities and recent developments. *Rev. Med. Virol.* (2021). doi:10.1002/rmv.2274.

60. Du, Z., Zhu, F., Guo, F., Yang, B., Wang, T. (2020). Detection of antibodies against SARS-CoV-2 in patients with COVID-19. *J. Med. Virol.* 92(10), 1735–1738. doi:10.1002/jmv.25820.

Chapter 7 Drug Repurposing and Novel Antiviral Drugs for COVID-19 Management

Shailendra Dwivedi, Aakanksha Rawat, Amit Ranjan, Ruchika Agrawal, Radhieka Misra, Sunil Kumar Gupta, Surekha Kishore, and Sanjeev Misra

7.1 INTRODUCTION

The threat of a deadly coronavirus outbreak was experienced in 2003 with the severe acute respiratory syndrome coronavirus (SARS-CoV) causing SARS. It was recognized as a highly infectious virus with propensity to spread rapidly. The first case was reported in China and later spread to five continents, with the calculated fatality rate of 9.6% during the outbreak period. As there were very few drugs to combat SARS, containment was the main strategy to stop its spread. Soon enough, in 2012, the second outbreak of the Middle East respiratory syndrome coronavirus (MERS-CoV) occurred on the Arabian Peninsula, with a fatality rate of about 34.4%. Again, the strategy was to prevent virus spread and the testing of some experimental drugs, plus containing the outbreak to a small geographical area. Then, in December 2019, the SARS-CoV-2 outbreak, which started in Wuhan, China and spread quickly around the world, was on March 11, 2020 declared the COVID-19 pandemic by the World Health Organization (WHO) [1, 2].

In the past, efforts have been made in the fields of immunology, genetics, medical biotechnology, molecular engineering, nutrition, nanotechnology, and regenerative medicine to answer the questions of origin, diagnosis, treatment and management of coronaviruses, but these initiatives were not focused. For this reason, management of the spread was again the main strategy at hand, and the lack of specific preventive guidelines contributed to the global spread of COVID-19. Integration of knowledge from different disciplines has therefore become important for the eradication of COVID-19.

Currently, the combination of symptomatic treatment and supportive measures have shown satisfactory responses in mild COVID-19 cases but in moderate to severe cases in patients with high risk, an effective disease-specific therapy is warranted. The process of *de novo* drug design and its approval is a time-consuming process so the alternative at hand is repurposing or re-profiling drugs already approved for human use for other indications. Drug repurposing by definition is a systematic method in drug discovery that aids in determining the new indications for an existing drug. With a known safety profile, pharmacokinetics, adverse effects, drug interactions etc. the time and expenditure in drug development is drastically reduced and in desperate times such as a pandemic this seems like a good choice.

We searched for published literature in PubMed, Google Scholar and EMBASE with the following search keywords:

coronavirus/COVID-19/SARS, CoV-2 with treatment/therapy/antiviral/hydroxychloroquine/ chloroquine/lopinavir/ritonavir/ Arbidol/azithromycin/remdesilvir/oseltamivir/steroid/medication/clinical trial/ interferon/novel antiviral therapy/stem cell therapy with COVID-19

We included studies in analysis, which met the following criteria:

1. Pre-clinical, clinical studies i.e., on confirmed COVID-19 human cases/cell lines and animal models

2. Original articles (clinical trials, case series, and case reports, etc.)

3. Where a specific existing therapeutic agent (drug) along with some outcome (clinical or virological) is mentioned

7.2 VARIOUS REPURPOSED DRUGS AND THEIR CHARACTERISTICS UTILIZED AGAINST COVID-19

Drug repurposing generally follows two concepts. Either a single drug interacts with several targets, which provide a way to investigate new target sites of action for the available compound, or targets associated with an illness are commonly relevant to a number of biological processes of pathogenesis. Thus the search for repurposing drugs was centered around the causal agent, which is a coronavirus, and common symptoms including inflammation, acute respiratory distress syndrome (ARDS) with many others.

7.2.1 Hydroxychloroquine (HCQ)/ Azithromycin (AZ)

Chloroquine (CQ) and its derivative HCQ are aminoquinoline compounds used for the treatment of malaria and systemic lupus erythematosus (SLE) [3]. Data on the antiviral potential of

DOI: 10.1201/9781003190394-7

CQ were generated from experiments on human immunodeficiency virus (HIV), hepatitis A, and influenza viruses [3]. HCQ is not a competitive blocker of the virus at the ACE-2 receptor inhibitor receptor. Rather, its antiviral activity is proposed to be related to a change in pH, and with increased acidity the viral spike protein degrades and the virus can neither bind to the ACE2 receptor nor can it survive and infect other cells. The in vitro evidence of efficacy of CQ on SARS-CoV-2 was presented as early as February 2020. It was observed that a with therapeutic dose of CQ, an effective concentration (EC90) value of 6.90 μM was achievable. These observations were subsequently strengthened by other authors, who showed that HCQ was more potent than CQ in attaining lower EC 50 values. This was postulated to be because of a higher intracellular concentration of HCQ. Along with HCQ, a combination therapy with Azithromycin (AZ), which acts through competitive binding at ACE2 receptors on the host cell, was proposed for the prophylaxis and treatment of mild to moderate COVID-19 infections.

During the initial spread of COVID-19 in France, two hospitals conducted an open-label non-randomized clinical trial that suggested combined treatment with HCQ and AZ was effective in patients [3]. Oral administration of 200 mg HCQ sulfate three times daily for 10 days along with 500 mg AZ on the first day followed by 250 mg per day for the next 4 days was given to PCR-confirmed COVID-19 patients aged >12 years in the intervention arm. On the sixth day post-inclusion, all patients treated with the HCQ-AZ combination were virologically cured as compared to 57.1% in patients treated with HCQ alone, and 12.5% in the control group ($P < 0.001$). Though labelled as a clinical trial this study sounded more like a trial-and-error attempt with retrospective analysis of treatment in desperate times. The study had a small sample size (total 36, intervention arm: 20, and control arm: 16) and was non-randomized, yet it provided a faint clue for research and treatment in the early days of the COVID-19 pandemic. Following the trend, another randomized control trial [4] with HCQ alone was conducted in China on 62 patients (31 in each arm), which reported significant improvement in recovery time for fever and cough in the HCQ group. The improvement rate of pneumonia in the HCQ arm (80.6%, 25 of 31) was much higher than in the control arm (54.8%, 17 of 31). However, this publication was not peer reviewed. A multi-center case series of 100 patients from 10 hospitals in China also showed that treatment with CQ phosphate at a therapeutic dose was effective in averting exacerbations of pneumonia, minimizing lung involvements in radio-imaging and accelerating virus-negative conversion thereby shortening the illness's course and severity, without any adverse effects [5].

However, further studies refuted many initial claims. In a multi-center, open label, randomized controlled trial [6] on HCQ with or without macrolide from different nations, no significant benefit of intervention over standard care in terms of intubation, mortality, survival, and negative virological outcome could be proven. In a few other studies [12] HCQ and non-HCQ groups were matched for their age and comorbid conditions (hypertension, diabetes, and chronic lung diseases, etc.). The HCQ groups reported adverse effects such as arrhythmia, cardiac arrest, other electrocardiogram (ECG) changes, and diarrhea. With similar results in other studies, there was a bias as HCQ was administered to the patients with a higher frequency of comorbidities. A multi-center randomized controlled clinical trial (RCT) conducted in the US reported therapeutic failure of HCQ among 1,309 asymptomatic COVID-19 patients. A study in China reported no significant improvement of HCQ treatment over placebo. Hence the noteworthy conclusion is that the efficacy of HCQ or CQ in COVID-19 treatment is unclear at the present time, and more clinical trials are needed to demonstrate efficacy and approval [7].

7.2.2 Lopinavir/Ritonavir

Protease inhibitors lopinavir and ritonavir are approved as antiretroviral drugs for HIV. In few in vitro studies lopinavir also showed inhibitory effect on both SARS-CoV and MERS-CoV. This inhibitory action was prolonged by combination therapy with ritonavir that competitively binds to the cytochrome P450-3A4 enzyme delaying the metabolism of lopinavir and prolonging plasma half-life.

In a study in Wuhan, 94 adult persons with confirmed cases of COVID-19 (100 cases in the control arm received standard care only) received lopinavir/ritonavir (400 mg and 100 mg) twice a day for 14 days. No significant benefit was observed in the intervention arm compared to the control arm (hazard ratio for median time to clinical improvement: 1.39; 95% CI: 1.00–1.91). In a retrospective study in 78 patients in China a significant decrease in viral shedding duration was observed when lopinavir/ritonavir treatment was started within 10 days of the onset of symptoms (median: 19 days versus 28.5 days, log-rank $P < 0.001$) [8]. Furthermore, in a randomized controlled study in China involving 86 patients, no clinical benefit of using lopinavir/ritonavir compared to umifenovir was seen among patients with mild to moderate COVID-19 [9]. A small retrospective case series reported improvement in viral load, radiography, and eosinophil count following the treatment with lopinavir, though the patients were on combination therapy with IFN- α2b atomization inhalation, Arbidol, methylprednisolone and immunoglobulin [9].

In an attempt to solve the puzzle, the WHO embarked on an ambitious global "megatrial" called SOLIDARITY in January 2020. In the trial, confirmed cases of COVD-19 were randomized to standard care or one of four active treatment arms (remdesivir, CQ or HCQ, lopinavir/ritonavir, or lopinavir/ritonavir plus interferon beta-1a). In early July 2020, the treatment arms in hospitalized patients that included HCQ, CQ, or lopinavir/ritonavir were discontinued. Interim results released in mid-October 2020 stated that the four aforementioned repurposed antiviral agents appeared to have little or no effect on hospitalized patients with COVID-19 in comparison to standard care, as indicated by overall mortality, initiation of ventilation, and duration of hospital stay [10]. With weak evidence and theoretically unfavorable pharmacodynamics the NIH Panel for COVID-19 Treatment Guidelines and Infectious Diseases Society of America (IDSA) did not recommend use of lopinavir/ritonavir or any other HIV protease inhibitors for the treatment of COVID-19 patients. IDSA also mentioned that CYP3A inhibition can result in increased risk of severe cutaneous reactions, QT prolongation, and potential drug interactions. Various combinations of methylprednisolone with umifenovir or lopinavir/ritonavir are still being studied to improve the treatment outcomes [11].

7.2.3 Umifenovir (Arbidol) versus Favipiravir

Umifenovir is an antiviral drug that binds to hemagglutinin protein. It is used in China and Russia to treat influenza. In a structural and molecular dynamics study, Vankadari corroborated that the drug target for umifenovir is the spike glycoprotein of SARS-CoV-2, similar to that of H3N2. A retrospective study of non-ICU hospitalized COVID-19 patients (n = 81) conducted in China did not show any improvement in viral clearance or prognosis. Another study (n = 86) that compared lopinavir/ritonavir or umifenovir monotherapy with standard care in patients with mild-to-moderate COVID-19 showed no statistical difference between the treatment groups [11].

Favipiravir (Avigan; Appili Therapeutics) is an oral antiviral drug approved for the treatment of influenza in Japan. It is approved in Russia for treatment of COVID-19. Favipiravir selectively inhibits RNA polymerase, which is necessary for viral replication. An adaptive, multi-center, open label, randomized, phase II/III clinical trial on favipiravir compared with standard of care in hospitalized patients with moderate COVID-19 was conducted in Russia. Both dosing regimens of favipiravir demonstrated similar virologic responses. Viral clearance on day 5 was achieved in 25/40 (62.5%) patients in the favipiravir group compared with 6/20 (30%) patients in the standard care group ($P = 0.018$). Viral clearance on day 10 was achieved in 37/40 (92.5%) patients treated with favipiravir compared with 16/20 (80%) in the standard care group ($P = 0.155$) [12].

A prospective, randomized, controlled, open-label multi-center trial compared the efficacy of umifenovir (Arbidol) to favipiravir among 240 (120 each drug) adult confirmed COVID-19 patients. Each patient received either umifenovir (Arbidol) as 200 mg thrice daily or favipiravir 1,600 mg twice daily on the first day followed by 600 mg twice daily for 10 days. On day 7 of follow-up, the clinical recovery rate did not differ significantly between the favipiravir group (61.2%) and the Arbidol group (51.6%). Favipiravir was associated with shorter latencies for recovery from fever (difference: 1.70 days, $P < 0.0001$) and cough (difference: 1.75 days, $P < 0.0001$). Rise in the level of serum uric acid was also reported in the favipiravir group. Otherwise, both drugs were found to be similarly effective so far and a clinical decision needs to be made based on the disease status and comorbidity of the patient [7] [REF: use original ref, not review].

7.2.4 Remdesivir

Remdesivir is a nucleoside analogue inhibitor of RNA polymerases with a large viral spectrum, exhibiting antiviral effects against filoviruses, paramyxoviruses, pneumoviruses, and coronaviruses originally developed for the treatment of Ebola virus disease,. This drug has been tested both in vitro and in vivo in mice and rhesus monkeys against SARS-CoV-2. Furthermore, clinical trials have been performed in SARS-CoV-2 infected adults and children at different dose ranges, demonstrating low toxicity. Additionally, double-blind, randomized, multi-center clinical studies observed a significant improvement in the reduction of viral load during the infection but without a considerable reduction in the mortality rate compared to patients who received placebo in the same period. Moreover, antiviral activity was demonstrated in Vero-E6 cells with an EC50 of 1.76 μM [13].

Remdesivir may have a place in treatment of patients with mild to moderate COVID-19 disease. Conversely, the initial studies with remdesivir failed to demonstrate clinical benefit over placebo; initially, daily doses of remdesivir for 10 days did not show any statistically significant improvement compared to standard care. However, a 5-day course showed improved outcomes compared to standard care, but the clinical impact was uncertain. On the other hand, Grein et al. (2020) found that 68% of the enrolled 61 patients with severe COVID-19 showed significant improvement after remdesivir treatment [14]. More recently, a US-based study conducted by the National Institutes of Health (NIH) with 1,062 COVID-19 patients showed encouraging results, including a reduction in recovery time and a trend towards lower mortality. This resulted in an emergency use authorization (EUA) by the US Food and Drug Administration (FDA) and an endorsement by the European Medicines Agency (EMA) and the National Health Service (NHS) in the UK. However, more recent evidence has caused the WHO no longer to recommend the use of remdesivir in hospitalized patients with COVID-19. This is based on reports that remdesivir could not reduce mortality, the need for mechanical ventilation, or the duration of hospital stay. Consequently, further large-scale randomized clinical trials are needed to better understand the role of remdesivir in the management of patients with COVID-19.

7.2.4.1 Remdesvir in Children
Remdesivir EUA includes pediatric dosing that was derived from pharmacokinetic data in healthy adults. Remedesivir has been available for compassionate use to children with severe COVID-19 since February 2020. A phase II/III trial (CARAVAN) of remdesivir was initiated in June 2020 to assess safety, tolerability, pharmacokinetics, and efficacy in children with moderate-to-severe COVID-19. CARAVAN is an open-label, single-arm study of remdesivir in children from birth to 18 years of age. Results were presented in July 2020 showing improvements in most of the 77 children with severe COVID-19. Clinical recovery was observed in 80% of children on ventilators or ECMO (Extracorporeal membrane oxygenation), and in 87% of those not on invasive oxygen support [15].

7.2.4.2 Remdesivir Use in Pregnant Women
The effect of Remedesivir was studied from March 21 to June 16, 2020 in 86 hospitalized pregnant women who had confirmed diagnosis (Real-Time PCR) of COVID-19. Remdesivir treatment was provided for 10 days (200 mg on day 1, followed by 100 mg for days 2–10, given intravenously). After 28 days of follow-up, the level of oxygen necessity decreased in 96% of pregnant women. Of pregnant women who were on mechanical ventilation, 93% were extubated, 93% recovered, and 90% were discharged. Remdesivir was well tolerated, with no severe complication of adverse events (AEs) [15].

7.2.5 Molnupiravir
Molnupiravir (MK-4482 [previously EIDD-2801]; Merck) is an oral antiviral agent that is a prodrug of the nucleoside derivative N4-hydroxycytidine. It elicits antiviral effects by introducing copying errors during viral RNA replication of the SARS-CoV-2. Preliminary results from the phase II dose-ranging MOVe-OUT study (n = 2,020) showed at an average of 10 days after symptoms onset, 24% of patients in the placebo group remained positive for infectious SARS-CoV-2, whereas no infectious virus could be detected in any molnupiravir-treated outpatient. The in-patient molnupiravir study (MOVe-IN) has been discontinued, but the phase III trial in outpatients who have at least one risk factor for poor outcomes (for example, advanced age, obesity, diabetes) is proceeding with patients receiving 800 mg molnupiravir orally twice daily [16].

7.3 OTHER MISCELLANEOUS AGENTS IN THERAPY AGAINST COVID-19

7.3.1 Interleukin Inhibitors
COVID-19–associated systemic inflammation and hypoxic respiratory failure can be associated with heightened cytokine release, as indicated by elevated blood levels of interleukin-6 (IL-6), C-reactive protein (CRP), D-dimer, and ferritin. It is hypothesized that modulating the levels of IL-6 or its effects may alter the course of disease. Several studies have indicated a "cytokine storm" with release of IL-6, IL-1, IL-12, and IL-18, along with tumor necrosis factor-alpha (TNFα) and other inflammatory mediators in COVID-19 patients as the main pathogenetic factor resulting in severe damage to lung tissues. The increased pulmonary inflammatory response may result in increased alveolar-capillary gas exchange, making oxygenation difficult in patients with severe illness. Interleukin inhibitors may ameliorate this damage caused by cytokine release. There are two classes of FDA-approved IL-6 inhibitors: anti-IL-6 receptor monoclonal antibodies (e.g., sarilumab, tocilizumab) and anti-IL-6 monoclonal antibodies (siltuximab). Currently, the NIH panel guidelines have recommended against the use of anti-IL-6 receptor monoclonal antibodies or anti-IL-6 monoclonal antibody for the treatment of COVID-19, except in a clinical trial [17].

7.3.1.1 Anti-Interleukin-6 Receptor Monoclonal Antibodies

7.3.1.1.1 Sarilumab

The efficacy and safety of sarilumab 400 mg IV and sarilumab 200 mg IV versus placebo were evaluated in patients hospitalized with COVID-19 in an adaptive Phase II and III, randomized (2:2:1), double-blind, placebo-controlled trial (ClinicalTrials.gov Identifier NCT04315298). Randomization was stratified by severity of illness (i.e., severe, critical, multisystem organ dysfunction) and use of systemic corticosteroids for COVID-19. The Phase II component of the trial verified that sarilumab reduces CRP levels at both 200 mg and 400 mg doses. The primary outcome for the Phase III part of the trial was changed on a seven-point ordinal scale, and this phase was modified to focus on the dose of 400 mg sarilumab among critically ill patients [18]. According to the latest information, the trial findings do not support a clinical benefit of sarilumab for any of the disease severity subgroups or dosing strategies studied.

7.3.1.1.2 Tocilizumab (TCZ)

Tocilizumab (TCZ) is another humanized monoclonal antibody that inhibits the IL-6 receptor. TCZ has been used successfully for the treatment of rheumatoid arthritis and other autoinflammatory processes. It has also been useful for the treatment of severe cytokine release syndrome (CRS) induced by the chimeric antigen receptor. Consequently, TCZ, an IL-6 receptor blocker, may be suitable for treating patients with severe pneumonia. A recent retrospective, observational study demonstrated that TCZ significantly reduced mortality among 630 COVID-19 patients admitted to an ICU [19]. Another study demonstrated that TCZ decreased mortality and duration of hospital stay in critically ill patients but seemed to have a high risk of serious infections [20]. Similar outcomes were reported in another related study involving 158 severe COVID-19 patients claiming significantly decreased mortality with TCZ [21]. Furthermore, in research carried out by Yale University School of Medicine, reduced need for mechanical ventilation and improved inflammatory biomarkers were noted in patients on TCZ [22]. A study in China revealed that TCZ significantly improved clinical outcomes and reduced mortality among patients with severe COVID-19 [23]. It also reduced the risk of cytokine storms among COVID-19 patients in another study. The abilities of the TCZ to relieve inflammation and cytokine storms among COVID-19 patients were further justified in many meta-analyses [24–26].

In contrast, Colaneri et al. (2020) reported that TCZ did not reduce mortality or the number of ICU admissions among 112 patients with severe COVID-19 [24]. Moreno Perez et al. (2020) also found that critically ill patients receiving TCZ appeared to have a high risk of severe infections [25]. Consequently, despite the promise shown by TCZ in relieving inflammation, decreased mortality, and shorter duration of hospital stay in some studies, we believe more research is needed before TCZ treatment is approved for patients with COVID-19.

TCZ is a recombinant humanized anti-IL-6 receptor monoclonal antibody that is approved by the FDA for use in patients with rheumatologic disorders and CRS induced by chimeric antigen receptor T cell (CAR-T) therapy. A press release on July 29, 2020 described the industry-sponsored Phase III COVACTA trial (ClinicalTrials.gov Identifier NCT04320615) in 450 adult patients with severe COVID-19–related pneumonia. The patients were randomized to receive TCZ or placebo. The primary outcome measured using a seven-point ordinal scale to assess clinical status based on the need for intensive care and/or ventilator use and the requirement for supplemental oxygen over a 4-week period thus depicting improved clinical status. Key secondary outcomes included 4-week mortality. Differences in the primary outcome between the TCZ and placebo groups were not statistically significant (OR 1.19; 95% CI, 0.81–1.76; $P = 0.36$). Consequently, despite the promise shown by TCZ in relieving inflammation, decreased mortality, and duration of hospital stay in some studies, we believe more research is needed before to the use of TCZ in the treatment of patients with COVID-19 [26].

7.3.1.1.3 Siltuximab

Siltuximab is a recombinant human–mouse chimeric monoclonal antibody that binds to IL-6 and is approved by the FDA for use in patients with Castleman's disease. Siltuximab prevents the binding of IL-6 to both soluble and membrane-bound IL-6 receptors, inhibiting IL-6 signaling [27]. Siltuximab has also been investigated as a potential drug for the treatment of severe COVID-19 [28].

7.3.1.1.4 Sarilumab

A study on sarilumab and standard of care in 28 patients showed no significant overall clinical improvement and mortality in patients with severe COVID-19. However, it demonstrated faster recovery in a subset of patients showing minor lung consolidation at baseline [28].

Preliminary results from the REMAP-CAP international adaptive trial evaluated efficacy of 8 mg/kg TCZ (n = 353), 400 mg sarilumab (n = 48), or standard care (n = 402) in adult critically ill hospitalized COVID-19 patients receiving organ support in intensive care. Hospital mortality at day 21 was 28% (98/350) for TCZ, 22.2% (10/45) for sarilumab, and 35.8% (142/397) for the control group. Of note, corticosteroids became part of the standard of care midway through the trial. Estimates of the treatment efficacy for patients treated with either TCZ or sarilumab and corticosteroids in combination were greater than for any single intervention [29]

7.3.1.2 Interleukin-1 Inhibitors

Endogenous IL-1 levels are elevated in individuals with COVID-19 and other conditions, such as severe CAR-T-cell-mediated cytokine-release syndrome. In June 2020, the NIH guidelines were against the use of interleukin (IL)-1 inhibitors, such as anakinra, for the treatment of COVID-19. A retrospective study in Italy reported that in patients with COVID-19 with moderate-to-severe ARDS, who received anakinra (5 mg/kg IV BID [high-dose] or 100 mg SC BID [low-dose]) plus standard treatment (i.e. HCQ 200 mg PO BID and lopinavir/ritonavir 400 mg/100 mg PO BID) showed reduced serum C-reactive protein levels and progressive improvements in respiratory function by 72% (21 of 29 patients) [30].

7.3.2 Interferon Alone or in Combination

A randomized, double-blind, placebo-controlled phase II pilot trial of nebulized interferon beta-1a was conducted in 101 adults admitted to hospital with COVID-19. It was observed that patients receiving nebulized interferon beta-1a had significantly greater odds of clinical improvement than those who received placebo, both on day 15/16 (odds ratio [OR] 2.32 [95% CI 1·07–5·04]; P = 0·033) and on day 28 (3.15 [1.39–7.14]; P = 0·006). However, there was no significant difference between treatment groups in the odds of hospital discharge by day 28: 39 (81%) of 48 patients had been discharged in the nebulized interferon beta-1a group compared with 36 (75%) of 48 in the placebo group (OR 1·84 [95% CI 0·64–5.29]; P = 0.26) [31].

Type 1 interferons are among the first cytokines produced during a viral infection and promote both innate and adaptive immunity. Interferon beta has shown an antiviral effect against SARS-CoV and MERS-CoV in in vitro studies and animal models. Clinical studies of SARS-CoV-2 found that a proportion of patients with severe COVID-19 had impaired type I interferon activity. However, preliminary results from the SOLIDARITY randomized clinical trial with 200 patients showed no efficacy of subcutaneous interferon alone or with lopinavir–ritonavir

[32]. This result contrasted with the findings from another study by Monk et al. 2021 [31], which supported the in vitro study results and suggested that the interferon pathway is an important inflammatory factor in SARS-CoV-2 infection, and IFN-β-1 may be considered as a safe and effective treatment against SARS-CoV-2 in the early phases of the illness.

7.3.3 Nitazoxanide

Nitazoxanide, a small-molecule (nitrothiazolyl-salicylamide) antiprotozoal drug marketed as tablets (500 mg) and suspension (100 mg/5 ml), is mainly indicated in protozoa *Cryptosporidium* or *Giardia* diarrhea in adults and children. In in vitro studies, the molecule has demonstrated a broad spectrum of antiviral efficacy against respiratory syncytial virus (RSV), parainfluenza virus, coronavirus (CoV), rotavirus, norovirus, hepatitis B virus (HBV), hepatitis C virus (HCV), Dengue virus (DENV), yellow fever virus (YFV), Japanese encephalitis virus (JEV), and human immunodeficiency virus (HIV). Few clinical trials have proved its role in gastroenteritis, hepatitis and influenza. A special quality is its ability to promote balance between pro-inflammatory and anti-inflammatory mediators in acute conditions and this is potentially helpful in management of hyper inflammatory cytokine storm in patients with COVID-19. Repurposing nitazoxanide against COVID-19 has been reported in many studies. Two phase III trials for prevention of COVID-19 in high-risk, elderly populations, and healthcare workers are ongoing [33, 34] Another multicenter, randomized, double-blind phase III study was initiated in August 2020 for the treatment of COVID-19 patients aged 12 years and older [35].

7.3.4 Niclosamide

Niclosamide (NIC) (FW-1002 [First Wave Bio]; ANA001 [ANA Therapeutics]) is a well-known anthelmintic agent used for tapeworm infestations. The action of niclosamide against SARS-CoV-2 is by S-phase kinase-associated protein 2 (SKP2)-inhibition preventing autophagy and blocking endocytosis, thus disrupting replication. This mode of action is thought to decrease the gut viral load. AzurRx BioPharma has started its Phase II clinical trial to evaluate safety and the potential of micronized oral NIC tablets to improve outcomes and reduce hospital stay in patients with COVID-19 gastrointestinal (GI) infections [36].

7.3.5 Corticosteroids

Corticosteroids have a definite anti-inflammatory property, but their immunosuppressant effects have caused problems in other viral epidemics, such as for infections of RSV, influenza virus, SARS-CoV, and MERS-CoV. Hence the use of corticosteroids is not generally recommended for treatment of viral pneumonia. However, definite evidence to support their use in COVID-19 patients is based on the randomized control trial RECOVERY in the UK with good sample size (n = 6,425) of hospitalized patients with COVID-19 for which differences in mortality rate at day 28 with dexamethasone (6 mg PO or IV daily for 10 days) compared to standard care alone were assessed. There was no significant difference between the two arms in general, but an important observation was that the incidence of death among patients receiving invasive mechanical ventilation was lower in the dexamethasone arm than in the standard care group (29.3% versus 41.4%) [37]. Several trials examining the use of corticosteroids in COVID-19 patients were halted following the publication of the RECOVERY trial results [38]. However, a prospective meta-analysis from the WHO rapid evidence appraisal for COVID-19 therapies (REACT) pooled data from 7 trials (for example, RECOVERY, REMAP-CAP, CoDEX, CAP COVID) and, based on that, prepared guidelines for the management of seriously ill patients [39]. It concluded that dexamethasone and hydrocortisone (glucocorticoids in general) reduced mortality in severe cases (32% absolute mortality for corticosteroids versus 40% assumed mortality for controls). Researchers at Henry Ford Hospital in Detroit used early, short-course, methylprednisolone 0.5–1 mg/kg/day divided into 2 IV doses for 3 days in patients with moderate to severe COVID-19. The primary outcome measure was a composite endpoint of escalation of care from ward to ICU, a new requirement for mechanical ventilation, or mortality. From the 213 eligible patients the composite endpoint was reached at a significantly lower rate in the post-corticosteroid group than in the pre-corticosteroid group (34.9% versus 54.3%; P = 0.005). Additionally, a significant reduction in median hospital length of stay was also observed in the post-corticosteroid group (8 versus 5 days; $P < 0.001$) [40]. A retrospective study at Montefiore Hospital, New York evaluated the role of early glucocorticoid treatment (within 48 hours of admission) in reduction of mortality rates or the need for mechanical ventilation in hospitalized patients with COVID-19. Of the 1,806 patients included in the study, 140 (7.7%) received glucocorticoid steroids. Patients with initial C-reactive protein (CRP) levels of 20 mg/dL or greater receiving glucocorticoids showed significant reduction in mortality or mechanical ventilation (OR, 0.23; 95% CI, 0.08–0.70). In contrast, patients with a CRP level of less than 10 mg/dL receiving glucocorticoid showed an increased risk of mortality or mechanical ventilation (OR, 2.64; 95% CI, 1.39–5.03) [41].

7.3.6 Convalescent Plasma

Convalescent plasma contains antibody-rich plasma products collected from eligible donors, who have recovered from COVID-19. In a US-based retrospective study of anti-SARS-CoV-2 IgG antibody levels in convalescent plasma and their effect in the treatment of hospitalized adults with COVID-19 was determined. The primary outcome was death within 30 days after plasma transfusion. Among patients hospitalized with COVID-19 who did not receive mechanical ventilation, transfusion of plasma with higher anti-SARS-CoV-2 IgG antibody titers was associated with a lower risk of death than transfusion of plasma with lower antibody levels. Among 3,082 patients in the analysis, death within 30 days occurred in 115 of 515 patients (22.3%) in the high-titer group, 549 of 2,006 patients (27.4%) in the medium-titer group, and 166 of 561 patients (29.6%) in the low-titer group. High plasma titer was defined as 250 or greater in the Broad Institute's neutralizing antibody assay or an S/C cut-off of 12 or higher in the Ortho VITROS IgG assay [42]. The FDA granted EUA on August 23, 2020, for use of convalescent plasma in hospitalized patients with COVID-19 [43].

7.3.7 Immune Modulator Trials

In October 2020, the NIH launched an adaptive phase III trial (ACTIV-Immune Modulators [IM]) to assess safety and efficacy of three immune modulator agents (infliximab (Remicade), abatacept (Orencia), and cenicriviroc) in hospitalized patients with COVID-19. Repurposing of these drugs would require a lot of RCT-based evidential support as the proposal of use in COVID-19 patients stems from retrospective observational studies of occurrence of COVID-19 in patients already receiving these drugs for other recommended indications. A summary of immune molecule-based trials is presented in Table 7.3.

7.3.7.1 Infliximab

Infliximab is a monoclonal antibody which binds a TNF-α receptor and prevents TNF-α activation (pro-inflammatory) by TNF-α signaling. Infliximab was initially approved in 1998 for the treatment of various chronic autoimmune inflammatory diseases (rheumatoid arthritis, psoriasis, inflammatory bowel diseases). The CLARITY study, recruited 6,935 patients with Crohn's disease and ulcerative colitis from 92 UK hospitals between September and December 2020, and noted that fewer than half of the people with inflammatory bowel disease who were treated with infliximab had detectable antibodies after SARS-CoV-2 infection [44].

7.3.7.2 Abatacept

Abatacept is a selective T cell costimulatory immuno-modulator with an extracellular domain of human cytotoxic T cell-associated antigen 4 fused to a modified immunoglobulin. It prevents full activation of T cells, resulting in inhibition of the downstream inflammatory cascade. An epidemiological survey performed in a large tertiary hospital in Barcelona, Spain, indicated that abatacept-treated patients (42 patients from a cohort of 959 patients treated with biological and synthetic disease-modifying antirheumatic drugs [DMARDs]) exhibited the lowest frequency of COVID-19–compatible symptoms [45]. Similar data were also obtained from a hospital in Madrid, Spain, where it was noted that none of the 27 abatacept-treated patients (among 802 DMARD-treated patients) were admitted to hospital with COVID-19 symptoms [46].

7.3.7.3 Cenicriviroc

Cenicriviroc (CVC), an immunomodulator that blocks the CCR2 and CCR5 chemokine receptors, is proposed to help in the respiratory sequelae in COVID-19 patients. In an in vitro study CVC was found to be a selective inhibitor of SARS-CoV-2 replication. The 50% effective concentrations of CVC were 19.0 and 2.9 μM, in the assays based on the inhibition of virus-induced cell destruction and viral RNA levels in culture supernatants of the infected cells, respectively [47]. The drug has now been included in the I-SPY COVID-19 clinical trial [48].

7.4 NOVEL STRATEGIES AGAINST COVID-19

This situation is like a novel clueless puzzle. From the first reported case of COVID-19 infection to the present date, several antiviral drugs have been used to tackle SARS-CoV-2, by means of the repurposing of drugs, but none have shown acceptable efficacy [49]. So relentless efforts are dedicated to the exploration of novel approaches to treat COVID-19 for the management of emerging viral outbreaks.

7.4.1 Stem Cell Therapy: Significance in COVID-19

Recently, stem cell therapy has emerged as one of the promising therapeutic strategies in management of several diseases [50] including viral diseases. However, the development and progress for cell-based therapies, especially application of pluripotent stem cells, has been quite slow because of limited sources and related ethical constraints. The choice to select MSCs (Mesenchymal Stem Cells) [51] may be related to the availability, high rate of multiplication, low invasive procedure, and no ethical issues.

The various benefits and characteristics of using MSC-based therapy are (i) MSCs are easily accessible and can be extracted from many tissues, for example from bone marrow, peripheral blood, and adipose tissues, such as abdominal fat, infrapatellar fat pad, and buccal fat pad. Other sites include neonatal birth-associated tissues such as placenta, umbilical cord, Wharton's jelly, amniotic fluid, and cord blood. Isolated MSCs can be stored for forthcoming promising applications; (ii) MSCs are multipotent stem cells, with the capacity to self-renew by division to evolve into multiple specialized cells; (iii) MSCs can easily be expanded to required clinical and scientific volumes in a suitable period of time; (iv) MSCs can be preserved for recurrent therapeutic applications; and (v) No severe adverse reactions to allogeneic MSC have been reported in any clinical trials to date.

In the context of viral diseases, it is well established that the innate and adaptive immunity defense becomes impaired during viral infections of high replicative and potent virulence power. There is a failure of orchestrated immune players, especially APCs (Antigen Presenting Cells: Dendritic cells, Macrophages etc.) to engulf, process and present antigens to adaptive immune players (T cells and B cells). This failure in innate and ultimately adaptive immune systems allow viruses to proliferate and aggravate the infection. It has been suggested that imbalance in innate and adaptive immune systems, which cause the mounting of an aggravated cytokine storm as in other infective diseases and cancer, can trigger similar phenomena after COVID-19 infection. This is mainly projected as being caused by excessive amounts of inflammatory factors such as interleukins [52–54]. The cytokine storm thus produced eventually impairs APCs and adaptive immune cells. Thus development of MSC-based therapy with either natural APCs or APCs is in progress to evoke appropriate immune responses, see Table 7.2.

Previous studies on viral diseases including COVID-19 have shown that MSCs retain immune-regulatory potential by modifying immune responses with the help of proliferation and function of numerous immune cells, such as inhibiting the differentiation of monocytes into dendritic cells (DCs), changing the cytokine profiles of DCs with upregulation of regulatory cytokines, and suppression of inflammatory cytokines. Thus MSCs also induce tolerant phenotypes of naive and effector T cells, constraining antibody production by B cells, and diminishing NK cell proliferation and NK cell-mediated cytotoxicity [55]. These immunomodulatory activities are mediated by both cell–cell communications and secreted cytokines including interferon- γ (IFN-γ), indoleamine 2,3-dioxygenase (IDO), transforming growth factor-β (TGF-β), IL-6, IL-10, and prostaglandin E2 [56]. Thus several COVID-19 trials on MSCs in the United States, China, Israel, Iran, Italy, and Iraq are in progress (Table 7.1).

Moreover, a recent case study was reported in which a 65-year-old female patient was diagnosed with severe COVID-19. The patient had an 87% increase in neutrophil count and a 9.8% decrease in lymphocyte count. Despite being treated with antiviral drugs such as lopinavir/ritonavir, IFN-α and oseltamivir, her condition worsened. The patient was treated three times with cord MSCs alone and with α1 thymosin 5×10^7 cells (not clear). The results of the study showed that after the second injection, serum albumin, CRP, and ALT/AST gradually decreased, and other vital signs improved. The patient was disconnected from life supporting devices and was able to walk. The number of white blood cells and neutrophils in the patient decreased to a normal level, while the number of lymphocytes increased to their normal level. Above all, CD3 + T cell, CD4 + T cell and CD8 + T cell numbers were significantly increased and based on CT images, the pneumonia resolved significantly after the third injection of UC-MSCs. Ultimately the patient was discharged from the ICU ward. This result also implied that UM-MSCs could be an attractive option alone or in combination with other immune modulators for the treatment of acute COVID-19 patients [55].

Recently researchers from China (Beijing, Shanghai, and Hubei) completed a study in which they successfully transplanted human MSCs [57] (Table 7.2). The study noted improvement in the outcome of seven treated patients with COVID-19 pneumonia in Beijing Youan Hospital, China, from January 23, 2020 to February 16, 2020. After MSC injection, the alterations in inflammatory, immune function levels as well as adverse effects of the patients were evaluated for 14 days. All seven patients showed significant improvements in pulmonary function and reduction in symptoms within two days of MSC transplantation without any adverse effects. After transplantation, peripheral lymphocyte counts increased, with a decrease in the C-reactive protein (infection and inflammatory marker). Moreover, it triggered cytokine secreting immune cells CXCR3 + CD4 + T cells, CXCR3 + CD8 + T cells, and CXCR3 + NK cells disappeared in 3–6 days. Increase in a group of CD14 + CD11c + CD11bmid regulatory DC population was also noticed. Additionally,

the level of pro-inflammatory TNF-α was reduced, and anti-inflammatory IL-10 levels were increased remarkably in the MSC treated group compared to the control placebo group. Thus the very first study of safe and effective intravenous transplantation of MSCs has opened new horizons for the treatment of patients with COVID-19 pneumonia [58].

Another trial on MSCs in March–April 2020 was reported by Pluristem Therapeutics Inc., a leading regenerative medicine company in Haifa, Israel. Successful treatment was obtained in patients suffering from COVID-19 complications in the United States [59]. The treatment was conducted according to the US FDA Single Patient Expanded Access Program, also called the Compassionate Use Program. This is part of the US Coronavirus Treatment Acceleration Program (CTAP), an emergency program for encouraging therapies that explore every existing method to move new treatments to patients as quickly as possible.

PLX cells are allogeneic mesenchymal-like cells that have immunomodulatory properties and are able to incite the immune system's natural regulatory T cells and M2 macrophages and. may pause or reverse the perilous aggravation of the immune system [60]. The incidence and\or severity of COVID-19 pneumonia and pneumonitis may potentially be reduced by PLX cells, which may lead to a better prognosis for patients. Before treatment with PLX, the patient was reported critically ill with respiratory failure resulting from ARDS and was on life support ventilation in ICU for three weeks. In order to explore PLX cell–based therapy for COVID-19, Pluristem Therapeutics is planning to work with the BIH Center for Regenerative Therapy (BCRT) and the Berlin Center for Advanced Therapies (BeCAT) at Charité University of Medicine, Berlin. Recently, a randomized, double-blind, placebo-controlled, multi-center, parallel-group phase II study to evaluate the efficacy and safety of intramuscular injections of PLX-PAD for the treatment of severe COVID-19 was registered by the company after being given FDA clearance. In this trial, 140 intubated and mechanically ventilated adult patients suffering from COVID-19 induced respiratory failure and ARDS will be treated. The primary efficacy endpoint of the study is the number of ventilator-free days from day 1 through day 28 of the study [61].

The above-mentioned and a few more stem cell–based trials are summarized in Table 7.3. The results from these MSC-based therapy trials will hopefully confirm that the strategy is a good option for the treatment of COVID-19 patients and potentially for other similar novel virus outbreaks.

Table 7.1 Major repurposed drugs and their proposed mechanism of action on COVID-19 infection

Name of Drug	Class/Type	Mechanism of Action	Name of Drug	Class/Type	Mechanism of Action
Chloroquine and Hydroxychloroquine	4-aminoquinoline	The post-translational alteration of newly synthesized proteins via glycosylation inhibition.	Lopinavir/Ritonavir	Protease inhibitors	Blocks viral cellular entry.
Zanamivir	Neuraminidase inhibitor	Zanamivir acts via inhibition of neuraminidase thus affects virus particle aggregation and release. The drug renders the influenza virus, and thus virus is unable to escape its host cell and infect others.	Amprenavir	Protease inhibitor (HIV)	It binds to the protease active site and inhibits the activity of the enzyme. This inhibition prevents cleavage of the viral polyproteins resulting in the formation of immature non-infectious viral particles.
Oseltamivir	Neuraminidase inhibitor	A selective inhibitor of influenza virus neuraminidase enzymes which is important for viral entry into uninfected cells, for the release of recently formed virus particles from infected cells.	Darunavir	Second-generation protease inhibitor	Darunavir can adapt to changes in the shape of a protease enzyme because of its molecular flexibility. It prevents HIV replication.
Favipiravir	RNA dependent RNA polymerase inhibitors	Favipiravir is a prodrug that is ribosylated and phosphorylated intracellularly to form the active metabolite favipiravir ibofuranosyl-5'-triphosphate, which competes with purine nucleosides and interferes with replication by incorporation into the virus RNA and thus potentially inhibiting the RNA-dependent RNA polymerase (RdRP) of RNA viruses.	Faldaprevir	Protease inhibitor	Pinpointed mechanism is still unknown, though it has been tried against chronic hepatitis C virus.
Nitazoxanide	Polymerase inhibitor	It inhibits replication of respiratory viruses in cell cultures, including SARS-CoV-2.	Galidesivir	Protease inhibitor Adenosine analogue	Initially developed for Zaire Ebolavirus, it binds to viral RNA polymerase in place of natural nucleotide, leading to disruption of viral RNA polymerase activity. Results in premature termination of the elongating RNA strand.
Baloxavir marboxil	RNA polymerase inhibitor (Endonuclease inhibitor)	It is a CAP endonuclease inhibitor. The influenza endonuclease is an essential subdomain of the viral RNA polymerase enzyme. CAP endonuclease processes host pre-mRNAs to serve as primers for viral mRNA and therefore has been a common target for studies of anti-influenza drugs. Inhibiting the activity of endonuclease can block the transcription of mRNA and inactivate the influenza virus.	Indinavir	Protease inhibitor	Indinavir inhibits the HIV viral protease enzyme which prevents cleavage of the gag-pol polyprotein, resulting in non-infectious, immature viral particles.

(Continued)

Table 7.1 (Continued) Major repurposed drugs and their proposed mechanism of action on COVID-19 infection

Name of Drug	Class/Type	Mechanism of Action	Name of Drug	Class/Type	Mechanism of Action
Ribavirin	Nucleoside analogue (guanine) –inhibits viral RNA-dependent RNA polymerase	It inhibits viral mRNA polymerase by binding to the nucleotide binding site of the enzyme, leading to a reduction in viral replication and it inhibits de novo synthesis of guanine nucleotides and decreased intracellular GTP pools, leading to a decline in viral protein synthesis.	Nelfinavir	Protease inhibitor	Nelfinavir inhibits the HIV viral proteinase enzyme which prevents cleavage of the gag-pol polyprotein, resulting in non-infectious, immature viral particles.
Sofosbuvir	Nucleotide analogue inhibitor and NS5B RNA-dependent RNA polymerase inhibitor	It is a nucleotide analogue inhibitor, which inhibits HCV NS5B protein, RNA-dependent RNA polymerase. After metabolism it is converted into uridine analogue triphosphate (GS-461203), it incorporates into HCV RNA by NS5B polymerase and acts as a chain terminator.	Tipranavir	Nonpeptidic protease inhibitor	It inhibits the processing of the viral gag and gag-pol polyproteins in HIV-1 infected cells, thus preventing formation of mature virions.
Remdesivir	Adenosine nucleotide analogues	It is metabolized into an active form known as GS-441524, an adenosine analogue. The GS-441524 interferes with the action of viral RdRP and evades proofreading by viral exoribonuclease (ExoN), thus decreasing viral RNA production.	Umifenovir	Fusion inhibitor	Viral fusion inhibition with the targeted membrane, which blocks virus entry into the cell.
Acyclovir	Nucleotide analogue	Acyclovir becomes acyclovir monophosphate through the action of viral thymidine kinase, and ultimately converted into acyclovir triphosphate, which has a higher affinity for viral DNA polymerase than cellular DNA polymerase, fits into the DNA and causes the DNA chain termination.	Thalidomide	Immunomodulatory	It has an anti-inflammatory action through its ability to speed up the degradation of messenger RNA in blood cells and thus reduce tumor necrosis factor-α (TNF-α). Thalidomide can increase the secretion of interleukins (IL), such as IL-12, and activate natural killer cells.
Entecavir	Guanine analogue (HCV)	Anti-Hepatitis B agent. By competing with the natural substrate deoxyguanosine triphosphate, entecavir functionally inhibits all three activities of HBV polymerase (reverse transcriptase, rt): (1) base priming, (2) reverse transcription of the negative strand from the pre-genomic messenger RNA, and (3) synthesis of the positive strand of HBV DNA.	Methylprednisolone	Corticosteroids	Prolongs the survival time and prevents complications of clinical cases through its anti-inflammatory and immunomodulatory action.

Drug	Class	Description	Mechanism
GS-441524	Adenosine nucleoside analogue		GS-441524 is phosphorylated 3 times to form the active nucleoside triphosphate, which is incorporated into the genome of virions, terminating its replication.
Tenofovir	Acyclic nucleoside analogue adenosine monophosphate		After activation, it acts as an antiviral acyclic nucleoside phosphonate. It is a potent inhibitor of the viral reverse transcriptase and it also has a role in the inhibition of viral polymerase causing chain termination and the inhibition of viral synthesis.
Niclosamide	Anti-helminthic agent		Niclosamide is thought to disrupt SARS-CoV-2 replication through S-phase kinase-associated protein 2 (SKP2)-inhibition, by preventing autophagy and blocking endocytosis.
Umifenovir	Direct-acting antiviral (DAA), host-targeting agent (HTA), and Hemagglutinin inhibitor (influenza)		Ability to interact with both viral proteins and lipids, it may also interfere with later stages of the viral life cycle.
Amantadine		Antiviral used in the prophylactic or symptomatic treatment of influenza A, and also used as an anti-parkinsonian agent	It helps in releasing dopamine, together with stimulation of norepinephrine response. It also has NMDA receptor antagonistic effects. The drug interferes with a viral protein, M2 (an ion channel), needed for the viral particle to become "uncoated" once it is taken inside the cell by endocytosis.
Interferon		Low molecular weight protein	The expression of the interferon-stimulated genes (ISGs) lead to development of an antiviral environment, thus inhibiting further viral replication. The interferons augment the immune system.
Pleconaril		Viral capsid inhibitor	It binds to a hydrophobic pocket in viral protein 1, the major protein which makes up the capsid (shell) of picornaviruses. This renders the viral capsid rigid and compressed, and prevents the uncoating of its RNA. As a result, the virus is stopped from attaching to the host cell and causing infection.

Source: https://go.drugbank.com/drugs.

Table 7.2 Stem cell therapy–based trials on COVID-19 patients (updated list on April 30, 2021 and removal of cancelled trials from the trials registry)

First Submitted Date/Date of Registration	Project Title	ID	Study Phase	Cell Type	Participants (Number, Age, Sex)	Intervention
2020-03-15	Treatment of COVID-19 patients using Wharton's jelly-mesenchymal stem cells.	NCT04313322	Phase 1	WJ-MSCs	Enrollment: 5 Age: 18 years to older Sex: All	WJ-MSCs will be derived from cord tissue of newborns, screened for HIV1/2, HBV, HCV, CMV, Mycoplasma, and cultured to enrich for MSCs. WJ-MSCs will be counted and suspended in 25 ml of saline solution containing 0.5% human serum albumin, and will be given to patients intravenously.
2020-01-27	Mesenchymal stem cell treatment for pneumonia patients infected with COVID-19.	NCT04252118	Phase 1	MSCs	Enrollment: 20 Age: 18–70 years Sex: All	Biological: MSCs 3 times of MSCs ($3.0 \times 10E7$ MSCs intravenously at Day 0, Day 3, Day 6).
2020-04-02	Clinical research of human mesenchymal stem cells in the treatment of COVID-19 pneumonia.	NCT04339660	Phase 1 Phase 2	UC-MSCs	Enrollment: 30 Age: 18–75 years Sex: All	Biological: UC-MSCs $1 \times 10E6$ UC-MSCs/kg body weight suspended in 100 ml saline Other: Placebo 100 ml saline intravenously.
2020-02-24	Treatment with mesenchymal stem cells for severe corona-virus disease 2019 (COVID-19).	NCT04288102	Phase 2	MSCs	Enrollment: 90 Age: 18–75 years Sex: All	Biological: MSCs 3 times of MSCs ($4.0 \times 10E7$ cells per time) intravenously at Day 0, Day 3, Day 6. Biological: Saline containing 1% Human serum albumin solution of MSC 3 times of placebo intravenously at Day 0, Day 3, Day 6.
2020-02-07	Umbilical cord (UC)-derived mesenchymal stem cells (MSCs) treatment for the 2019-novel coronavirus (nCOV) pneumonia.	NCT04269525	Phase 2	UC-MSCs	Enrollment: 10 Age: 18–75 years Sex: All	Biological: UC-MSCs After enrollment, each subject will receive UC-MSC infusion intravenously on Day 1, Day 3, Day 5, and Day 7.
2020-04-13	Use of UC-MSCs for COVID-19 patients.	NCT04355728	Phase 1 Phase 2	UC-MSCs	Enrollment: 24 Age: 18 years to older Sex: All	Biological: Umbilical cord mesenchymal stem cells UC-MSC will be administered at 100×10^6 cells/infusion administered intravenously in addition to the standard of care treatment. Other: Standard of care Standard of Care treatment per the treating hospital protocol.

Date	Phase	NCT	Title	Intervention	Population	Description
2017-02-01	Phase 1 Phase 2	NCT03042143	Repair of acute respiratory distress syndrome by stromal cell administration (REALIST) (COVID-19).	Human UC-MSCs CD362 enriched	Enrollment: 75 Age: 16 years to older Sex: All	Biological: Human umbilical cord derived CD362 enriched MSCs Infusion of human umbilical cord derived CD362 enriched MSCs Biological: Placebo (Plasma-Lyte 148) infusion of placebo.
2020-04-20	Phase 2 Phase 3	NCT04366063	Mesenchymal Stem Cell Therapy for SARS-CoV-2-related acute respiratory distress syndrome.	MSCs	Enrollment: 60 Age: 16-65 years Sex: All	Biological: Cell therapy protocol 1. Cell therapy protocol 1(n = 20). Patients will receive two doses of MSCs 100 × 10e6 (±10%) at Day 0 and Day 2 plus conventional treatment. Biological: Cell therapy protocol 2 Patients will receive two doses of MSCs 100 × 10e6 (±10%) at Day 0 and Day 2, intravenously plus two doses of EVs at Day 4 and Day 6 plus conventional treatment.
2020-03-29	Phase 1 Phase 2	NCT04333368	Cell therapy using umbilical cord-derived Mesenchymal Stromal Cells in SARS-CoV-2-related ARDS.	UC-MSCs	Enrollment: 60 Age: 18 years to older Sex: All	Biological: Umbilical cord Wharton's jelly-derived human umbilical cord Wharton's jelly-derived human MSC (at the dose of 1 million/kg) will be administered via a peripheral or central venous line over 30–45 minutes, using tubing with a 200-μm filter. Cells, in a 150 ml volume, will be delivered at D1 – D3 – D5. Other: NaCl 0.9% NaCl 0.9% (150 ml) given via an intravenous route at D1 – D3 – D5.
2020-02-14	– (No information on trial registry)	NCT04273646	Study of human umbilical cord mesenchymal stem cells in the treatment of severe COVID-19.	Human UC-MSCs	Estimated Enrollment: 48 Age: 18-65 years Sex: All	Biological: UC-MSCs 4 times of UC-MSCs (0.5 × 10E6 UC-MSCs/kg body weight intravenously at Day 1, Day 3, Day 5, Day 7). Drug: Placebo 4 times of cell-free stem cell suspension (saline containing 1% human albumin) intravenously at Day 1, Day 3, Day 5, Day 7).
2020-02-27	Phase 1	NCT04302519	Novel coronavirus induced severe pneumonia treated by dental pulp mesenchymal stem cells.	Dental pulp mesenchymal stem cells	Enrollment: 24 Age: 18-75 years Sex: All	Biological: Dental pulp mesenchymal stem cells. On the basis of clinical standard treatment, the injection of dental mesenchymal stem cells was increased on Days 1, 3 and 7 of the trial.

(Continued)

Table 7.2 (Continued) Stem cell therapy–based trials on COVID-19 patients (updated list on April 30, 2021 and removal of cancelled trials from the trials registry)

First Submitted Date/Date of Registration	Study Phase	ID	Project Title	Cell Type	Participants (Number, Age, Sex)	Intervention
2020-02-18	Phase 1 Phase 2	ChiCTR2000029990	Clinical trials of mesenchymal stem cells for the treatment of pneumonitis caused by novel coronavirus pneumonia (COVID-19).	MSCs	Enrollment: 120 Age: 18 years and 95 years Sex: All	Experimental group: MSCs Control group: Saline
2020-04-08	(Not available on trial registry)	ChiCTR2000031735	Clinical study for natural killer (NK) cells from umbilical cord blood in the treatment of novel coronavirus pneumonia (COVID-19).	NK cells	Enrollment: 20 Age: 18 years and older Sex: All	Experimental group: NK cells were injected by intravenous drip once a day for 2 to 3 times in total, each dose was 4×10^7 pieces/kg body weight, 100 ml normal saline suspension. Control group: 100 ml normal saline intravenous drip.
2020-03-27	(Not available on trial registry)	ChiCTR2000031319	Safety and efficacy study of allogeneic human dental pulp mesenchymal stem cells to treat severe novel coronavirus pneumonia (COVID-19) patients.	hDPSC	Enrollment: 20 Age: 18–65 years Sex: All	hDPSCs group: Routine treatment + intravenous injection of human dental pulp stem cells Control group: Routine treatment + placebo.
2020-03-22	(Not available on trial registry)	ChiCTR2000031139	Safety and effectiveness of human embryonic stem cell-derived M cells (CAStem) for pulmonary fibrosis correlated with novel coronavirus pneumonia (COVID-19).	Human embryonic stem cell-derived M cells	Enrollment: 20 Age: 18–80 years Sex: All	Case series: The cell dose was 3×10^6 cells/kg. It was intravenously infused twice in a row. The interval between each infusion was 1 week (+/−2 days). If the investigator considered it necessary, an additional infusion could be performed. Infusion interval 1 week (+/−2 days) from the previous time.
2020-03-18	Phase 1	ChiCTR2000030944	Clinical study of human NK cells and MSCs transplantation for severe novel coronavirus pneumonia (COVID-19).	NK cells and MSCs	Enrollment: 20 Age: 4–80 years Sex: All	Experimental group: On the basis of the current clinical treatment of SNCP, NK cells and MSCs were increased. Control group: current clinical treatment of SNCP.
2020-02-24	(Not available on trial registry)	ChiCTR2000030173	Key techniques of umbilical cord mesenchymal stem cells for the treatment of novel coronavirus pneumonia (COVID-19) and clinical application demonstration.	UC-MSCs	Enrollment: 60 Age: 18–70 years Sex: All	Experimental group: Umbilical cord mesenchymal stem cells Control group: Conventional treatment.

Date	Phase	Registry ID	Title	Cell type	Enrollment	Intervention
2020-02-24	Phase 2	ChiCTR2000030138	Clinical trial for human mesenchymal stem cells in the treatment of severe novel coronavirus pneumonia (COVID-19).	UC-MSCs	Enrollment: 60 Age: 16–75 years Sex: All	Experimental group: Intravenous injection of human umbilical cord mesenchymal stem cells (UC-MSC). Control group: Routine treatment + placebo.
2020-02-23	– (Not available on trial registry)	ChiCTR2000030116	Safety and effectiveness of human umbilical cord mesenchymal stem cells in the treatment of acute respiratory distress syndrome of severe novel coronavirus pneumonia (COVID-19).	MSCs	Enrollment: 16 Age: 16–75 years Sex: All	Two groups: Different stem cell doses.
2020-02-22	– (Not available on trial registry)	ChiCTR2000030088	Umbilical cord Wharton's jelly-derived mesenchymal stem cells in the treatment of severe novel coronavirus pneumonia (COVID-19).	Wharton's jelly MSCs	Enrollment: 40 Age: 18–80 years Sex: All	Experimental group: Iv injection of Wharton's jelly mesenchymal stem cells (1×10^6/kg), cell suspension volume: 40 ml Control group: Iv 40 ml saline.
2020-02-20	– (Not available on trial registry)	ChiCTR2000030020	The clinical application and basic research related to mesenchymal stem cells to treat novel coronavirus pneumonia (COVID-19).	MSCs	Enrollment: 20 Age: 18–70 years Sex: All	Case series: Mesenchymal stem cells therapy.
2020-02-07	– (Not available on trial registry).	ChiCTR2000029606	Clinical study for human menstrual blood-derived stem cells in the treatment of acute novel coronavirus pneumonia (COVID-19).	Human menstrual blood-derived stem cells preparations	Enrollment: 63 Age: 1–99 years Sex: All	Experimental group A: Conventional treatment followed by intravenous infusion of human menstrual blood-derived stem cells preparations. Control group A: conventional treatment Experimental group B1: Artificial liver therapy + conventional treatment. Experimental group B2: Artificial liver therapy followed by Intravenous infusion of Human Menstrual Blood-derived stem cells preparations + conventional treatment. Control group A: Conventional treatment.

(Continued)

Table 7.2 (Continued) Stem cell therapy–based trials on COVID-19 patients (updated list on April 30, 2021 and removal of cancelled trials from the trials registry)

First Submitted Date/Date of Registration	Study Phase	ID	Project Title	Cell Type	Participants (Number, Age, Sex)	Intervention
2020-02-05	– (Not available on trial registry)	ChiCTR2000029580	Severe novel coronavirus pneumonia (COVID-19) patients treated with ruxolitinib in combination with mesenchymal stem cells: a prospective, single blind, randomized controlled clinical trial.	Mesenchymal stem cells	Enrollment: 70 Age: 18–75 years Sex: All	Experimental group: Ruxolitinib combined with mesenchymal stem cell. Control group: Routine treatment.
2020-02-05	– (Not available on trial registry)	ChiCTR2000029572	Safety and efficacy of umbilical cord blood mononuclear cells in the treatment of severe and critically novel coronavirus pneumonia (COVID-19): a randomized controlled clinical trial.	Umbilical cord blood mononuclear cells	Enrollment: 30 Age: 18 years to older Sex: All	Experimental group: Conventional treatment combined with umbilical cord blood mononuclear cells group Control group: Conventional treatment.
2020-02-04	– (Not available on trial registry)	ChiCTR2000029569	Safety and efficacy of umbilical cord blood mononuclear cells conditioned medium in the treatment of severe and critically novel coronavirus pneumonia (COVID-19): a randomized controlled trial.	Umbilical cord mesenchymal stem cells	Enrollment: 30 Age: 18 years to older Sex: All	Experimental group: Conventional treatment combined with umbilical cord mesenchymal stem cell conditioned medium group. Control group: Conventional treatment.

Source: NIH: http://cli.nicaltrials.gov, http://www.coronavirus.gov, Chinese clinical trial registry http://www.chictr.org.cn/ and also based on institutional websites.

Table 7.3 Miscellaneous interventions in COVID-19 patients

First Submitted Date/Date of Registration	Study Phase/ Recruitment Status	ID	Project Title		Participants (Number, Age, Sex)	Intervention
2020-04-27	Phase 1 Phase 2	NCT04368728	Study to describe the safety, tolerability, immunogenicity, and potential efficacy of RNA vaccine candidates against COVID-19 in healthy adults.	RNA	Enrollment: 7600 Age: 18–85 years Sex: All	Biological:BNT162a1 0.5 ml intramuscular injection. Biological: BNT162b1 0.5 ml intramuscular injection Biological: BNT162b2 0.5 ml intramuscular injection. Biological: BNT162c2 0.5 ml intramuscular injection. Other: placebo 0.5 ml intramuscular injection.
2020-02-21	Phase 1	NCT04283461	Safety and immunogenicity study of 2019-nCoV vaccine (mRNA-1273) for prophylaxis of SARS-CoV-2 infection (COVID-19)	mRNA	Enrollment: 105 Age: 18–99 years Sex: All	Biological: mRNA-1273 Lipid nanoparticle (LNP) dispersion containing an mRNA that encodes for the prefusion stabilized spike protein 2019-nCoV. mRNA-1273 consists of an mRNA drug substance that is manufactured into LNPs composed of the proprietary ionizable lipid, SM-102, and 3 commercially available lipids, cholesterol, DSPC, and PEG2000 DMG.
2020-03-05	Phase 1	NCT04299724	Safety and immunity of COVID-19 aAPC vaccine.	artificial antigen presenting cells (aAPC)	Enrollment: 100 Age: 6 months to 80 years Sex: All	Biological: Pathogen-specific aAPC. The subjects will receive three injections of 5×10^6 each COVID-19/aAPC vaccine via subcutaneous injections.
2020-04-03	Phase 1	NCT04336410	Safety, tolerability and immunogenicity of INO-4800 for COVID-19 in healthy volunteers.	INO-4800 (DNA)	Enrollment: 40 Age: 18–50 years Sex: All	Drug: INO-4800 INO-4800 will be administered ID on Day 0 and Week 4.

7.4.2 Synthetic Nano Stem Cell–Based Therapy

LIF (leukemia inhibitory factor) is documented in an animal-based study as an essential factor to neutralize the cytokine storm in lungs during viral pneumonia [62]. MSCs are known to release LIF, but the costs of processing and maintaining MSCs is too high to be generally applicable and affordable for common patients. Introduction of LIFNano offers a plausible solution to this. It involves the application of nanotechnology-based synthetic stem cells as "LIFNano" which are a thousand times more potent than soluble LIF [63]. As a cutting-edge technology, LIFNano could be utilized as an alternative to cell-based therapy, for replacement of the need for high volume and off-the-shelf therapeutic agents. Thus this therapy may be able to rejuvenate injured tissues and suppress cytokine storms in pneumonia.

7.5 CONCLUSIONS

In summary, extensive data from in vitro and in vivo studies in cell lines and animal models, and clinical trials on more than 25 drugs and compounds can support the correct clinical management of COVID-19 patients. Additionally, we hope that this might facilitate future prophylactic studies in large clinical settings. Many compounds, including FDA approved drugs and drug-like molecules subjected to repurposing for COVID-19 have been included. This amalgamation of in silico, in vitro, in vivo screenings and experimentation, and data from clinical trials can help in the design and development of new antiviral drugs for various stages of the current pandemic. Furthermore, this chapter presents the concomitant use of drugs associated with polypharmacy, which can lead to significant adverse effects, sometimes with toxic and degenerative drug interactions for humans. The role of MSCs in lowering the inflammation through activation of APCs could be a major breakthrough representing an entirely new biological approach to the treatment of COVID-19 patients, and to raise the awareness of better preparation for future emerging outbreaks.

ACKNOWLEDGEMENTS

SD is thankful to the department staff: LDC Rohit Nigam, and office attendants Daulat Singh and Shubham Kumar for their help while preparing this chapter.

REFERENCES

1. Mackenzie, J.S., Smith, D.W. (2020). COVID-19: A novel zoonotic disease caused by a coronavirus from China: What we know and what we don't. *Microbiol. Aust.* doi:10.1071/MA20013. PMCID: PMC7086482.

2. Maurya, C.K., Misra, R., Sharma, P., et al. (2020). Novel stem cells and nucleic acid-based vaccine trials against viral outbreak: A systematic evaluation during COVID-2019 pandemic. *Ind. J. Clin. Biochem.* 35. doi:10.1007/s12291-020-00907-4. PMCID: PMC7347658.

3. Gautret, P., Lagier, J.-C., Parola, P., et al. (2020). Hydroxychloroquine and azithromycin as a treatment of COVID-19: Results of an open-label non-randomized clinical trial. *Int. J. Antimicrob. Agents* doi:10.1016/j.ijantimicag.2020.105949. PMCID: PMC7102549.

4. Chen, J., Liu, D., Liu, L., et al. (2020). A pilot study of hydroxychloroquine in treatment of patients with moderate COVID-19. *Zhejiang Da Xue Xue Bao Yi Xue Ban.* doi:10.3785/j.issn.1008-9292.2020.03.03. PMID: 32391667.

5. Gao, J., Tian, Z., Yang, X., et al. (2020). Breakthrough: Chloroquine phosphate has shown apparent efficacy in treatment of COVID-19 associated pneumonia in clinical studies. *Biosci. Trends.* doi:10.5582/bst.2020.01047. PMID: 32074550.

6. Tang, W., Cao, Z., Han, M., et al. (2020). Hydroxychloroquine in patients with mainly mild to moderate coronavirus disease 2019: Open label, randomised controlled trial. *BMJ.* doi:10.1136/bmj.m1849. PMCID: PMC7221473.

7. Abubakar, A.R., Sani, I.H., Godman, B., et al. (2020). Systematic review on the therapeutic options for COVID-19: Clinical evidence of drug efficacy and implications. *Infect. Drug Resist.* doi:10.2147/IDR.S289037. PMCID: PMC7778508.

8. Yan, D., Liu, X.-Y., Zhu, Y.-N., et al. (2020). Factors associated with prolonged viral shedding and impact of lopinavir/ritonavir treatment in hospitalised non-critically ill patients with SARS-CoV-2 infection. *Eur. Respir. J.* doi:10.1183/13993003.00799-2020. PMCID: PMC7241115.

9. Liu, F., Xu, A., Zhang, Y., et al. (2020). Patients of COVID-19 may benefit from sustained Lopinavir-combined regimen and the increase of Eosinophil may predict the outcome of COVID-19 progression. *Int. J. Infect. Dis.* doi:10.1016/j.ijid.2020.03.013. PMCID: PMC7193136.

10. Khan, S.A., Xu, A., Zhang, Y., et al. (2021). Patients of COVID-19 may benefit from sustained Lopinavir-combined regimen and the increase of Eosinophil may predict the outcome of COVID-19 progression. *J. Infect. Public Health.* doi:10.1016/j.jiph.2020.10.012. PMCID: PMC7590838.

11. Li, Y., Xie, Z., Lin, W., et al. (2020). Efficacy and safety of lopinavir/ritonavir or arbidol in adult patients with mild/moderate COVID-19: An exploratory randomized controlled trial. *Med.* doi:10.1016/J.Medj.2020.04.001.

12. Ivaschenko, A., Dmitriev, K.A., Vostokova, N.V., et al. (2021). AVIFAVIR for treatment of patients with moderate coronavirus disease 2019

(COVID-19): Interim results of a phase II/III multicenter randomized clinical trial. *Clin. Infect. Dis.* 73, 531–534.

13. Andrade, B.S., de Souza Rangel, F., Santos, N.O., et al. (2020). Repurposing approved drugs for guiding COVID-19 prophylaxis: A systematic review. *Front. Pharmacol.* doi:10.3389/fphar.2020.590598. PMCID: PMC7772842.

14. Grein, J., Ohmagari, N., Shin, D., et al. (2020). Compassionate use of Remdesivir for patients with severe COVID-19. *Engl. J. Med.* doi:10.1056/NEJMoa2007016. PMID: 32275812.

15. Burwick, R.M., Yawetz, S., Stephenson, K.E., et al. (2020). Compassionate use of Remdesivir in pregnant women with severe coronavirus disease 2019. *Clin. Infect. Dis.* doi:10.1093/cid/ciaa1466.

16. Wahl, A., Gralinski, L.E., Johnson, C.E., et al. (2021). SARS-CoV-2 infection is effectively treated and prevented by EIDD-2801. *Nature.* doi:10.1038/s41586-021-03312-w.

17. Ulhaq, Z.S., Soraya, G.V. (2020). Anti-IL-6 receptor antibody treatment for severe COVID-19 and the potential implication of IL-6 gene polymorphisms in novel coronavirus pneumonia. *Med. Clin.* doi:10.1016/jmedcli.2020.07.002.

18. Lescure, F.X., Honda, H., Fowler, R.A., et al. Sarilumab in patients admitted to hospital with severe or critical COVID-19: A randomised, double-blind, placebo-controlled, phase 3 trial. *Lancet Respir. Med.* 2021. PMID: 33676590.

19. De Rossi, N., Scarpazza, C., Filippini, C., et al. (2020). Early use of low dose tocilizumab in patients with COVID-19: A retrospective cohort study with a complete follow-up. *EClinical Medicine* 25 100459. doi:10.1016/J.Eclinm.2020.100459.

20. Somers, E., Eschenauer, G., Troost, J.P., et al. 2020. Tocilizumab for treatment of mechanically ventilated patients with COVID-19. *Clin. Infect. Dis.* Ciaa954. doi:10.1093/Cid/Ciaa954.

21. Biran, N., Ip, A., Ahn, J., et al. (2020). Tocilizumab among patients with COVID-19 in the intensive care unit: a multicentre observational study. *Lancet. Rheumatol.* 2, e603–e612.

22. Price, C., Altice, F., Shyr, Y., et al. (2020). Tocilizumab treatment for cytokine release syndrome in hospitalized COVID-19 patients: Survival and clinical outcomes. *Chest* S0012-3692(20), 31670–31676. doi:10.1016/J.Chest.2020.06.006.

23. Xu, X., Han, M., Li, T., et al. (2020). Effective treatment of severe COVID-19 patients with tocilizumab. *Proc. Natl. Acad. Sci. U.S.A.* 117, 10970–10975.

24. Colaneri, M., Bogliolo, L., Valsecchi, P., et al. (2020). Tocilizumab for treatment of severe COVID-19 patients: Preliminary results from SMAtteo COvid19 REgistry (SMACORE). *Microorganisms* doi:10.3390/microorganisms8050695. PMCID: PMC7285503.

25. Moreno-Pérez, O., Andres, M., Leon-Ramirez, J.-M., et al. (2020). Experience with tocilizumab in severe COVID-19 pneumonia after 80 days of follow-up: A retrospective cohort study. *J. Autoimmun.* doi:10.1016/j.jaut.2020.102523. PMCID: PMC7365106.

26. Lan, S., Lai, C.-C., Huang, H.-T., et al. (2020). Tocilizumab for severe COVID-19: A systematic review and meta-analysis. *Int. J. Antimicrob. Agents.* doi:10.1016/j.ijantimicag.2020.106103. PMCID: PMC7377685.

27. Della-Torre, E., Campochiaro, C., Cavalli, G., et al. (2020). Interleukin-6 blockade with sarilumab in severe COVID-19 pneumonia with systemic hyperinflammation: An open-label cohort study. *Ann. Rheum. Dis.* doi:10.1136/annrheumdis-2020-218122. PMCID: PMC7509526.

28. van Rhee, F., Wong, R.S., Munshi, N., et al. (2014). Siltuximab for multicentric Castleman's disease: a randomised, double-blind, placebo-controlled study. *Lancet Oncol.* 15, 966–974.

29. Palanques-Pastor, T., López-Briz, E., Andrés, J.L.P., et al. (2020). Involvement of interleukin 6 in SARS-CoV-2 infection: siltuximab as a therapeutic option against COVID-19. *Eur. J. Hosp. Pharm.* 27, 297–298.

30. Gordon, A.C., Mouncey, P.R., Al-Beidh, F., et al. (2021). Interleukin-6 receptor antagonists in critically Ill patients with COVID-19. *N. Engl. J. Med.* doi:10.1056/NEJMoa2100433. PMCID: PMC7953461.

31. Franzetti, M., Forastieri, A., Borsa, N., et al. (2021). IL-1 receptor antagonist Anakinra in the treatment of COVID-19 acute respiratory distress syndrome: A retrospective, observational study. *J. Immunol.* doi:10.4049/jimmunol.2001126. PMCID: PMC7980530.

32. Monk, P.D., Tear, V.J., Brookes, J., et al. (2021). Safety and efficacy of inhaled nebulised interferon beta-1a (SNG001) for treatment of SARS-CoV-2 infection: A randomised, double-blind, placebo-controlled, phase 2 trial. *Lancet Respir. Med.* doi:10.1016/S2213-2600(20)30511-7. PMCID: PMC7836724.

33. WHO Solidarity Consortium. (2020). Repurposed antiviral drugs for COVID-19 – Interim WHO SOLIDARITY trial results. *medRxiv.* doi:10.1101/2020.10.15.20209817.

34. Lokhande, A.S., Devarajan, P.V. (2021). A review on possible mechanistic insights of Nitazoxanide for repurposing in COVID-19. *Eur. J. Pharmacol.* doi:10.1016/j.ejphar.2020.173748. PMCID: PMC7678434.

35. ClinicalTrials.gov. (2020). Trial to evaluate the efficacy and safety of Nitazoxanide (NTZ) for post-exposure prophylaxis of COVID-19 and other viral respiratory illnesses in elderly residents of long-term care facilities (LTCF). Apr 16. Available at https://clinicaltrials.gov/ct2/show/NCT04343248?term=nitazoxanide&recrs

=ab&cond=COVID&draw=2&rank=6. Accessed April 28, 2020.

36. Romark Pharmaceuticals. Romark initiates new phase 3 clinical trial of NT-300 for the treatment of COVID-19. 2020, Aug 11. Available at https://www.romark.com/romark-initiates-new-phase-3-clinical-trial-of-nt-300-for-the-treatment-of-covid-19/.

37. Businesswire. (2020). ANA therapeutics begins phase 2/3 clinical trial of proprietary oral niclosamide formulation to treat COVID-19. Oct 26. Available at https://www.businesswire.com/news/home/20201026005569/en/ANA-Therapeutics-Begins-Phase-23-Clinical-Trial-of-Proprietary-Oral-Niclosamide-Formulation-to-Treat-COVID-19.

38. RECOVERY Collaborative Group, Horby, P., Lim, W.S. et al. (2021). Dexamethasone in hospitalized patients with COVID-19. N. Engl. J. Med. doi:10.1056/NEJMoa2021436.

39. World Health Organization. (2020). [Guideline] WHO. Corticosteroids for COVID-19 – Living guidance. Sep 2. Available at https://www.who.int/publications/i/item/WHO-2019-nCoV-Corticosteroids-2020.1. Accessed: September 3, 2020.

40. Fadel, R., Morrison, A.R., Vahia, A., et al. (2020). Early short-course corticosteroids in hospitalized patients with COVID-19. Clin. Infect. Dis. doi:10.1093/cid/ciaa601. PMCID: PMC7314133.

41. Keller, M.J., Kitsis, E.A., Arora, S., et al. (2020). Effect of systemic glucocorticoids on mortality or mechanical ventilation in patients with COVID-19. J. Hosp. Med. doi:10.12788/jhm.3497. PMCID: PMC7518134.

42. Joyner, M.J., Carter, R.E., Senefeld, J.W., et al. (2021). Convalescent plasma antibody levels and the risk of death from COVID-19. N. Engl. J. Med. doi:10.1056/NEJMoa2031893. PMCID: PMC7821984.

43. US Food and Drug Administration. (2020). Fact sheet for health care providers - Emergency use authorization (EUA) of COVID-19 convalescent plasma for treatment of COVID-19 in hospitalized patients. Aug 23. Available at https://www.fda.gov/media/141478/download. Accessed August 23, 2020.

44. Kennedy, N.A., Goodhand, J.R., Bewshea, C., et al. (2021). Anti-SARS-CoV-2 antibody responses are attenuated in patients with IBD treated with infliximab. Gut. doi:10.1136/gutjnl-2021-324388. PMCID: PMC7992387.

45. Michelena, X., Borrell, H., López-Corbeto, M., et al. (2020). Incidence of COVID-19 in a cohort of adult and paediatric patients with rheumatic diseases treated with targeted biologic and synthetic disease-modifying anti-rheumatic drugs. Semin. Arthritis Rheum. doi:10.1016/j.semarthrit.2020.05.001.

46. Fernandez-Gutierrez, B., Leon, L., Madrid, A., et al. (2021). Hospital admissions in inflammatory rheumatic diseases during the peak of COVID-19 pandemic: incidence and role of disease-modifying agents. Adv. Musculoskeletal. Dis. doi:10.1177/1759720X20962692. PMCID: PMC7869066.

47. Okamoto, M., Toyama, M., Baba, M. (2020). The chemokine receptor antagonist cenicriviroc inhibits the replication of SARS-CoV-2 in vitro. Antiviral Res. doi:10.1016/j.antiviral.2020.104902.

48. ClinicalTrials.gov. (2020). I-SPY COVID-19 TRIAL: An adaptive platform trial for critically ill patients (I-SPY_COVID). Aug 12. https://clinicaltrials.gov/ct2/show/NCT04488081. Accessed: August 25, 2020.

49. Dwivedi, S., Yadav, S.S., Singh, M.K., et al. (2013). Pharmacogenomics of Viral Diseases. Springer, New Delhi. doi:10.1007/978-81-322-1184-6_28.

50. Dwivedi, S., Sharma, P., (2018). Stem cell biology: A new hope in regenerations and replenishments therapy. Ind. J. Clin. Biochem. doi:10.1007/s12291-018-0792-4.

51. Golchin, A., Farahany, T.Z., Khojasteh, A., et al. (2019). The clinical trials of mesenchymal stem cell therapy in skin diseases: An update and concise review. Curr. Stem Cell Res. Ther. doi:10.2174/1574888X13666180913123424. PMID: 30210006.

52. Cronkite, D.A., Strutt, T.M. (2018). The regulation of inflammation by innate and adaptive lymphocytes. J. Immunol. Res. doi:10.1155/2018/1467538.

53. Dwivedi, S., Singh, S., Goel, A., et al. (2015). Pro-(IL-18) and anti-(IL-10) inflammatory promoter genetic variants (intrinsic factors) with tobacco exposure (extrinsic factors) may influence susceptibility and severity of prostate carcinoma: A prospective study. Asian Pac. J. Cancer Prev. doi:10.7314/apjcp.2015.16.8.3173.

54. Dwivedi, S., Shukla, K.K., Gupta, G., et al. (2013). Non-invasive biomarker in prostate carcinoma: A novel approach. Ind. J. Clin. Biochem. doi:10.1007/s12291-013-0312-5.

55. Spaggiari, G.M., Capobianco, A., Abdelrazik, H., et al. (2006). Mesenchymal stem cell-natural killer cell interactions: Evidence that activated NK cells are capable of killing MSCs, whereas MSCs can inhibit IL-2-induced NK-cell proliferation. Blood. doi:10.1182/blood-2005-07-2775. PMID: 16239427.

56. Mehta, P., McAuley, D.F., Brown, M., et al. (2020). COVID-19: Consider cytokine storm syndromes and immunosuppression. Lancet. doi:10.1016/S0140-6736(20)30628-0. PMCID: PMC7270045.

57. Bing, L., Chen, J., Li, T., et al. (2020). Clinical remission of a critically ill COVID-19 patient treated by human umbilical cord mesenchymal stem cells. ChinaXiv. doi:10.12074/202002.00084.

58. Leng, Z., Zhu, R., Hou, W., et al. (2020). Transplantation of ACE2 - Mesenchymal stem cells improves the outcome of patients with COVID-19 pneumonia. *Aging Dis.* doi:10.14336/AD.2020.0228. PMCID: PMC7069465.

59. Papait, A., Vertua, E., Magatti, M., et al. (2020). Mesenchymal stromal cells from fetal and maternal placenta possess key similarities and differences: Potential implications for their applications in regenerative medicine. *Cells* 9, 127.

60. Barkama, R., Mayo, A., Paz, A., et al. (2020). Placenta-derived cell therapy to treat patients with respiratory failure due to coronavirus disease 2019. *Crit. Care Explor.* 2(9), e0207. doi:10.1097/CCE.0000000000000207. PMID: 32984833; PMCID: PMC7498138.

61. U.S. FDA clears Pluristem's IND application for phase II COVID-19 study. https://www.pluristem.com/wp-content/uploads/2020/05/FDA-Clearance-COVID-19-FINAL.pdf. Accessed: May 25, 2020.

62. Foronjy, R.F., Dabo, A.J., Cummins, N., et al. (2014). Leukemia inhibitory factor protects the lung during respiratory syncytial viral infection. *BMC Immunol.* doi:10.1186/s12865-014-0041-4. PMCID: PMC4189665.

63. Metcalfe, S.M., Strom, T.B., Williams, A., et al. (2015). Multiple sclerosis and the LIF/IL-6 axis: Use of nanotechnology to harness the Tolerogenic and reparative properties of LIF. *Nanobiomedicine (Rij).* doi:10.5772/60622. PMCID: PMC5997376.

Chapter 8   Convalescent Plasma and Antibody Therapy in COVID-19

Didem Rıfkı, Eymen Ü. Kılıç, and Şükrü Tüzmen

8.1 INTRODUCTION

SARS-CoV-2 is defined as the etiological agent that caused the COVID-19 pandemic at the end of 2019. Considering its dramatic consequences on people's health, economics, daily life, education, and politics, scientists all over the world have been working hard to understand the physiopathology of this disease in order to develop efficient treatment strategies. Immunomodulation has gained importance as a potential therapeutic strategy for this disorder, as the main battle of care is the cytokine storm. Specific and nonspecific immunotherapies, such as convalescent plasma (CP) and specific immunoglobulins, are being investigated for the treatment of extreme COVID-19 disease, but no conclusive proof of their efficacy has yet been found, with the exception of the approval of Regeneron's monoclonal antibody (mAb) cocktails. CP therapy is focused on the concept of using antibodies produced from naturally recovered individuals to prevent and cure COVID-19. It has also decreased viral antigen levels, improved blood oxygen saturation, and increased lymphocyte ratio [1]. CP treatment, which involves transfer of antibodies to the recipient, provides both antiviral and immunomodulatory activities through anti-inflammatory cytokines and antibodies [1].

After plasma transfer, the National People's Health Commission of the People's Republic of China (NHCPRC) recorded a substantial decrease in symptoms such as fever, cough, sputum, muscle pain, and weakness [1]. A clinical trial investigating the efficacy and effectiveness of CP in patients with mild to moderate COVID-19 symptoms admitted to a hospital emergency unit has been suspended by the National Institutes of Health after showing no benefits at all. The independent Data and Safety Monitoring Board (DSMB) decided on February 25, 2021, that while the CP intervention did not cause any harm, it was unlikely to help this group of patients. CP has the best chance of demonstrating efficacy for the early treatment of patients who are at the greatest risk of serious disease and mortality [2].

Zhikun Zeng et al. in 2020 [34] published the first study on specific anti-SARS-COV-2 antibodies, detecting SARS-CoV-2 specific IgM and IgG at days 9 and 15, respectively, after the onset of the disease [1]. Anti-SARS-CoV-2 IgG can be detected on day 11, or 18–21 days after infection, according to another study [3]. Until symptomatic recovery, serum levels of IgM and IgG antibodies that can neutralize SARS-CoV-2 were also identified. SARS-CoV-2 anti-spike (S) protein receptor-binding domain (anti-RBD) IgG/IgM seropositivity and anti-nucleoprotein (anti-NP) IgG/IgM seropositivity were detected 14 days or later after disease onset, and anti-NP/RBD IgG levels correlated with virus neutralization titers [1].

Despite the demonstrated therapeutic efficacy of immunoglobulins against COVID-19, the efficacy of single agent therapy has yet to be fully established. Remdesivir (RDV) in combination with an mAb may improve outcomes over single-agent therapy by causing less weight loss, lower virus lung titers, less acute lung injury, and improved pulmonary function, thereby extending the therapeutic window [4].

8.2 EFFECTS OF COVID-19 ON THE IMMUNE SYSTEM

The SARS-CoV-2 replicates in the early stages of COVID-19. In the later stages, known as the "cytokine storm", the host's immune response to viral infection becomes uncontrolled, marked by sharp increases in proinflammatory cytokines such as the interleukins IL-1β, IL-1RA, IL-2, IL-4, IL-6, IL-7, IL-8, IL-10, interferon-γ (IFN-γ), granulocyte macrophage-colony stimulating factor (GM-CSF), and tumor necrosis factor-α (TNF-α). The condition worsens, progressing from a mild infection to a systemic inflammatory response and, eventually, to multi-system organ failure [5].

IFNs (IFN-I, IFN-α/β) provide a form of natural antiviral protection during the early stages of viral infection. In the later stages of the disease, the number of proinflammatory interleukins (IL-1 β, IL-6), TNF-α, and C-C motif chemokine ligands (CCL-2, CCL-3, and CCL-5) increase while IFNs decrease. Along with the decreased secretion of IFN, antiviral responses are also hampered by the reduced IFN secretion, which in return is accompanied by a rise in chemokine release attracting a large number of inflammatory cells, such as monocytes and neutrophils. This will result in an excessive inflammatory

DOI: 10.1201/9781003190394-8

response. Mononuclear macrophages are activated by the delayed release of IFN-α/β via receptors on their surfaces. CCL2, CCL7, and CCL12, which are monocyte chemoattractants, are released by activated mononuclear macrophages, causing an increase in the number of mononuclear macrophages, which leads to increased levels of proinflammatory cytokines (IL1-, IL-6, and TNF-α) [5].

Inflammatory cytokines activate the development of GM-CSF, which functions as a co-regulator alongside TNF-α, IL-6, and IL-1 in a positive feed-forward inflammatory loop involving monocytes/macrophages, fibroblasts, endothelial cells, dendritic cells, and T helper cells. The GM-CSF receptor (GM-CSFR), which consists of a basic ligand-binding α-chain and a signal-transducing β-chain, mediates GM-CSF signals [6].

The downstream signaling of GM-CSFR is mediated by Janus kinase 2 (JAK2)/signal transducer and activator of transcription 5 (STAT5), nuclear factor kappa-light-chain-enhancer of activated B cells (NF-κB), extracellular signal-regulated kinase (ERK), and the phosphoinositide 3-kinase (PI3K)-Akt pathway. Higher levels of GM-CSF were observed in the early stages (1–3 days), with a steady decrease in the late stages (day 14). GM-CSF may also have unintended consequences. As activated neutrophils play a major role in the microvascular injury that contributes to lung damage, they may contribute to acute respiratory distress syndrome (ARDS) by suppressing neutrophil apoptosis [6].

Proinflammatory cytokines cause cell death of cytotoxic T lymphocytes, preventing viral particle clearance. IFN-α/β and IFN-γ trigger apoptosis of alveolar and airway epithelial cells, resulting in hypoxemia throughout the body. Furthermore, IL-6 forms a complex with its receptor, activating the IL-6-sIL-6R-Janus Kinase (JAK)-Signal Transducer and Activator of Transcription 3 (STAT3) signaling pathway. This causes endothelial cells to secrete VEGF, MCP-1, IL-8, and additional IL-6, as well as leading to a decrease in E-cadherin expression. The cytokine storm is aggravated by increased vascular permeability and leakage as a result of this chain of events. Multiple organ failure is caused by leakage in the systemic circulation [5].

8.3 IMMUNOTHERAPY

A variety of drugs approved for other indications as well as various investigational agents have been repurposed for the treatment of COVID-19 in clinical trials around the world. Despite the large amount of data from clinical trials, the results are insufficient to draw firm conclusions about the effectiveness and safety of potential therapeutics.

Many unknowns surround the application of immunotherapy, including dosage adjustments for patients with organ failures or those who need extracorporeal equipment, as well as the possible consequences and safety of combination therapies. Agents that modulate immune responses are being investigated as adjunctive therapies for the management of moderate to serious COVID-19 disease, because of the hyperactive inflammatory effects of extreme COVID-19 disease. Human blood–derived products and immunomodulators are potential agents. Individuals who have recovered from SARS-CoV-2 infections can provide certain COVID-specific and COVID-nonspecific human blood-derived products such as CP and immunoglobulin products.

8.3.1 Convalescent Plasma

8.3.1.1 Definition, Extraction, and Applications of Plasma in Viral Infections

Passive immunization by transfer of antibodies from recovered patients is a century-old technique for treating bacterial/viral infections dating back before the discovery of antibiotics and vaccines. In principle, plasma from recovered patients is the source of antibodies for a particular viral infection at sufficient titers. The aim is to transfer the same immunity to new patients, ensuring exposure to a particular virus. It has been revealed that plasma transfusions into sick patients elicit neutralizing antibodies as well as the ability to manage excessive inflammatory cascades from infectious agents [7].

The CP treatment reemerged for the prevention and management of COVID-19 because of the lack of sufficient antiviral drugs or vaccines at the beginning of the pandemic. Compared to convalescent blood products such as mAbs and intravenous immunoglobulins, CP can be procured in simpler terms as a first-choice emergency treatment as it has been used widely in earlier coronavirus outbreaks [7].

Clinical application and criteria for CP donation eligibility show differences internationally, while newly updated regulations are released by the FDA for donor recruitment in workflow protocols. Recently, the FDA updated their issuance with a new guidance on February 11, 2021, to provide recommendations for healthcare providers during the public health emergency. CP is not an approved therapy but only under Emergency Use Authorization (EUA) and Investigational New Drug (IND) regulation. Donors have to be tested for the presence of antibodies against virus following 14 days of confirmed infection as well as a negative molecular test to guarantee safety, though the number of days is relaxed since antibody titer seroconversion becomes available around 8–21 days after the onset of symptoms, ideally confirmed with CLIA certified validated tests such as ELISA. Moreover, antibody testing brings its own complications to the equation in the context of eligibility to become a donor, as the question remains unanswered as to whether total antibody or subclasses are most relevant [8, 9].

8.3.1.2 Efficacy and Safety

FDA-authorized (non-approved) use of CP therapy came into operation for hospitalized patients upon EUA in the emergence of COVID-19 on April 23, 2020. Application of CP began as early immediate interventions in COVID-19 patients. However, in recent randomized, double-blind, placebo clinical trials and meta-analysis (RECOVERY, PLACID), conclusive benefits from CP have not been confirmed [10, 11]. Decisive factors from recent research reemerged related to the effectiveness of CP therapy. Ahead of these multi meta-analysis studies, proof of benefit was inconsistent. The RECOVERY trial independent Data Monitoring Committee (DMC) discontinued CP trials on January 14, 2021, after seeing no convincing evidence of the conclusive proof of worthwhile mortality benefits either in normal overall care or in any pre-specified subgroup. Moreover, NIH announced in a press release the halting of clinical trials of COVID-19 CP(C3PO) in emergency patients on February 25, 2021 (launched in August 2020), also claiming CP therapy caused no harm but neither did it offer any benefits [10, 12].

Previously, observational evidence pointed to the effectiveness of CP in "standard of care" against precedent viral infections but in such nonrandomized studies, the patients were also administered additional treatments such as steroids, antivirals, and other drugs simultaneously with CP treatment, consequently causing inferential complications. In an FDA sponsored study involving 100,000 patients, efficacy of CP did not meet with a clear prospect. While many patients showed clinical improvement, the study could not provide answers as to which treatments the patients were responding [13].

CP therapy remains an official treatment in the COVID-19 pandemic, as seen in prior infectious diseases. With respect to other drugs/preventive measures, CP will likely continue to be a relevant treatment at times of first responses to a possible pandemic outbreak prior to antivirals and vaccines becoming available. Nevertheless, there are still some issues to consider in making the final decision on the advisability of CP transfusion programs. The fact that CP consists of more than just antibodies makes it a difficult therapeutic choice since it is essentially blood plasma from recovered patients, whereas mAbs are solitary products. Hence, CP contains complex components, which may possibly also contribute to immune response. Such elaborate prophylaxis measures will most likely cease to be necessary once a certain level of immunity is reached within the population, depending on how soon vaccines will fulfil the expectation of herd immunity. The scientific committees have delivered mixed opinions and results. Angus et al. called out clinical research and enterprise setups by comparing them to a marketplace where researchers face each other in terms of competing for funding, hence recommend facilitating national data sharing and interoperability between research and clinical care for optimal operation [14]. Despite competition from trials, further multi-center-controlled trials are needed to implement the optimal conditions (timing and dose) in case of proven efficacy [14].

8.3.2 Immunoglobulins
8.3.2.1 Non-SARS-CoV-2 Specific

Yun Xie et al. [15] announced the first study of administration of intravenous immunoglobulin (IVIG) combined with a glucocorticoid adjuvant treatment to 58 patients with extreme COVID-19. Within 48 hours of admission of patients to the ICU, this treatment decreased the use of mechanical ventilation and reduced the length of hospital stay, resulting in substantial clinical efficacy and a reduction in 28-day mortality [1]. The effectiveness of IVIG in the management of COVID-19 and MIS-C (Multisystem inflammatory syndrome in children) is still being investigated.

8.3.2.2 SARS-CoV-2 Specific

SARS-CoV-2 immunoglobulins (human mAbs) are produced from plasma obtained from recovered COVID-19 patients. This method of immunization using virus-specific concentrated antibodies has previously been applied safely and effectively for viral infections. IL-6, IL-1RA, IL8, IL-1, IL-17A, IL-33, IFN-γ, TNF-α, CTGF, plasma kallikrein, TNFSF14, GM-CSF, CSF-1R, CD14, CD147, VEGF, PD-1, human factor XIIa, complementary protein 5, NKG2A, HER2, ILT7 receptor, C5aR, and viral attachment to the human cell are among the targets for immunoglobulins under investigation.

8.3.2.2.1 Interleukin-6 Inhibitors

The IL-6 cytokine is the most studied cytokine that has been linked to viral load, incidence, severity, and prognosis in COVID-19 patients. Many clinical trials have focused on IL-6 for the treatment of extreme stages of COVID-19. As a result, tocilizumab is thought to be the most promising candidate for cytokine storm control in COVID-19 [5]. Tocilizumab blocks the IL-6 receptor signaling pathway. It has been tested in COVID-19 patients alone or in combination with other antiviral therapies including hydroxychloroquine, remdesivir, and favipiravir, as well as a broad-spectrum of antibiotics and dexamethasone to treat ARDS. It has been approved by the FDA for the treatment of cytokine storm caused by a variety of diseases [5].

The safety of the tocilizumab and dexamethasone combination for immunocompromised patients is unknown. In addition to this, the risk of superinfection when including steroids in the therapy must be kept in mind [5]. Initial studies resulted in conflicting conclusions because of standardization problems, while other trials with chronically ill patients yielded mixed findings. Tocilizumab therapy, on the other hand, was found to reduce the frequency or length of stay in intensive care units (ICU) and hospitals, as well as the composite rate of mechanical ventilation or death in some studies. Tocilizumab or sarilumab is used to minimize mortality and length of stay in the ICU, as well as to increase the number of organ-support-free days. It has been demonstrated that intravenous administration of tocilizumab at an 8 mg/kg dose results in lower serum IL-6 levels and rapid clinical improvement in patients with COVID-19 pneumonia with ARDS [17].

Chimeric antigen receptor (CAR) T-cell therapy can greatly reduce the rate of cytokine release syndrome (CRS). CRS is characterized by a systemic inflammatory response caused by a large cytokine release, such as IL-6, GM-CSF, and IFN-γ. Tocilizumab, an IL-6 receptor inhibitor, has been approved for the treatment of extreme CRS following CAR T-cell therapy because of its association with rapid improvement of clinical manifestations and a decrease in cytokines, as well as low CAR T-cell toxicity [18].

Sarilumab is a human mAb that binds to the IL-6 receptor and blocks it. The efficacy and protection of sarilumab in adult COVID-19 patients with severe complications is currently being studied in a phase II/III trial [19]. Tocilizumab can cause acute pancreatitis, hypertriglyceridemia, cytopenia, hypofibrinogenemia, elevated ferritin levels, and lactate dehydrogenase in COVID-19 patients. Sarilumab and tocilizumab can cause a dose-dependent increase in liver enzymes in long-term use, which are temporary and/or reversible (occurring during the use of medication) (Table 8.2). Thrombocytopenia and neutropenia are uncommon complications. Long-term use of these medications has also been linked to severe bacterial or fungal infections, and bowel perforation [20].

Siltuximab, another mAb, blocks IL-6 signaling by preventing IL-6 from binding to both soluble and membrane-bound IL-6 receptors. This drug is currently being tested in four clinical trials in COVID-19 patients [21].

8.3.2.2.2 Casirivimab and Imdevimab Combination

Casirivimab and imdevimab (together called REGN-COV2), an mAb combination, are currently being tested in a Phase-III clinical trial. The aim is to stop SARS-CoV-2 in its early stages by focusing on the S protein on the viral surface [22]. Casirivimab and imdevimab bind to non-overlapping epitopes of the SARS-CoV-2 S protein RBD. The combination of casirivimab and imdevimab prevents the SARS-CoV-2 from binding to the host cell ACE2 receptor. The FDA released an EUA on November 21, 2020, for the casirivimab and imdevimab combination available for the treatment of non-hospitalized COVID-19 patients, adults and children aged 12 years or over and weighing 40 kg, who are at high risk of developing serious disease and/or in need of hospitalization (Table 8.2). Safety protocols for casirivimab and imdevimab can be found in Table 8.1.

The combination of casirivimab and imdevimab is not considered standard of care treatment. However, if the clinicians believe that the potential value of the drug combination outweighs the potential harm, it should not be withheld from pregnant women with disorders that put them at high risk of developing serious COVID-19. At both low and high doses, the safety profile was stated to be close to that of placebo. Because of the small number of patients in early phase trials and the low number of hospitalizations or ICU treatment, the clinical value of this combination therapy is not yet recognized [23].

In patients hospitalized due to COVID-19, there was no benefit seen of treatment with the casirivimab and imdevimab combination. Furthermore, mAbs, including casirivimab and imdevimab, have been linked to worse clinical results in hospitalized COVID-19 patients, who need high-flow oxygen or mechanical ventilation.

8.3.2.2.3 Bamlanivimab

Bamlanivimab (also known as LY-CoV555 and LY3819253) is an mAb that targets the RBD of the SARS-CoV-2 S protein. This drug can prevent SARS-CoV-2 from infecting host cells. The FDA released an EUA on November 9, 2020, to make bamlanivimab available for the treatment of non-hospitalized patients with mild to moderate COVID-19 in adults and children who are at high risk of developing serious disease and/or requiring hospitalization. According to

Table 8.1 Safety protocols for casirivimab-imdevimab and bamlanivimab

For casirivimab and imdevimab, individuals classified as high risk under the EUA must meet at least one of the following criteria [23]:

- Body mass index (BMI) of 35 or less
- Kidney failure (chronic)
- Diabetes mellitus
- Conditions that weaken the immune system
- Currently undergoing immunosuppressive therapy
- **65 years of age or older**

55 years old and older, and have:

- Cardiovascular disease (CVD), or
- Hypertension (high blood pressure), or
- COPD (chronic obstructive pulmonary disease) or another chronic respiratory condition

Between the ages of 12 and–17 years and have:

- BMI in the 85th percentile for their age and gender; or
- Sickle cell disease; or
- Heart disease either congenital or acquired; or
- Neurodevelopmental conditions, such as cerebral palsy; or
- A medical-based technical reliance, such as tracheostomy, gastrostomy, or positive pressure ventilation (not related to COVID-19); or
- Asthma, allergic airway disease, or any chronic respiratory disease that necessitates regular medication.

Casirivimab and imdevimab are not authorized for use in patients:

- Hospitalized as a result of COVID-19; or
- Under oxygen therapy as a result of COVID-19; or
- Who need an improvement in baseline oxygen flow rate as a result of COVID-19; or
- On chronic oxygen therapy as a result of an underlying non-COVID-19 associated comorbidity.

For bamlanivimab, individuals under the age of 12 who have one of the following conditions are considered high risk according to the EUA [24]:

- BMI≥35
- Chronic kidney disorder
- Diabetes mellitus
- Disease-inhibiting immune system
- Patients presently receiving immunosuppressive treatment
- People ≥65 years

People ≥55 years who have:

- Heart disease; or
- High blood pressure; or
- COPD (chronic obstructive pulmonary disease) or another chronic respiratory condition.

People between the ages of 12 and 17 who have:

- BMI ≥ 85th percentile based on their age and gender; or
- Sickle cell anemia; or
- Heart disease, either congenital or acquired; or
- A neurodevelopmental condition, cerebral palsy, for example; or
- A medically induced technical dependency, such as tracheostomy, gastrostomy, or positive pressure ventilation (not linked to COVID-19); or
- Asthma, allergic airway disease, or any chronic respiratory disease that necessitates regular medication.

previous reports, among those who received bamlanivimab there were fewer ICU visits and fewer deaths within 28 days of treatment than among those who received placebo. The safety profile of bamlanivimab at all three doses was reportedly close to that seen after placebo treatment. The currently available evidence on the effects of bamlanivimab is insufficient, and because of the lack of demonstration of clinical benefit in hospitalized patients, bamlanivimab should not be considered as the standard of care treatment for COVID-19 patients [24] (Table 8.2).

Table 8.2 mAbs, target, findings, and development stages

mAb	Target	Finding	Stage of Development	References
Tocilizumab	IL-6 inhibition	Maximum clinical studies are on tocilizumab among all the mAbs candidates, as well as mAbs targeting IL-6. Tocilizumab is considered to be the most promising candidate for the management of cytochrome storm in COVID-19. Tocilizumab intervention was frequently associated with improved outcomes and reduced mortality.	Eighty-one concurrent planned/in-process clinical trials are underway. Under evaluation of clinical trials and currently recruiting for REMAP-CAP trials (NCT02735707) in phase IV studying mortality.	[5, 12, 37]
Sarilumab	IL-6 inhibition	Evidence for the efficacy in COVID-19 is currently insufficient, and adequately powered high-quality randomized clinical studies are urgently needed. A single sarilumab RCT demonstrated that intervention was associated with improved outcomes and reduced hospital stays. The data for a trial of sarilumab are not yet available, but press releases indicated no benefit in the whole population, but there was a trend towards reduced mortality in the critically ill group and a trend towards harm in a subgroup not mechanically ventilated.	Currently recruiting for REMAP-CAP trials (NCT02735707) in Phase IV.	[12, 37]
Siltuximab	IL-6 inhibition	Evidence for the efficacy in COVID-19 is currently insufficient and adequately powered high-quality randomized clinical studies are urgently needed. No randomized studies were identified for siltuximab.	Up to now, 4 clinical trials of this drug are underway in COVID-19 patients with one that is testing for Efficacy and Safety at phase II (NCT04329650).	[1, 12]
Casirivimab – Imdevimab	Non-overlapping epitopes of Spike Protein RBD	In patients hospitalized because of COVID-19, there was no benefit of treatment with the casirivimab and imdevimab combination. Furthermore, mAbs including casirivimab and imdevimab have been linked to worse clinical results in hospitalized COVID-19 patients who need high-flow oxygen or mechanical ventilation.	This monoclonal antibody combination is currently being tested in a Phase-III clinical trial.	[13, 16]
Bamlanivimab	RBD of S protein	Because of a lack of demonstration of clinical benefit in hospitalized patients, bamlanivimab should not be considered the standard of care treatment for COVID-19 patients, and safety profile reports close to placebo effect.	Currently 13 clinical trials reported for COVID-19 patients, 3 of them are at phase IV.	[14]

(Continued)

Table 8.2 (Continued) mAbs, target, findings, and development stages

mAb	Target	Finding	Stage of Development	References
Anakinra	Recombinant human IL-1R antagonist	The high-dose Anakinra group survival rate: 90% standard treatment group (did not receive anakinra) survival rate: 56%. (Evidence for the efficacy in COVID-19 is currently insufficient, and adequately powered high-quality randomized clinical studies are urgently needed.)	A randomized Phase 2 and 3 clinical trial of intravenous anakinra in COVID-19 (NCT04324021) have terminated and other 27 out of 35 trial phases are ongoing.	[12]
Canakinumab	Inflammation with IL-1β inhibition	The treatment was associated with: • Rapid reduction in systematic inflammatory response • Increase in oxygenation • Reduced need for intrusive mechanical ventilation and earlier hospital discharge	Two Phase III non-small cell lung cancer clinical trials are ongoing in first-line and adjuvant settings.	[15, 22]
Emapalumab	IFN-γ Neutralizer	Anakinra is tested in COVID-19 patients combined with Emapalumab targeting Interferon gamma to block binding to cell surface receptors and activation of inflammatory signals.	One multi-center randomized clinical trial (NCT04324021) is currently being terminated after Phase 3.	[24]
TJ003234(TJM2)	Anti-GM-CSF	Directly bind GM-CSF with the final common result of blocking the intracellular signaling. Based on current knowledge, this agent can be used to reduce the hyperinflammation caused by SARS-CoV-2 in the course of the disease.	I-Mab Announces IND Clearance from FDA for TJM2 to Treat Cytokine Release Syndrome (CRS) Associated with Severe Coronavirus Disease. Currently at Phase II and III (Placebo).	[6]
Mavrilimumab	Anti-GM-CSF	Improved oxygenation and reduced hospitalization in COVID-19 patients as a result of binding to GM-CSF receptor. It was also well received by the patients, showing clinical benefits in these patients.	Five ongoing placebo trials are currently at Phase II.	[25]
Lenzilumab	Anti-GM-CSF	GM-CSF neutralization with lenzilumab was safe and associated with clinical benefits related to oxygen demand, and cytokine storm in high-risk patients with serious pneumonia.	Two Phase III are currently being studied for evaluation efficacy and safety of Lenzilumab in COVID-19 patients (NCT04351152).	[27]
Gimsilumab	Anti GM-CSF, CSF2	No worthwhile finding yet from solitary trial.	The only registered clinical trial (NCT04351243) was completed on April 1, 2021, with no shared results.	[28]
Meplazumab	Anti-CD147	One study (NCT04275245) reported that giving meplazumab to patients with COVID-19 may lead to a decrease of CRP, increase the virological clearance rate while boosting lymphocytopenia, and result in recovered chest radiography.	A new Safety and Efficacy trial is in Phase 3 (NCT04275245), due to be completed in September 2021.	[1, 30]

Bamlanivimab should not be provided to COVID-19 patients who are not enrolled in a clinical trial. When mAbs such as bamlanivimab are provided to hospitalized COVID-19 patients who need high-flow oxygen or mechanical ventilation, they can have worse clinical outcomes. Bamlanivimab, on the other hand, should not be withheld from pregnant women who have diseases with high risk of progressing to extreme COVID-19 and where clinical evaluation indicates that possible advantages of the drug outweigh the risk. The EUA requires healthcare providers to prescribe and administer bamlanivimab as a single intravenous dose. Anaphylaxis and infusion-related reactions, nausea, diarrhea, dizziness, headache, itching, and vomiting are all possible side effects [24].

Bamlanivimab has been approved by the FDA for the care of non-hospitalized adults and children aged 12 years and above and weighing 40 kg who are at high risk of developing extreme COVID-19 or requiring hospitalization. Safety protocols for bamlanivimab can be found in Table 8.1.

8.3.2.2.4 *Anakinra*

Anakinra is an antagonist for the interleukin IL-1 receptor. This recombinant antibody is used to treat autoinflammatory disorders by blocking the action of IL-1α and IL-1β (proinflammatory cytokines). Anakinra has the advantage of a shorter half-life compared to other cytokine blockers and is therefore suitable for the treatment of critically ill patients [25]. Treatment with high-dose Anakinra was linked to lower serum C-reactive protein levels and improved respiratory function over time (72%) in a retrospective longitudinal analysis of COVID-19 patients with ARDS and hyperinflammation [26]. In addition, the high-dose anakinra group had a survival rate of 90%, while the standard treatment group showed a survival rate of 56% [26] (Table 8.2).

Treatment with anakinra after non-response to corticosteroids or corticosteroids-tocilizumab combination therapy may be a choice for patients with moderate hyperinflammation associated with extreme COVID-19 pneumonia and may result in improved prognosis [27]. Additional studies showed no improved condition from patients with mild to moderate COVID-19 pneumonia treated with anakinra [28].

8.3.2.2.5 *Canakinumab*

Subcutaneous canakinumab administration (against human IL-1) was associated with a rapid reduction in the systemic inflammatory response and an increase in oxygenation without causing any serious side effects [29]. It was also associated with a reduced need for intrusive mechanical

ventilation, earlier hospital discharge, and a better prognosis than standard of care, according to previous studies [29] (Table 8.2). As a result, it represents a therapeutic alternative for adult hospitalized patients with moderate to serious non-ICU complications [30].

8.3.2.2.6 *Emapalumab*

Emapalumab is an anti-IFN-γ antibody that works by preventing IFN-γ from binding to cell surface receptors and activating inflammatory signals. Emapalumab combined with anakinra is being tested in COVID-19 patients currently in a Phase II/III multi-center randomized clinical trial (NCT04324021) [31] (Table 8.2).

8.3.2.2.7 *GM-CSF Inhibitors Gimsilumab, Otilimab, Namilumab, Lenzilumab, TJ003234*

CSL311 targets the GM-CSF receptor, which is the common receptor for GM-CSF, IL-3, and IL-5. TJ003234 (also known as TJM2), received FDA approval to begin a COVID-19 clinical trial [18] (Table 8.2).

Since GM-CSF is widely recognized as a key mediator in inflammation and is secreted by a variety of cells, a single intravenous dose of mavrilimumab improved oxygenation and reduced hospitalization in COVID-19 patients. Thirteen non-mechanically ventilated patients with median age of 57 years (IQR 52–58) were given mavrilimumab. Compared to the control group of 26 patients with similar characteristics who did not receive mavrilimumab, the thirteen treated patients showed earlier improvement. The study concluded the result of eight days mean time to improvement in patients treated with mavrilimumab. The treatment was well received, as mavrilimumab therapy presented clinical benefits in patients with serious COVID-19 pneumonia and systemic hyperinflammation [32].

Lenzilumab was approved by the FDA for compassionate use in COVID-19 patients with moderate or serious COVID-19 pneumonia. Lenzilumab, was authorized to be used as a first-line care alternative in hospitalized patients [33]. GM-CSF neutralization with lenzilumab was safe and associated with clinical benefits related to oxygen demand, and cytokine storm in high-risk patients with serious pneumonia [34].

Gimsilumab (MORAb-022) is a fully human IgG1 mAb, which has been studied for its ability to treat a variety of inflammatory diseases and cancers. In a Phase II clinical trial, gimsilumab was studied for lung injury or ARDS caused by COVID-19 (NCT04351243). The research was carried out in an adaptive design with a planned interim review with no results yet available [35] (Table 8.2).

Meplazumab is an anti-CD147 antibody that has been humanized. Since CD147 is a spike protein receptor for proinflammatory factor Cyclophilin A, meplazumab can prevent virus invasion and replication in host cells by inhibiting viral replication and suppressing inflammation storm. The proinflammatory factor Cyclophilin A binds to the CD147 receptor (CyPA). Since CD147 attracts leukocytes to the stimulated site, it is the intended target for binding inhibition. As a result, meplazumab can protect against cytokine storm [36] (Table 8.2).

According to Huijie Bian et al., adding meplazumab reduced C-reactive protein levels, increased viral clearance rates, facilitated lymphocytopenia, and improved chest radiography recovery [37].

8.4 CONCLUSIONS

REGN-COV2 (casirivimab and imdevimab combination) showed reduced viral load in patients with uninitiated immune response, and subcutaneous administration, reduced the risk of symptomatic infection by 81% in those who were not infected when entering the trial [38, 39]. These results supported the FDA to provide an EUA for REGN-COV2. Other success reports from mAbs are also emerging from recent interim trials. Tocilizumab, for example, is considered to be the most promising among mAbs, with reports indicating significantly reduced mortality rates [5].

Immunology itself is a highly complicated field, and recently has been one of the main topics of research globally. The deadly COVID-19 pandemic further accelerated the studies on understanding immunopathology of many diseases, thus consequently leading to various possible treatment methods. More in-depth studies are required to understand the mechanism of COVID-19 immunopathogenesis in order to implement the most successful immunotherapy strategies [1]. Until now there has been no single molecule or antibody sufficient on its own for the treatment of COVID-19 disease. Moreover, each COVID-19 case needs to be evaluated individually to assess the prognosis and progress of the disease, and to design the immunotherapy accordingly, whether monotherapy or combination therapies.

REFERENCES

1. Masoomikarimi, M., Garmabi, B., Alizadeh, J., Kazemi, E., Azari Jafari, A., Mirmoeeni, S. et al. (2021). Advances in immunotherapy for COVID-19: A comprehensive review. *Int. Immunopharmacol.* 93, 107409. https://doi.org/10.1016/j.intimp.2021.107409.

2. National Institutes of Health (NIH). (2021). NIH halts trial of COVID-19 convalescent plasma in emergency department patients with mild symptoms. Retrieved April 30, 2021, from https://www.nih.gov/news-events/news-releases/nih-halts-trial-covid-19-convalescent-plasma-emergency-department-patients-mild-symptoms.

3. Lee, N., Li, C., Tsai, H., Chen, P., Syue, L., Li, M. et al. (2020). A case of COVID-19 and pneumonia returning from Macau in Taiwan: Clinical course and anti-SARS-CoV-2 IgG dynamic. *J. Microbiol. Immunol. Infect.* 53(3), 485–487. https://doi.org/10.1016/j.jmii.2020.03.003.

4. Martinez, D., Schaefer, A., Leist, S., Li, D., Gully, K., Yount, B. et al. (2021). Prevention and therapy of SARS-CoV-2 and the B.1.351 variant in mice. *Cell Reports* 36, 109450.

5. Patel, S., Saxena, B., Mehta, P. (2021). Recent updates in the clinical trials of therapeutic monoclonal antibodies targeting cytokine storm for the management of COVID-19. *Heliyon* 7(2), e06158. https://doi.org/10.1016/j.heliyon.2021.e06158.

6. Bonaventura, A., Vecchié, A., Wang, T., Lee, E., Cremer, P., Carey, B. et al. (2020). Targeting GM-CSF in COVID-19 pneumonia: Rationale and strategies. *Front. Immunol.* 11. https://doi.org/10.3389/fimmu.2020.01625.

7. Khan, S., Ali, S., Lohana, N. (2020). Convalescent plasma therapy and its century-old untapped potential for COVID-19. *Scimed. J.* 2(4), 234–242. https://doi.org/10.28991/scimedj-2020-0204-6.

8. Wood, E., Estcourt, L., McQuilten, Z. (2021). How should we use convalescent plasma therapies for the management of COVID-19? *Blood* 137(12), 1573–1581.

9. FDA. (2021). Convalescent plasma EUA letter of authorization. Retrieved April 30, 2021, from https://www.fda.gov/media/141477/.

10. Wood, E., Estcourt, L., McQuilten, Z. (2021). How should we use convalescent plasma therapies for the management of COVID-19. *Blood*, 137(12), 1573–1581.

11. Recoverytrial.net. (2021). RECOVERY trial closes recruitment to convalescent plasma treatment for patients hospitalised with COVID-19 – RECOVERY Trial. Retrieved April 29, 2021, from https://www.recoverytrial.net/news/statement-from-the-recovery-trial-chief-investigators-15-january-2021-recovery-trial-closes-recruitment-to-convalescent-plasma-treatment-for-patients-hospitalised-with-covid-19.

12. National Institutes of Health (NIH). (2021). NIH halts trial of COVID-19 convalescent plasma in emergency department patients with mild symptoms. Retrieved April 30, 2021, from https://www.nih.gov/news-events/news-releases/nih-halts-trial-covid-19-convalescent-plasma-emergency-department-patients-mild-symptoms.

13. FDA. (2021). Convalescent plasma EUA letter of authorization. Retrieved April 15, 2021, from https://www.fda.gov/media/141477/.

14. Angus, D., Gordon, A., Bauchner, H. (2021). Emerging lessons from COVID-19 for the US clinical research enterprise. *JAMA* 325(12), 1159. https://doi.org/10.1001/jama.2021.3284.

15. Xie, Y., Cao, S., Dong, H., Li, Q., Chen, E., Zhang, W. et al. (2020). Effect of regular intravenous immunoglobulin therapy on prognosis of severe pneumonia in patients with COVID-19. *J. Infect.* 81(2), 318–356. https://doi.org/10.1016/j.jinf.2020.03.044.

16. Patel, S., Saxena, B., Mehta, P. (2021). Recent updates in the clinical trials of therapeutic monoclonal antibodies targeting cytokine storm for the management of COVID-19. *Heliyon* 7(2), e06158.

17. Samaee, H., Mohsenzadegan, M., Ala, S., Maroufi, S.S., Moradimajd, P. (2020). Published online September 16, 2020. Tocilizumab for treatment patients with COVID-19: Recommended medication for novel disease. *Int. Immunopharmacol.* 89, 107018.

18. Bonaventura, A., Vecchié, A., Wang, T., Lee, E., Cremer, P., Carey, B. et al. (2020). Targeting GM-CSF in COVID-19 pneumonia: Rationale and strategies. *Front. Immunol.* 11. https://doi.org/10.3389/fimmu.2020.01625.

19. Sancho-Lopez, A., Caballero-Bermejo, A.F., Ruiz-Antorán, B., Rubio, E.M., Gasalla, M.G., Buades, J., et al. (2021). Efficacy and safety of Sarilumab in patients with COVID-19 pneumonia: A randomized, Phase III Clinical Trial (SARTRE Study). *Infect. Dis. Ther.* 10, 2735–2748.

20. Khan, F., Stewart, I., Fabbri, L., Moss, S., Robinson, K., Smyth, A., Jenkins, G. (2021). Systematic review and meta-analysis of anakinra, sarilumab, siltuximab and tocilizumab for COVID-19. *Thorax* 1(13). https://doi.org/10.1136/thoraxjnl-2020-215266.

21. Palanques-Pastor, T., López-Briz, E., Andrés, J.L.P. (2020). Involvement of interleukin 6 in SARS-CoV-2 infection: Siltuximab as a therapeutic option against COVID-19. *Eur. J. Hosp. Pharm.* 27, 297–298.

22. Aomar-Millán, I., Salvatierra, J., Torres-Parejo, Ú., Faro-Miguez, N., Callejas-Rubio, J., Ceballos-Torres, Á. et al. (2021). Anakinra after treatment with corticosteroids alone or with tocilizumab in patients with severe COVID-19 pneumonia and moderate hyperinflammation: A retrospective cohort study. *Intern. Emerg. Med.* 16. https://doi.org/10.1007/s11739-020-02600-z

23. FDA.gov. (2021). Fact sheet for health care providers emergency use authorization (EUA) of casirivimab and imdevimab. Retrieved April 30, 2021, from https://www.fda.gov/media/143892/download.

24. U.S. Food and Drug Administration. (2021). Coronavirus (COVID-19) update: November 9, 2020. Retrieved April 30, 2021, from https://www.fda.gov/news-events/press-announcements/coronavirus-covid-19-update-november-9-2020.

25. Cavalli, G., Dinarello, C. (2018). Anakinra therapy for non-cancer inflammatory diseases. *Front. Pharmacol.* 9(1157). https://doi.org/10.3389/fphar.2018.01157.

26. Cavalli, G., De Luca, G., Campochiaro, C., Della-Torre, E., Ripa, M., Canetti, D. et al. (2020). Interleukin-1 blockade with high-dose anakinra in patients with COVID-19, acute respiratory distress syndrome, and hyperinflammation: A retrospective cohort study. *Lancet Rheumatol.* 2(6), e325–e331. https://doi.org/10.1016/s2665-9913(20)30127-2.

27. Aomar-Millán, I., Salvatierra, J., Torres-Parejo, Ú., Faro-Miguez, N., Callejas-Rubio, J., Ceballos-Torres, Á. et al. (2021). Anakinra after treatment with corticosteroids alone or with tocilizumab in patients with severe COVID-19 pneumonia and moderate hyperinflammation: A retrospective cohort study. *Intern. Emerg. Med.* 1(10). https://doi.org/10.1007/s11739-020-02600-z.

28. Tharaux, P., Pialoux, G., Pavot, A., Mariette, X., Hermine, O., Resche-Rigon, M. et al. (2021). Effect of anakinra versus usual care in adults in hospital with COVID-19 and mild-to-moderate pneumonia (CORIMUNO-ANA-1): A randomised controlled trial. *Lancet Respir. Med.* 9(3), 295–304. https://doi.org/10.1016/s2213-2600(20)30556-7.

29. Ucciferri, C., Auricchio, A., Di Nicola, M., Potere, N., Abbate, A., Cipollone, F. et al. (2020). Canakinumab in a subgroup of patients with COVID-19. *Lancet Rheumatol.* 2(8), e457–e458. https://doi.org/10.1016/s2665-9913(20)30167-3.

30. Katia, F., Myriam, D., Ucciferri, C., Auricchio, A., Di Nicola, M., Marchioni, M. et al. (2021). Efficacy of canakinumab in mild or severe COVID-19 pneumonia. *Immun. Inflam. Dis.* 1(7). https://doi.org/10.1002/iid3.400.

31. Magro, G. (2020). COVID-19: Review on latest available drugs and therapies against SARS-CoV-2. Coagulation and inflammation crosstalking. *Virus Res.* 286, 198070. https://doi.org/10.1016/j.virusres.2020.198070.

32. De Luca, G., Cavalli, G., Campochiaro, C., Della-Torre, E., Angelillo, P., Tomelleri, A. et al. (2020). GM-CSF blockade with mavrilimumab in severe COVID-19 pneumonia and systemic hyperinflammation: A single-centre, prospective cohort study. *Lancet Rheumatol.* 2(8), e465–e473. https://doi.org/10.1016/s2665-9913(20)30170-3.

33. Temesgen, Z., Assi, M., Shweta, F., Vergidis, P., Rizza, S., Bauer, P. et al. (2020). GM-CSF neutralization with lenzilumab in severe COVID-19 pneumonia. *Mayo Clin. Proc.* 95(11), 2382–2394. https://doi.org/10.1016/j.mayocp.2020.08.038.

34. Temesgen, Z., Assi, M., Vergidis, P., Rizza, S., Bauer, P., Pickering, B. et al. (2020). First clinical

use of lenzilumab to neutralize GM-CSF in patients with severe and critical COVID-19 pneumonia. https://doi.org/10.1101/2020.06.08.20125369.

35. Clinicaltrials.gov. A study to assess the efficacy and safety of gimsilumab in subjects with lung injury or acute respiratory distress syndrome secondary to COVID-19 (BREATHE): Full text view. Retrieved April 30, 2021, from https://clinicaltrials.gov/ct2/show/NCT04351243.

36. Bian, H., Zheng, Z., Wei, D., Zhang, Z., Kang, W., Hao, C. et al. (2020). Meplazumab treats COVID-19 pneumonia: An open-labelled, concurrent controlled add-on clinical trial. https://doi.org/10.1101/2020.03.21.20040691.

37. REMAP-CAP Investigators. (2021). Interleukin-6 receptor antagonists in critically ill patients with COVID-19. *N. Engl. J. Med.* 384(16), 1491–1502. https://doi.org/10.1056/nejmoa2100433.

38. Roche.com. (2021). Phase III prevention trial showed subcutaneous administration of investigational antibody cocktail casirivimab and imdevimab reduced risk of symptomatic COVID-19 infections by 81%. [online]. Retrieved from https://www.roche.com/media/releases/med-cor-2021-04-12.htm [Accessed May 11, 2021].

39. O'Brien, M.P., Forleo-Neto, E., Musser, B.J., et al. Subcutaneous REGEN-COV2 antibody combination to prevent COVID-19. *N. Engl. J. Med.* 385(13), 2021. 1184–1195.

Chapter 9 Application of Stem Cell and Exosome-Based Therapy in COVID-19

Suleyman Gokhan Kara and Ayla Eker Sariboyaci

9.1 WHAT IS COVID-19? PATHOGENESIS, IMMUNE RESPONSE, AND THERAPEUTIC STRATEGIES

COVID-19 is an infectious disease caused by SARS-CoV-2. The transmission occurs mainly through respiratory droplets, and results in respiratory tract infection. The spectrum of the disease ranges from asymptomatic to critical illness. Patients with mild illness have mild symptoms such as fever, cough, and fatigue. The severe form of COVID-19 progresses rapidly to acute respiratory distress syndrome (ARDS) because of the infiltration of monocytes and macrophages, diffused alveolar damage, and cellular fibromyxoid exudates. ARDS is a life-threatening condition characterized by acute onset of respiratory failure, unexplained volume overload, severe hypoxemia requiring ventilation support, and diffuse opacities in chest radiography. In ARDS, the lung will have some injuries such as diffused alveolar and endothelium damage, and vascular permeability will be increased, causing poor oxygenation. Most of the severe COVID-19 patients develop ARDS. Patients with severe illness develop dyspnea, have a respiratory rate of 30/min, SaO2 <93%, PaO2/FiO2 <300, and/or lung infiltrates >50% within 24–48 hours [1]. In critical cases, respiratory failure, septic shock, and/or multiple organ dysfunction are additionally seen [1].

In COVID-19 patients, the SARS-CoV-2 infects type II pneumocytes and other cells that express ACE2. The SARS-CoV-2 binds to host cell ACE2 receptors via its Spike (S) protein and interferes with the host's immune response via nucleocapsid (N) and envelope (E) proteins. The immune response against SARS-CoV-2 occurs as a combination of cell-mediated immunity and antibody production. Chemokines secreted from infected cells cause the influx of neutrophils, macrophages, and T cells. The accumulation of inflammatory cells causes the production of a large number of pro-inflammatory cytokines, which in turn induce a cytokine storm. IL-1, IL-2, IL-6, TNF-α, and IFN-γ, are components of normal immune responses which unintentionally trigger the cytokine storm. The cytokine storm may lead to death via the immune reaction, and it can cause ARDS and multiple organ failures. Cytokine storms are the main reason for the progress of ARDS in COVID-19 patients.

Glucocorticoids, remdesivir, baricitinib, tocilizumab, hydroxychloroquine/chloroquine, favipiravir, and interferons are medicines used for the treatment of COVID-19. Despite all these available drugs, mortality has remained high, especially in severe and critically ill patients. Anti-inflammatory treatment has been proposed but challenged with the dilemma of balancing the risk of secondary infections. The use of immunosuppressant agents has been associated with an increased risk of severe disease of other respiratory infections. Therefore effective treatment methods are needed. Theoretically, the critical role of mesenchymal stem cell (MSC)-based treatment of COVID-19 is that it creates an anti-inflammatory effect without causing secondary infections. MSCs and MSCs-derived exosomes are being tested in clinical trials for treating COVID-19, and the results are promising.

9.2 MESENCHYMAL STEM CELLS (MSCs) AND MSC-DERIVED EXOSOMES

MSCs were first mentioned in 1867 by the pathologist Julius Friedrich Cohnheim. While MSCs were described long ago in the literature, their first use in clinical trials was in 1995. The main characteristics of MSCs that made them attractive for therapeutic use are self-renewal, regeneration, multidirectional differentiation, immunomodulation, antimicrobial effect, and homing properties. MSCs are thought to have possibilities for broad clinical applications, including the treatment of ARDS. MSCs are effective in treating ARDS because they increase alveolar fluid clearance and regulate pulmonary vascular endothelial permeability. Similarly, MSC-derived exosomes have also demonstrated a strong ability to repair, regenerate, and immunomodulate organ damage, which also play essential roles in treating ARDS. MSCs migrate to the damaged area because of the homing effect, and studies are ongoing to increase this effect. Pre-treatment of MSCs with hypoxia, activation of the FAK/ERK signaling pathway, binding CD90 to specific integrins b3 and b5, activation of integrin b1 and b5, and using nanotechnological carriers represent attempts to increase the effect. However, despite all these approaches, the efficacy of MSC engraftment is still unsatisfactory.

DOI: 10.1201/9781003190394-9

Engraftment rates in lung injury models were less than 1%. Therefore studies have focused on the ability of MSCs to secrete paracrine factors such as antiapoptotic, angiogenic, immunoregulatory, and cell migration factors. The beneficial effects of MSCs are thought to be mainly as a result of paracrine mechanisms.

MSCs can be isolated from various sources of tissue, such as bone marrow, umbilical cord, adipose tissue, dental pulp, and other tissues. MSCs from different sources have significant similarities, but some studies have shown that minor differences have been discovered depending on the MSC source. Therefore it is essential to indicate the source from which MSCs are isolated in studies.

Minimal criteria for defining MSCs were established by ISCT (International Society for Cell & Gene Therapy) in 2006. MSCs must ensure adherence to plastic, and they are characterized by the presence of cell surface markers ($\geq$95% must expresses CD105, CD73, CD90, and $\leq$2% must lack expression of CD45, CD34, CD14 or CD11b, CD79α or CD19, and HLA class II). Additionally, MSCs must differentiate into osteoblasts, adipocytes, and chondroblasts under standard in vitro–differentiating conditions [2].

Both allogeneic and autologous MSCs are used in clinical studies. Many studies have shown that allogeneic MSC treatments do not stimulate significant alloimmune reactions, and do not show more severe side effects than autologous MSC treatments. The main advantage of the allogeneic treatment is that it can be used immediately in acute cases without waiting for the production process.

MSC-derived exosomes have recently been used in clinical trials. Since exosomes cannot replicate, they cannot transform into malignant cells. Furthermore, they are less likely to trigger an immunogenic response, have no teratogenic activity, cannot be infected with microbes, and they contain no adventitious agents. Also, exosomes have been used for immunomodulation. MSC-derived exosomes overcome most limitations of MSC treatment. Exosomes have similar functions to their origin cells, and they carry the cell's genomic components. Exosomes are produced by all cell types, particularly by MSCs. Accordingly, exosomes could provide an alternative treatment strategy for MSC-based therapies, since the MSC-based therapies still have hurdles to overcome, including unintentional differentiation of cells, large-scale production, reconstitution limitations of cryopreserved cells, storage of cells, gene mutations, immune rejection, and tumorigenesis or tumor promotion. The use of MSCs has shown promise as they target multiple pathways such as regeneration, immunomodulation, and antimicrobial effects.

9.3 CHARACTERISTICS OF MSCs AND MSC-DERIVED EXOSOMES IN COVID-19: CLINICAL EFFICACY

9.3.1 Immunomodulation

The term immunomodulation is used to restore the immune response and maintain homeostasis. Immunomodulators are used as immunosuppression in autoimmune diseases and organ transplant rejection. Moreover, they can be used for immunostimulation in cancer and immunodeficiency. Immunosuppressants inhibit the immune response, whereas immunostimulants increase the immune response.

In clinical studies, MSC-based treatment interventions have been used for years for immunomodulation. First, in 2002, MSCs were demonstrated to modulate immunosuppression, In particular, the suppression of mixed lymphocyte response in vitro, and prevention of rejection in a baboon skin allograft model in vivo were demonstrated [3]. In 2006, they were used in steroid-refractory GvHD in humans, and promising results were obtained [4]. Since then, MSCs have been tested as immunomodulators for many diseases. Consequently, MSC-mediated immunomodulation has been approved for GvHD, type 1 diabetes, and Crohn's disease in New Zealand, Canada, and Japan [5].

The balance of the immune reaction in sepsis is crucial. When immunosuppression is dominant, the infection increases, and when immunostimulation is dominant, life-threatening systemic inflammatory syndromes develop, such as cytokine storm and ARDS. Therefore, the use of immunomodulators in infectious diseases is essential. ARDS and secondary bacterial infections are among the most common causes of death in COVID-19 patients; because of the immunomodulation effect of MSCs, these life-threatening situations can be prevented.

MSCs can modulate the entire immune system, including both innate and adaptive immune responses. In particular, they can reduce the inflow and aggregation of neutrophils, can suppress pro-inflammatory cells (CD4 T helper cells, CD8 cytotoxic T cells, and macrophages), induce their differentiation into anti-inflammatory variants (regulatory T cells (Treg), and M2 macrophages), and inhibit the activity of dendritic cells (DCs) and natural killer (NK) cells, as well as inhibiting the proliferation of T cells, B cells, DCs, and NK cells [6–9].

MSC-mediated immunomodulation is regulated through cell-to-cell contact and various soluble factors. It has been found that the stimulation of the surface receptors of MSCs by RNA viruses leads to immunomodulation. The immunomodulation of MSCs is mediated by TLRs (mainly TLR3 and TLR4) present on the surface of MSCs [10]. RNA viruses activate these TLRs, which leads to secretion of chemokines (MIP-1α, MIP-1β, CXCL9, CXCL10, CXCL11, and RANTES), and these initiate the anti-inflammatory immune response [10]. This response can be beneficial in a cytokine storm, where a hyper-proinflammatory response is triggered by SARS-CoV-2 in COVID-19 patients.

Hypersecretion of pro-inflammatory cytokines stimulates MSCs to release IL-10, and soluble factors such as PGE2, NO, and IDO. MSCs decrease the production of TNF-α and IL-12 by secreting IL-10, which mediates cell cycle arrest by repressing the transcription of STAT-5 in T-cells, and decreasing the proliferation of activated T-cells. Similarly, PGE2 acts with IDO to alter the proliferation of T cells and NK cells, as IDO leads to apoptosis of the activated T-cells, and PGE2 leads to the suppression of T cells, NK cells, and macrophages [11].

MSCs are also effective for fibrosis treatment. MSCs have strong antifibrotic effects and can alleviate lung fibrosis. Remarkably, the immunomodulation effect of MSCs prevents fibrosis by inhibition of the TGF-β1 pathway and the reduction of oxidative stress.

9.3.2 Regeneration and Repair

MSCs have the properties of regeneration and repair by reducing inflammation, decreasing cell death, the secretion of cell-protective substances, anti-oxidative effects, regulating the microenvironment, and performing regeneration of irreversible damage.

Oxidative stress, which is the primary cause of cell damage, is reduced by MSCs in several ways. MSCs can transfer their mitochondria to damaged cells. So, the damaged cell reduces reactive oxygen species (ROS) levels and shifts the metabolism to oxidative phosphorylation, promoting cell survival, and reducing cell death. Moreover, MSCs activate antioxidant signaling pathways such as AKT/pAKT and ERK1/2/pERK in damaged cells. Though the mechanisms are not completely clear, the regulation of the microenvironment and the released mediators make MSCs responsible for therapy. MSC-based therapeutic applications are currently being tested in clinical trials on neurodegenerative diseases because of their oxidative-stress-reducing effects, and the results of these trials are promising.

The homing effect of MSCs is much lower than expected. So, how can it repair tissue without migrating sufficiently to the damaged area? The answer is the paracrine effect; MSCs can release soluble factors for repair-damaged cells. The best-known factors secreted from MSCs are fibroblast growth factor-2 (FGF2), hepatocyte growth factor (HGF), keratinocyte growth factor (KGF), insulin-like growth factor (IGF), vascular endothelial growth factor (VEGF), pigmented epithelium-derived factor (PEDF), placental growth factor (PLGF), stromal cell-derived factor-1 (SDF1), tumor necrosis factor-inducible gene 6 protein (TSG6), matrix metalloproteinases (MMP), tissue inhibitor of metalloproteinases (TIMP), angiogenin, angiopoietin-1 (Ang-1), and thrombospondin-1. These factors have many functions, including cell repair, microenvironment regulation, promoting regeneration, tissue vascularization, prevention of fibrosis, reduction in inflammation, and anti-apoptotic effects. In addition to these factors, because exosomes carry genomic elements of the MSCs, the MSC-derived exosomes stimulate gene-mediated repair.

If the cell damage is irreversible or the cell is dead, regeneration is the only option. MSCs are used in regeneration because of their multipotency and differentiation properties. MSCs were first tried in experiments because of their regenerative properties. Initially, the focus was on the ability of MSCs to differentiate in vivo and transform into musculoskeletal system cells such as osteoblasts, chondrocytes, adipocytes, and myoblasts. Accumulated experience confirmed that the regeneration ability of MSC is effective even in neurons that are thought to be non-regenerative.

MSCs that migrate to the damaged areas can regenerate tissue by differentiation into the target cells. Regeneration can occur even when stem cell transplantation cannot be applied directly to the damaged tissue. The reason is that MSCs can differentiate themselves into tissue cells as well as stimulate local stem cells in the tissue to differentiate. MSC-derived exosomes, which are not cellular structures and therefore cannot differentiate, regenerate tissue in this way. For example, it has been shown that lung stem cells (LSC) play an active role in lung regeneration, and that regeneration is promoted by exogenous stem cell transplantation.

MSCs are being tested in lung damage caused by COVID-19 through their ability of endothelial and epithelial repair, bacterial and alveolar fluid clearance, and their anti-inflammatory and anti-apoptotic effects. COVID-19 pneumonia occurs because of damage to the alveoli. It is necessary to know alveolar histopathology to understand the mechanism of damage. The alveolar epithelium consists of Type I and Type II pneumocytes. Type I pneumocytes occupy 95% of the alveolar surface and are responsible for gas exchange, while Type II pneumocytes secrete surfactant, reduce alveolar surface tension, and protect from alveolar collapse. In COVID-19 pneumonia, Type II pneumocytes become infected by the virus, and cell death occurs. The decrease in surfactant causes alveolar collapse. The migration of inflammatory cells and mediators into the alveoli results in the development of alveolar oedema. As a result of these events, cell death also occurs in Type I pneumocytes. Lung alveolar epithelium has limited regeneration. Type I pneumocytes are unable to replicate. In the event of damage, Type II pneumocytes can proliferate and differentiate into Type I pneumocytes. The function of this repair mechanism changes according to the extent of the damage. When alveolar damage is mild, a repair mechanism preserves lung function. However, if there is extensive alveolar damage, fibrosis or emphysema develops, and the alveoli lose their function.

Inflammation in the alveoli also damages the capillary vessels. VEGF and HGF released from MSCs stabilize endothelial barrier function by restoring pulmonary capillary permeability. MSCs protect the lung endothelial barrier by inhibiting capillary endothelial cell apoptosis, and enhance VE-cadherin recovery. MSCs also secrete FGF7 and Ang-1 for the clearance of alveolar fluid [12]. Also, Ang-1 restores epithelial and endothelial permeability. MSCs can promote the regeneration of Type II pneumocytes by secreting KGF, VEGF, and HGF to repair the alveolar epithelial barrier in injured lung tissue and prevent the apoptosis of endothelial cells in COVID-19 patients. Alveolar damage in COVID-19 pneumonia can cause permanent lung damage to the patient. The treatment strategy should be to prevent permanent damage to the alveoli and to regenerate the damage. For these reasons, MSCs are promising in COVID-19 pneumonia.

9.3.3 Antimicrobial Activity

MSC-based therapy has already shown promise in viral infections such as HIV, hepatitis B virus, virus-associated ARDS, influenza, and coronavirus-associated lung injuries. The effectiveness of MSC-based treatments in virus-associated ARDS is the reason why it is used for COVID-19 studies. MSCs have been thought to neutralize free virus particles by producing antibiotic proteins such as LL37, which bind to virus and lung cell-binding sites [13]. LL37 can also inhibit neutrophil intravasation and NET formation, favoring bacterial clearance [14]. MSCs show most of their antimicrobial effect by immunomodulation. MSCs increase phagocytosis and support bacterial clearance by modulating M1 macrophages [14].

9.4 CLINICAL TRIALS USING MSCs AND MSC-DERIVED EXOSOMES

Since the COVID-19 pandemic started, many strategies have been tried to treat the disease. Among these treatment strategies, MSC-based therapy has been used in the clinical trials of ARDS since 2014, which has attracted attention. These treatment methods, which were previously only cell-based, went down to the level of vesicles with the advancement of medicine and have been tried in clinical studies. Both MSCs and MSC-derived exosomes as a cell-free approach, have been subjected to clinical trials. The MSC-derived exosomes have hypoimmunogenic properties and are enclosed in a lipid bilayer, which make them extraordinarily stable and suitable for transport to the target organ rather than via accumulation through the bloodstream. MSC-derived exosomes could attenuate the inflammatory response, switch it to a reparative phenotype, heal the alveolar epithelium, implement its regeneration, repair lung vascular damage, ameliorate and prevent pulmonary fibrosis. For these reasons, MSC-derived exosomes can be beneficial to treat lung injury.

Recent studies have demonstrated the importance of stem cells in the restoration of lung function. Thus the published data where stem cells were applied to treat virus-related ARDS point to a possible role of MSC-based therapies for COVID-19 [14]. Some case reports on the safety and efficacy of stem cells in COVID-19 have shown that stem cell–based therapies reduce inflammation by lowering cytokine levels without causing allergic reactions. Consequently, these reports have provided the opportunity for large-scale studies. While the results of clinical trial data are motivating, it will still be too early to predict the potential therapeutic role of MSCs in COVID-19. Therefore, large-scale trials of MSC therapy should be conducted to confirm their clinical efficacy. Considering the properties of MSCs and their exosomes, they are theoretically suitable for ARDS treatment. However, because of the lack of large-scale clinical studies, the MSC-based approach still cannot be used as routine therapy. Sufficiently robust clinical trials are urgently needed to test clinical outcomes in patients with COVID-19, and should use well-characterized MSC products with documented safety profiles from FDA-approved studies.

There are many studies where MSCs and MSC-derived exosomes are used in the treatment of COVID-19 (Table 9.1). The mechanisms behind MSC therapy and MSC-derived exosome therapy in COVID-19 are illustrated in Figure 9.1.

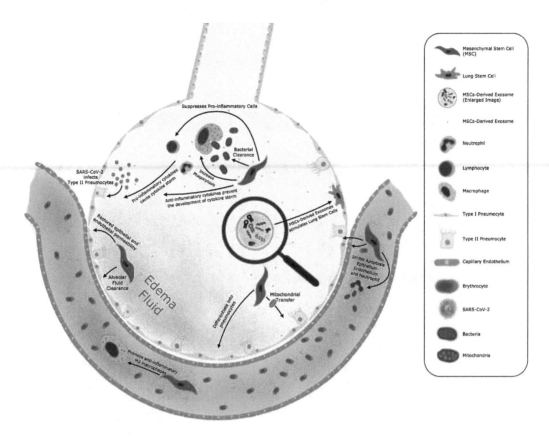

Figure 9.1.   Graphical illustration of mechanisms behind MSC-therapy and MSC-derived exosome therapy in COVID-19. As a result of SARS-CoV-2 infecting Type II pneumocytes, neutrophils, lymphocytes, and macrophages migrate to the alveoli. Cytokine
storm occurs as a result of excessive release of pro-inflammatory cytokines such as
IL-1, IL-2, IL-6, TNF-a, and IFN-y. Pneumocytes and capillary endothelium are damaged, and as a result of impaired permeability, intra-alveolar edema fluid develops.
Bacteria can cause secondary infections. MSCs suppress pro-inflammatory cells by
secreting soluble factors such as IL-10, PGE2, NO, IDO. MSCs indirectly increase the
release of anti-inflammatory factors by promoting the transformation of cells of anti-
inflammatory phenotypes such as M2 macrophage and Treg. MSCs maintain bacterial clearance by secreting LL-37 and by inducing phagocytosis of neutrophils and
macrophages. Fibroblast growth factor-2 (FGF2), hepatocyte growth factor (HGF),
keratinocyte growth factor (KGF), insulin-like growth factor (IGF), vascular endothelial growth factor (VEGF), pigmented epithelium-derived factor (PEDF), placental
growth factor (PLGF), stromal cell-derived factor-1 (SDF1), tumor necrosis factor-
inducible gene 6 protein (TSG6), matrix metalloproteinases (MMP), tissue inhibitor
of metalloproteinases (TIMP), angiogenin, and angiopoietin-1 (Ang -1) regulate epithelial and endothelial permeability by secreting thrombospondin-1. MSCs suppress
apoptosis of epithelium, endothelium, and neutrophils and transfer their mitochondria to damaged cells. MSCs differentiate into cells and provide regeneration. The
immunomodulation and antimicrobial effects of MSCs occur through the exosomes
they secrete. MSC-derived exosomes also support regeneration by stimulating lung
stem cells. MSC: Mesenchymal stem cells. COVID-19: Coronavirus disease. SARS-
CoV-2: Severe acute respiratory syndrome coronavirus 2.

Table 9.1 Clinical trials of stem cell–based therapy in COVID-19

Study Type	Aim	Study Groups	Design	Intervention/ Details of Stem Cell Use	Outcomes	Conclusion	References
A prospective non-randomized open-label cohort study	Safety and efficacy of exosomes derived mesenchymal stem cells for the treatment in COVID-19	24 severe COVID-19 patients	Patients who received MSC-derived exosomes were evaluated for safety and efficacy from days 1–14	ExoFlo™, Exosomes derived from allogeneic human bone marrow mesenchymal stem cells, Commercial product, 15 ml	The survival rate was 83.71% patients recovered, 13% patients remained critically ill, 16% of patients expired. Patients' PaO2/FiO2 increase of 192%. Lymphocyte counts increased. CRP, ferritin, and D-dimer reduced	ExoFlo is safe and effective in COVID-19	[15]
Open-label, individually randomized, standard treatment-controlled trial	Safety and efficacy of hUC-MSCs for the treatment in COVID-19	Total: 41 COVID-19 patients Treatment Group: 12 severe COVID-19 patients Control Group: 29 severe COVID-19 Patients	Progression of disease, mortality, CRP, lymphocyte number, and IL-6, and imaging changes were observed	hUC-MSCs were suspended in 100 ml of normal saline, and the total number of transplanted cells was calculated as 2×10^6 cells/kg.	28-day mortality rate was 0 in the treatment group, while the mortality rate was 10.34% in the control group. In the treatment group, the time to clinical improvement was shorter than control. CRP and IL-6 levels were lower from day 3 and lymphocyte count return to the normal range, and lung inflammation absorption was shorter on CT imaging in the treatment group than the control	Intravenous transplantation of hUC-MSCs is safe and effective in severe COVID-19.	[16]
The Non-randomized parallel trial, Phase 1 trial	To show UC-MSCs are safe for use in moderate and severe COVID-19 patients	Total: 18 COVID-19 patients Treatment Group: 5 moderate, 4 severe COVID-19 patients Control Group: 5 moderate, 4 severe COVID-19 patients	Side effects have been evaluated	Received intravenous infusion of allogeneic 3×10^7 UC-MSCs cells infusion on days 0, 3, and 6	UC-MSC has not been found effective but is safe	The use of UC-MSCs to treat COVID-19 is safe	[17]
Randomized, double-blind, and placebo-controlled Phase 2 trial	To assess the efficacy and safety of UC-MSCs to treat severe COVID-19 patients with lung damage	Total: 100 severe COVID-19 patients Treatment group: 65 patients Placebo Group: 35 patients	Lung lesions and capacity were monitored from baseline to day 28	4×10^7 UC-MSCs cells per intravenous infusion Receive treatment or placebo on days 0, 3, and 6	UC-MSCs reduced lesion volume in the lung compared with placebo. Lung capacity increased in patients treated with UC-MSCs. The adverse events were similar in the two groups	UC-MSCs treatment is safe and effective in COVID-19	[18]

Phase 1 Trial	To demonstrate the effects and safety of stem cell therapies	11 patients critically ill COVID-19-induced ARDS	Mortality, clinical symptom improvement, laboratory and imaging changes were observed	The patients received three intravenous infusions 2×10^8 cells every other day for a total of 6×10^8 MSCs UC-MSCs; 6 cases PL-MSCs; 5 cases	No serious adverse events reported. Reduced dyspnea and increased SpO_2 after treatment in 7 patients. Of these 7 patients, 5 were discharged from the ICU in 4 days, one patient was discharged from the ICU on day 18, and one patient suddenly developed cardiac arrest on day 7. Four patients died on day 10.	Multiple infusions of MSCs are safe and effective in critically ill COVID-19–induced ARDS patients	[19]
Phase 1 Trial	Investigate whether MSC transplantation improves the outcome in COVID-19 patients	Total: 10 COVID-19 patients Treatment Group: 7 patients Placebo Group: 3 patients	Patients were followed for 14 days	1×10^6 cells per kg MSCs in 100 ml normal saline for intravenous infusion. The type of MSC is not described in the article, but it has been reported as ACE2- and TMPRSS2	The pulmonary function and symptoms improved in 2 days after MSC transplantation. Lymphocytes were increased, CRP decreased, and overactivated cytokine-secreting immune cells disappeared. TNF-α was decreased, while IL-10 increased	The intravenous transplantation of MSCs was safe and effective for treatment in COVID-19	[20]

Note: Clinical trials that have been completed and published in the literature are shown in the table.
Abbreviations: MSC: Mesenchymal stem cell; CRP: C-reactive protein; UC-MSC: Umbilical cord-derived mesenchymal stem cell; IL-6: Interleukin-6; hUC-MSC: Human umbilical cord-derived mesenchymal stem cell; CT: Computerized tomography; ARDS: Acute respiratory distress syndrome; PL-MSC: Placenta-derived mesenchymal stem cell; SpO$_2$: Pulse oximetry; ICU: Intensive care unit; ACE2: Angiotensin-converting enzyme 2; TMPRSS2: Transmembrane protease serine 2; TNF-α: Tumor necrosis factor-α; IL-10: Interleukin-10.

9.5 UNIQUE CHALLENGES OF MSCs AND MSC-DERIVED EXOSOME THERAPY FOR COVID-19

Chemical agents are used primarily in the treatment of diseases. Unlike other treatments, MSC treatments are cell-based, but the use of living cells generates many problems. Unfortunately, as time passes, cells may become less effective because of senescence. If appropriate conditions are not provided, the cells can die and lose their effectiveness completely. Storage conditions at low temperatures such as –196°C are required for cell preservation. It may not be easy to provide these conditions everywhere. Also, after thawing the cryopreserved cells, it is necessary to evaluate their viability.

For MSCs to be used in clinical trials, they must be of human origin and produced under sterile conditions according to GMP laboratory standards. It is not always possible to follow these standards.

Stem cells can be isolated from different sources. They may show different effectiveness depending on the isolated tissue. Also, the age of the isolated source can affect the efficiency of the cells. For example, fetal stem cells have a greater differentiation capacity than adult stem cells. That is why it is essential to specify the source of stem cells used in studies.

Different doses of cells have been used in different studies [21]. Generally, the applied doses were based on those demonstrated effective and safe in previous studies. There is no consensus on the appropriate dosage. A study that is ineffective because of an insufficient dose use, or a study that is found not to be safe because of high doses may distract us from MSC-based treatments. Therefore, Phase 1 studies are of great importance and they should be designed for treatment safety, focusing explicitly on pharmacokinetics and pharmacodynamics. It is crucial to establish the therapeutic index to study the safety of MSCs as a drug, so the amount of MSCs that provides the therapeutic effect does not cause toxicity.

Another difficulty encountered with MSC-based treatments is the optimal route of administration. MSCs can be applied directly to the target tissue, or by intravenous administration expected to reach the target tissue via the bloodstream. In COVID-19 clinical trials, MSC-based therapies were administered both intravenously and by inhalation. While MSC-based therapies in COVID-19 studies have been reported to be efficacious with both intravenous and inhalation routes, both have advantages and disadvantages. The inhalation route has the benefit of delivering the MSC-based treatment topically, without the possible risk of diluting the MSCs and their exosomes throughout the body. However, if the MSC-based treatment is delivered in an aerosolized form, there is a risk that MSCs and their exosomes would localize primarily in the proximal airways without sufficiently reaching the lower airways, which are more affected. However, the direct effect of intravenously administered MSCs on inflamed lungs is uncertain, as MSCs have limited ability of homing on target tissue. The activity seen may be caused by the paracrine effect of MSCs. It is not easy to determine if the origin of the effect is paracrine or cell–cell contact.

COVID-19 also affects organs other than the lung. MSC-based clinical trials have so far focused on treatment only of the lung, and other organs have not been evaluated. MSC therapy has been shown to be beneficial on lung tissue. However, these results were shown depending on the records taken during the patient's treatment. Long-term results of the studies are not available.

The current COVID-19 pandemic has demonstrated the potential of SARS-CoV-2 to mutate as a number of multi-mutant variants have appeared in different parts of the world. The efficacy and safety of MSC-based therapies in relation to the novel SARS-CoV-2 variants have not yet been investigated.

9.6 FUTURE PERSPECTIVES

MSC-based therapies have been used extensively in many fields, which has enabled us to understand the mechanisms of action of stem cells. In the context of the COVID-19 pandemic, accelerated clinical trials have allowed analysis of the efficacy and safety of stem cell–based therapy. If studies continue at this speed, stem cells will be included in the treatment guidelines for most diseases soon. It is predicted that stem cells will alter most treatment modalities. Significantly, the immunomodulatory effects of stem cells are promising for the treatment of inflammatory diseases.

On the other hand, exosomes are seen as the future approach for MSC-based treatments. The therapeutic efficacy of MSC-derived exosomes has been shown in the lung, brain, kidney, heart, muscle, skin, and many tissues. Exosomes can be manipulated by preconditioning of MSCs. CRISPR/Cas9, a genome editing technology, can also be applied to improve the therapeutic efficacy of MSC-derived exosomes. For these reasons, we will most likely see plenty of activities related to MSC- and exosome-based therapy in the coming years.

9.7 CONCLUSIONS

The use of MSC-based therapies in clinical trials for the treatment of COVID-19 has increased remarkably. There is a real possibility that it will be common clinical practice in the near future. In this way, it is estimated that many diseases can be included in the treatment practices. If we can improve the mechanisms of action of MSCs and develop appropriate treatment methods, it will play an important role in routine clinical practice. It is fascinating that MSCs are effective even in such respiratory failure as ARDS caused by COVID-19. We believe that current evidence from clinical evaluations has confirmed the potential of MSC-based therapies use for the treatment of COVID-19 patients.

ACKNOWLEDGMENTS

Ethics Committee: This chapter does not require approval by the ethics committee.

Declaration of Interest: The authors report no conflicts of interest. The authors alone are responsible for the content and writing of the paper.

REFERENCES

1. Wu, Z., McGoogan, J.M. (2020). Characteristics of and important lessons from the coronavirus disease 2019 (COVID-19) outbreak in China: Summary of a report of 72 314 cases from the Chinese Center for Disease Control and Prevention. *JAMA* 323(13), 1239–1242.

2. Dominici, M.L., Le Blanc, K., Mueller, I., et al. (2006). Minimal criteria for defining multipotent mesenchymal stromal cells: The International Society for Cellular Therapy position statement. *Cytotherapy* 8(4), 315–317.

3. Bartholomew, A., Sturgeon, C., Siatskas, M., et al. (2002). Mesenchymal stem cells suppress lymphocyte proliferation in vitro and prolong skin graft survival in vivo. *Exp. Hematol.* 30(1), 42–48.

4. Ringdén, O., Uzunel, M., Rasmusson, I., et al. (2006). Mesenchymal stem cells for treatment of therapy-resistant graft-versus-host disease. *Transplantation* 81(10), 1390–1397.

5. Galipeau, J., Sensébé, L. (2018). Mesenchymal stromal cells: Clinical challenges and therapeutic opportunities. *Cell Stem Cell* 22(6), 824–833.

6. Özdemir, R.B.Ö., Özdemir, A.T., Sarıboyacı, A.E., et al. (2019). The investigation of immunomodulatory effects of adipose tissue mesenchymal stem cell educated macrophages on the CD4 T cells. *Immunobiology* 224(4), 585–594.

7. Demircan, P.C., Sariboyaci, A.E., Unal, Z.S., et al. (2011). Immunoregulatory effects of human dental pulp-derived stem cells on T cells: Comparison of transwell co-culture and mixed lymphocyte reaction systems. *Cytotherapy* 13(10), 1205–1220.

8. Özdemir, A.T., Özdemir, R.B.Ö., Kırmaz, C., et al. (2016). The paracrine immunomodulatory interactions between the human dental pulp derived mesenchymal stem cells and CD4 T cell subsets. *Cell. Immunol.* 310, 108–115.

9. Sariboyaci, A.E., Demircan, P.C., Gacar, G, et al. (2014). Immunomodulatory properties of pancreatic islet-derived stem cells co-cultured with T cells: Does it contribute to the pathogenesis of type 1 diabetes? *Exp. Clin. Endocrinol. Diab.* 122(03), 179–189.

10. Dandekar, A.A., Perlman, S. (2005). Immunopathogenesis of coronavirus infections: Implications for SARS. *Nat. Rev. Immunol.* 5(12), 917–927.

11. Jiang, W., Xu, J. (2020). Immune modulation by mesenchymal stem cells. *Cell Prolif.* 53(1), e12712.

12. Chan, M.C., Kuok, D.I., Leung, C.Y., et al. (2016). Human mesenchymal stromal cells reduce influenza A H5N1-associated acute lung injury in vitro and in vivo. *Proc. Natl. Acad. Sci. U.S.A.* 113(13), 3621–3626.

13. Krasnodembskaya, A., Song, Y., Fang, X., et al. (2010). Antibacterial effect of human mesenchymal stem cells is mediated in part from secretion of the antimicrobial peptide LL-37. *Stem Cells* 28(12), 2229–2238.

14. Xiao, K., Hou, F., Huang, X., et al. (2020). Mesenchymal stem cells: Current clinical progress in ARDS and COVID-19. *Stem Cell Res. Ther.* 11(1), 1–7.

15. Sengupta, V., Sengupta, S., Lazo, A., et al. (2020). Exosomes derived from bone marrow mesenchymal stem cells as treatment for severe COVID-19. *Stem Cells Dev.* 29(12), 747–754.

16. Shu, L., Niu, C., Li, R., et al. (2020). Treatment of severe COVID-19 with human umbilical cord mesenchymal stem cells. *Stem Cell Res. Ther.* 11(1), 1–11.

17. Meng, F., Xu, R., Wang, S., et al. (2020). Human umbilical cord-derived mesenchymal stem cell therapy in patients with COVID-19: A phase 1 clinical trial. *Signal Transduct. Target. Ther.* 5(1), 1–7.

18. Shi, L., Huang, H., Lu, X., et al. (2021). Effect of human umbilical cord-derived mesenchymal stem cells on lung damage in severe COVID-19 patients: A randomized, double-blind, placebo-controlled phase 2 trial. *Signal Transduct. Target. Ther.* 6(1), 1–9.

19. Hashemian, S.M.R., Aliannejad, R., Zarrabi, M., et al. (2021). Mesenchymal stem cells derived from perinatal tissues for treatment of critically ill COVID-19-induced ARDS patients: A case series. *Stem Cell Res. Ther.* 12(1), pp. 1–12.

20. Leng, Z., Zhu, R., Hou, W., et al. (2020). Transplantation of ACE2-mesenchymal stem cells improves the outcome of patients with COVID-19 pneumonia. *Aging Dis.* 11(2), 216.

21. Lee, O.J., Luk, F., Korevaar, S.S., et al. (2020). The importance of dosing, timing and in(activation) of adipose tissue-derived mesenchymal stromal cells on their immunomodulatory effects. *Stem Cells Dev.* 29, 38–48.

Chapter 10 Host and Pathogen-Specific Drug Targets in COVID-19

Bruce D. Uhal, David Connolly, Farzaneh Darbeheshti, Yong-Hui Zheng, Ifeanyichukwu E. Eke, Yutein Chung, and Lobelia Samavati

10.1 INTRODUCTION

A number of pharmacologic therapies for COVID-19 have either been approved for use, are currently in clinical trials or undergoing various stages of development. These are designed to act through a wide variety of targets on the SARS-CoV-2 virus as well as within the host. Drug targets include the primary viral receptor ACE-2, alternative receptors, sialic acids, viral and host proteases, the furin cleavage site within the SARS-CoV-2 spike (S) protein, and the viral replication machinery. Other drug targets are under study, but because of space limitations the discussion here is limited to the targets mentioned above.

10.2 ACE-2

Angiotensin-converting enzyme-2 (ACE-2) has been widely accepted as the primary receptor to which both SARS-CoV and SARS-CoV-2 bind and use to cross the plasma membrane of epithelial cells in the respiratory tract and other organs [1–3]. In humans, ACE-2 is a membrane-bound carboxypeptidase which modulates the renin-angiotensin system (RAS) by converting the octapeptide angiotensin-II to the heptapeptide angiotensin 1-7 via its large extracellular enzymatic domain [4]. Angiotensin 1-7 is protective against injury to lungs and other organs [4], and thus the effect of SARS-CoV-2 binding to ACE-2 on its normally protective activity is also implicated in the pathogenesis of COVID-19 organ damage in the lungs, heart, kidney, and other organs [5].

The SARS-CoV-2 spike protein (S protein) contains key domains that enable high affinity binding to ACE-2, including the receptor-binding domain (RBD). The RBD of the S protein binds to two "hotspots" in the extracellular domain of ACE-2: Lys31 and Lys353 [1, 6]. It therefore stands to reason that compounds, which inhibit or interfere with SARS-CoV-2 binding to ACE-2 might inhibit the entry of the virus into host cells. Accordingly, a number of *in silico* drug discovery studies have attempted to identify candidate inhibitors of SARS-CoV-2-ACE-2 interaction that might be druggable [7, 8].

In addition, the administration of exogenous ACE-2 could potentially be a viable strategy to inhibit SARS-CoV-2 binding and/or host cell entry. Systemic administration of exogenous ACE-2 would be expected, at least theoretically, to provide a "decoy" receptor to bind the virus and thereby inhibit its entry into host cells. At the time of writing, there were several ongoing clinical trials utilizing ACE-2-based products as potential pharmacologic therapies for COVID-19. One such clinical trial, being conducted by Apeiron Biologics (ClinicalTrials.gov ID: NCT04335136) [9], utilizes intravenous administration of recombinant human ACE-2 (rhACE-2) to treat patients infected with SARS-CoV-2. The hypothesis of this trial is that the exogenous, soluble rhACE-2 will act as a "decoy" to bind the circulating SARS-CoV-2 virion. In this way, the RBD of the S protein would be occupied, and therefore could not infect human cells. In support of this hypothesis, a recent study showed that entry of SARS-CoV-2 pseudovirions into HEK293 cells was significantly decreased if the pseudovirions were pre-incubated with soluble human ACE-2, and suggested that soluble rhACE-2 could be a valuable inhibitor of SARS-CoV-2 infection [10].

This interpretation is complicated, however, by the documented presence of soluble ACE-2 in the serum [11], which is believed to be a cleaved form of the enzyme released from cells by the action of various proteases such as the disintegrin and metalloproteinase domain 17 (ADAM-17). Serum-borne soluble ACE-2 (sACE-2) is believed to be capable of binding SARS-CoV-2 as tightly as cellular ACE-2 [12], and thus might be expected to compete with cell-bound ACE-2 for available virions. Moreover, sACE-2 has shown elevated levels in patients with known risk factors for poor outcome in COVID-19, such as hypertension and obesity [13]. Thus it is difficult to predict the overall effect of adding exogenous ACE-2 to a system that is already composed of both cell-associated and soluble, serum-borne forms of the main viral receptor.

Adding to this complexity and uncertainty, a recent cell culture study indicated that soluble ACE-2 enhanced, rather than inhibited, SARS-CoV-2 infection in human cell lines [14]; the data suggested that soluble ACE-2 may facilitate infection via receptor-mediated endocytosis. Indeed, these experiments indicated that inhibition of ADAM17 "sheddase" – thereby decreasing the concentration of soluble ACE-2 – suppressed infection of human kidney cell lines,

DOI: 10.1201/9781003190394-10

rather than enhancing it as might be expected [14]. In light of these surprising findings, there is clearly a need for further research to determine the effect that soluble recombinant human ACE-2 would have on SARS-CoV-2 entry and infection in the human body. In addition to ACE-2 and the S protein domains that bind to it, other domains in the S protein facilitate viral entry, as do other host factors such as proteases, sialic acids, and gangliosides [6], as discussed below.

10.3 OTHER PUTATIVE VIRAL RECEPTORS AND CELL ENTRY COFACTORS

While ACE-2 is known to be the primary receptor for SARS-CoV-2 that exhibits high affinity binding to the viral S protein, host cell entry by the virus has been shown to be mediated, in some cell types, by other molecules that can act as cofactors with ACE-2, or in some cases, as alternative receptors in the absence of ACE-2. For example, heparan sulfate proteoglycans (HSPGs) can bind to both the prefusion and ACE-2 bound conformations of the SARS-CoV-2 S protein [15]. Indeed, Kim et al. [16] showed that various preparations of heparin can block SARS-CoV-2 interactions with ACE-2 and cell infection *in vitro*, suggesting that such preparations might have potential as therapeutics. The roles of host cell sialic acid interactions with HSPGs will be discussed in the next section.

Neutropilin-1 (NRP-1) has been shown to function as a "detour receptor", in the absence of ACE-2, for Epstein-Barr virus infection of olfactory neuronal cells of the nasal epithelium. Since the SARS-CoV-2 S protein contains the C-terminal sequence 676-TQTNSPRRAR-685, the binding site for NRP-1 [17], it seems likely that SARS-CoV-2 may also be capable of NRP-1-dependent cell entry, but at the time of writing no strategies for inhibiting this pathway have yet entered the drug pipeline. Another pathway for viral cell entry is that mediated by C-type lectin receptors (CLRs), which are specialized for pathogenic interactions with sialic acid [18, 19], as discussed in the next section.

10.4 SIALIC ACIDS

Sialic acids are a family of monosaccharides attached to various glycolipids and glycoproteins on epithelial cell membranes. That is why sialic acids are considered a highly accessible cell membrane component for receptor–ligand and protein–ligand interactions. In the context of virology, sialic acids were the first characterized receptors promoting the viral entry process [20]. Viral entry through the sialic acid-dependent manner has been shown in

several types of coronaviruses based on enzymatic activities of hemagglutinin esterase [21]. Concerning SARS-CoV-2, specific sialic acids [22] on the respiratory tract's epithelium could be employed as co-receptors for the S protein so that virus clustering is facilitated. Moreover, ACE2, as the primary receptor for SARS-CoV-2 attachment, is heavily sialylated on N- and O-linked sugar chains. Consequently, the sialic acid-mediating targeted therapies may inhibit SARS-CoV-2 invasion by inhibiting virus–host cell interaction and modulation of endocytosis. However, the host sialome could also play a protective role against viral infections by providing a large layer of sialylated residues on mucosal cell surfaces and interfering with virus entry by offering an alternative binding site. This section aims to summarize the potential sialic acid-mediating targeted therapies in COVID-19 and provides insight into their molecular mechanisms (Figure 10.1).

Sialic acid-blocking drugs: Chloroquine (CLQ) and hydroxychloroquine (HCQ) could interfere with the viral pre-entry step by inhibiting the biosynthesis of sialic acid [23]. CLQ inhibits the quinone reductase 2 enzyme and consequently prevents terminal glycosylation. Structural and molecular modeling has revealed a new mechanism of action of CLQ and HCQ against SARS-CoV-2 infection through direct interaction with the N-terminal domain of the S protein, hence interfering with high-affinity S protein binding to sialylated ganglioside GM1 [24].

This drug has been used for several years in malaria therapy with acceptable safety and efficacy. In the current global crisis, CLQ and HCQ were among the early options of repurposing drugs. Several clinical trials investigated the therapeutic potential of CLQ and HCQ in COVID-19 patients. The results indicated inconsistent outcomes, and the randomized controlled trials have failed to confirm its therapeutic usefulness in patients [25, 26]. Moreover, some reports imply probable cardiomyopathy as a severe adverse effect caused by CLQ. HCQ remains among the available candidates to prevent the severity of SARS-CoV-2 infections in humans, and additional clinical and molecular observations are needed to identify relevant subgroups that may benefit from HCQ, if any such groups exist. This seems unlikely, as the study of Elavarasi et al. [27], based on a systematic meta-analysis of 12 observational and 3 randomized trials including 10,659 patients, revealed that HCQ did not generate a significant reduction in mortality, time to fever resolution, or clinical deterioration or development of acute respiratory distress syndrome (ARDS).

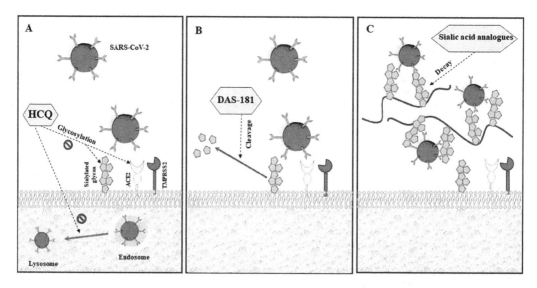

Figure 10.1 Sialic acid-targeted therapeutic strategies in SARS-CoV-2 infection. (A) Sialic acid-blocking drugs through inhibition of terminal glycosylation; (B) Sialic acid decomposing drugs by cleavage of sialic acid residues; (C) Sialic acid mimicking drugs through competition for cell surface receptors; HCQ, hydroxychloroquine.

Sialic acid decomposing drugs: One of the potentially broad-spectrum groups of antiviral drugs is decomposing sialic acid agents that target the virus entry pathway. The most common isoform of sialic acid in humans is N-acetylneuraminic acid (Neu5Ac). DAS-181, also known as Fludase, is a recombinant neuraminidase, which consists of a sialidase catalytic domain and a glycosaminoglycan-binding tag. The FDA has approved DAS181 as a therapeutic approach in hypoxic patients with lower respiratory tract parainfluenza infection.

It is proposed that inhalation of nebulized DAS181 could cleave sialic acids in the lung epithelium and interfere with the entry of viruses targeting sialic acid glycoconjugates [27]. Therefore SARS-CoV-2 could be sensitive to DAS181. The results from a pilot study of a small case series of patients indicated the potential clinical benefit of DAS181 in COVID-19 patients [28]. It seems that more investigations in double-blind, randomized controlled studies are needed to clarify the effects of DAS181 on clinical recovery, inflammatory markers, and adverse events. Notwithstanding these concerns, DAS-181 is currently the only medication to tackle COVID-19 by targeting the sialic acid receptor itself.

Sialic acid mimicking drugs: Another strategy to inhibit the virus attachment to cell surface receptors is sialic acid mimicking compounds as a decoy, thereby competing with the host cell receptors to bind the virus. The first investigated sialic acid–receptor analogues are exogenous mucins and surfactant proteins, which are part of the innate immune system. These compounds are naturally secreted by respiratory epithelial cells and contain a wide variety of phospholipids and carbohydrates, including sialic acid. The next generation of sialic acid–receptor analogues are synthetic sialic acid compounds which are optimized by nanoparticle or liposome formulations. The concept of sialic acid mimicking antiviral drugs is promising, and some studies have been conducted to investigate their possibility for treating viral infections, especially influenza virus. So far, this concept has not been investigated for COVID-19. Some groups are investigating the effects of surfactant administration on the outcome of patients with COVID-19 (ClinicalTrials.gov IDs: NCT04375735, NCT04362059, NCT04384731). It is suggested that using exogenous surfactant in COVID-19 patients with acute respiratory distress syndrome (ARDS) and on mechanical ventilation could improve their outcome by restoring surfactant damaged by lung infection, reducing pulmonary edema, and blocking spread of the virus particles to healthy cells in the lung [29]. Overall, the results of ongoing trials could indicate if this therapy is effective for COVID-19 patients or not. It should be noted that more in vitro and in vivo studies are needed to evaluate the benefits of nanotechnology in sialic acid–receptor analogues, e.g. sialic acid–functionalized dendrimers, for treatment strategies against COVID-19 [30].

Collectively, at the current level of knowledge, it can neither be confirmed nor excluded that sialic acid-mediating targeted therapies could reduce COVID-19 clinical manifestations. Profound knowledge about the role of the human sialome in this pandemic could result in developing the combined therapies to reduce viral load and inflammation. However, whether or not manipulation of sialic acids has clinical significance in COVID-19 patients remains to be determined.

10.5 VIRAL AND HOST PROTEASES

10.5.1 SARS-CoV-2–Specific Viral Proteases

While many of the protease-inhibitor based antiviral drugs exert their effects on multiple viruses, it is still important to design more specific inhibitors targeting SARS-CoV-2 proteases. This is especially important because many of the popular effective inhibitors such as ganciclovir, ribavirin, and peramivir, while effective in containing influenza virus, failed to show any effectiveness against SARS-CoV-2 [31, 32]. Despite significant progress in understanding the SARS-CoV-2 genome and specific viral proteins, there is still limited knowledge on SARS-CoV-2-specific proteases. In fact, most of our understanding about proteases is based on SARS-CoV. To better design therapeutics to target SARS-CoV-2, we first must understand what is known about specific proteases and their functions in SARS-CoV-2 virions. Two viral proteases, Mpro and PLpro, stand out,

and knowledge about their function may provide insights for better design of SARS-CoV-2 therapeutics.

Mpro: The SAS-CoV-2 main protease, Mpro, also known as chymotrypsin-like or 3CL protease or non-structural protein 5 (NSP5), is a member of the cysteine protease family. Upon SARS-CoV-2 entry and translation of the viral polyprotein complex, Mpro is one of the first viral NSPs that are released from the complex [33] (see Figure 10.2). On release from the polyprotein complex, Mpro dimerizes with itself and becomes enzymatically active [34]. Activated Mpro has 11 known cleavage sites on the viral polyprotein [35]. It also cooperates with another viral protease Papain-like protease (PLpro) to release the NSP7-10 complex [36]. This is important, since NSP7-10 contains the critical domains for the assembly of the viral replication-transcription complex (RTC), which is vital for replication of the SARS-CoV-2 genome and the transcription of viral genes. Mpro is a 306 amino acid protein and is structurally conserved between SARS-CoV and SARS-CoV-2.

I. **Entry.** SARS-COV-2 binds the host ACE2 receptor via the S protein. Host proteases ADAM17 and TMPRSS2 cleave ACE2 at the ecto and intracellular domain, respectively, allowing viral entry into endosome. Host proteases cathepsin and furin further break down the S protein to allow endosomal fusion and release of the viral genome into the cytoplasm.

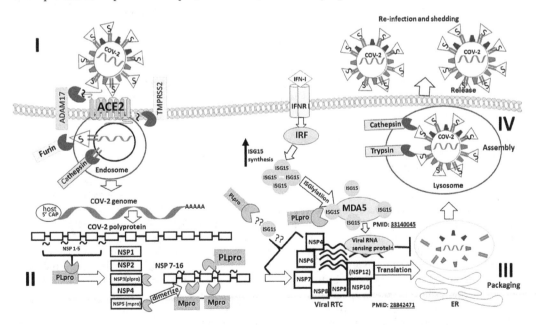

Figure 10.2   Critical pathways of the SARS-COV-2 infection cycle and key proteases involved: The four stages of SARS-COV-2 infection cycle.

II. **Polyprotein synthesis/processing.** The viral genome is capped at the 5′ end, contains a poly-A tail at the 3′ end and is translated to a viral polyprotein complex by the host. NSP3/PLpro cleaves and frees viral NSPs 1-5. Freed NSP5/Mpro dimerizes and becomes activated. Activated Mpro partners with PLpro to process NSPs to form the viral replication and transcription complex (RTC).

III. **Viral genome and protein synthesis.** RTC synthesizes the viral genome allowing production and packaging of virions in the host ER. Viral PLpro down-regulates the host IFN-1 signaling cascade by preventing ISGlylation of viral RNA sensing/binding proteins such as MDA5. (It is unknown whether direct ISGlylation occurs on the RTC and whether PLpro directly inhibits it.

IV. **Viral assembly and release.** Packaged virions enter host lysosomes where they mature and are released to the surface to re-infect host cells and spread of viral infection.

Some progress has been made on identifying specific inhibitors against Mpro. Computer models based on X-ray crystallography showed that Mpro has three functional domains. Domains one and two contain a chymotrypsin-like domain [37], implying that the alpha-ketoamide-based protease inhibitor effective against viral 3CL-family proteases [38], may be a candidate for SARS-CoV-2 as it effectively binds to Mpro [39, 40]. Additionally, Mpro contains docking sites for HIV protease inhibitors such as lopinavir, ritonavir, and saquinavir. In fact, remdesivir, the viral RNA polymerase inhibitor can also bind to the docking site [41]. Indole-based inhibitors such as GRL-1720 are known to both interact with Mpro molecularly and to inhibit the viral infectivity of cultured cells [42]. In silico analysis identified a synthetic octopeptide AT1001 (Larazotide acetate) to interact with Mpro, which showed inhibition of this protease [43]. AT1001 is an investigational drug for ARDS [43]. Many inhibitors contain a carboxyl group, commonly seen in the design of anti-HIV proteases [44]. Recently, a GC-376 analogue was discovered with inhibitory activity against Mpro. This analogue is also active against human cathepsin L, a host protease that is important for viral entry [45]. N3, a synthetic Aza-peptide Michael acceptor inhibitor, irreversibly competes with the Mpro substrate-binding site [46]. Other candidate protease inhibitors such as ebselen, disulfiram, armofur, and PX-12 are currently being tested and have shown positive binding results with Mpro [47, 48]. Given their cost-effectiveness in production, these small molecule–based protease inhibitors may prove to be beneficial candidates in treating SARS-CoV-2 in the near future.

Alongside synthetic inhibitors, natural-forming inhibitors have also been investigated. Several plant-based compounds such as quercetin show crystal structure homology to Mpro as well as binding affinity [49]. Molecular docking assay screening of phytochemicals against SARS-COV-2 proteases showed over 50 potential candidates of plant-based compounds with the ability to bind to Mpro with the potential of inhibition [50]. These include procyanidins, flavornoids found in berries, and rutin, a flavornoid found in buckwheats. In fact, some of these phytochemicals contain hydroxyl groups similar to the synthetic inhibitors, exerting similar functions in inhibiting Mpro. Extracts from herbal medicine Crofton weed, *A. adenophora*, has also been shown to bind and inhibit SARS-CoV-2 Mpro [51]. These findings indicate a potential of herbal-based medicine as effective SARS-CoV-2 therapies.

PLpro: The aforementioned "partner" of Mpro, papain-like protease (PLpro) aka NSP3, is another important SARS-CoV-2 specific protease involved in processing of the viral polyprotein. Similar to Mpro, PLpro needs to be released from pro-enzyme complexes. Studies on SARS-CoV revealed PLpro to be the first protease, which is released from the polyprotein complex. PLpro cleaves the NSP1-NSP2, NSP2-NSP3 while the NSP3-NSP4 junction still remains in the complex form. However, NSP3/PLpro is free from the complex. PLpro then cleaves the NSP 4-6 domain to release NSP5/Mpro [52]. PLpro then coordinates with Mpro in the initial release of other viral NSPs to form the viral RTC. Therefore, like Mpro, PLpro is another potential target for antiviral therapies for SARS-CoV-2

Unlike Mpro, fewer candidate inhibitors seem to be known for PLpro. Anti-HIV drugs such as lopinavir and darunavir seem to have some inhibitory effect on PLpro [53]. Interestingly, docking site computer simulation has implicated CLQ, the controversial malaria drug, as one of the potential candidates [54]. Recently, the small molecule GRL0617 was shown to be a promising inhibitor for PLpro [55]. Molecular docking studies revealed that available clinically approved protease inhibitors nafamostat and VR23 bind to the inhibitor sites of both PLpro and Mpro [56].

Besides being a viral protease, PLpro has been shown to exert its effects on the host antiviral immunity. It was discovered that PLpro functions as a deubiquitinating agent (DUB). This was further validated since both GRL0617 and Z93, another potential inhibitor for PLpro, were used as inhibitors for human ubiquitin carboxyl-terminal hydrolase 2 (USP)-2 [57]. However, PLpro shows more homology to the USP18 and its primary target is the host Ubiquitin-Like Protein interferon stimulated gene ISG15. ISG15 is induced by type I interferon (IFN-I) signaling via interferon-response factor (IRF) and functions like ubiquitination processing K48 [58], a process known as ISGlylation [59]. ISGlylation has two major antiviral functions. It can be directed to viral transcriptases/replicases to inhibit viral protein synthesis. Examples of that are seen for the influenza virus, where ISGylation of the replication complex protein NS1 shuts down virion production [59]. ISGlylation of host viral RNA sensors RIG-1 and MDA5 provides positive feedback of IFN-I responses as well as directly inhibits viral replication [60]. PLpro has been demonstrated to be a de-ISGlylation agent which directly cleaves ISG15 [61] (Figure 10.1). The role of PLpro and how it downregulates ISG15 was starting to merge, as a protease beside cleaving viral polyprotein, alternatively it antagonizes IFN-1-induced antiviral activities [58, 62, 63]. This implies that targeted drugs that inhibit PLpro are very important, as they are not only controlling viral replication but also restoring host responses to viral infections. Currently, it is not clear whether ISGlylation occurs directly at the SARS-CoV-2 RTC complex. Nevertheless, the role of PLpro and its antagonism on ISGlylation needs to be further studied.

10.5.2 Host Cell Proteases in SARS-CoV-2 Infection

Most of these host proteases affect viral entry/binding to the cell surface, providing targets for inhibiting the early stages of viral infection. Host proteases are also important, since some of the antiviral drugs (i.e. aprotinin) also affect host proteases. Since the beginning of the COVID-19 pandemic, several studies have been conducted on host protease candidates and how they may interplay with the viral proteases as potential therapeutics [64].

TMPRSS2: One of the best studied host proteases involved in RNA virus infection is the Type II transmembrane serine protease (TMPRSS2). This trypsin-like enzyme expressed on plasma membranes, functions by cleaving the intracellular domains of host receptors and is critical for SARS-CoV-2 infections [65]. Later, TMPRSS2 was identified as a therapeutic target for coronavirus and influenza virus infections [66]. TMPRSS2 was identified to be associated with SARS-CoV infected primate airways and its expression is increased after viral infection [67, 68]. The enzymatic cleavage of ACE2 by TMPRSS2 is critical for viral internalization. Such a cleavage of the ACE2 ectodomain facilitates the intracellular uptake of SARS-CoV-2. Furthermore, TMPRSS2 antagonizes ADAM17, an ecto-domain sheddase (discussed below), by preventing the ectodomain shedding of ACE2. In fact, camostat, the inhibitor of TMPRSS2, is known to inhibit replication of influenza virus in vitro [69] and was one of the first drugs discovered to have inhibitory effects against SARS-CoV-2. Recently, molecular modeling and crystallography showed camostat to bind directly to TMPRSS2. Besides camostat, nafamostat is another potential TMPRSS2 inhibitor and it has been shown in cell culture studies to block SARS-CoV-2 infection [70]. TMPRSS2 is also known to cleave the SARS-CoV-2 S protein directly, thus affecting the free/unbound virus. This cleavage by TMPRSS2 gives the virus two advantages: first it allows better fusion with host cell membranes, and second, better immune evasion by host immunoglobulins [71]. Therefore, TMPRSS2 involvement in SARS-CoV-2 pathogenesis is two-fold. Inhibitors against TMPRSS2 should both block viral binding/entry as well as improve humoral responses against the virus.

ADAM17 is a transmembrane protease that functions as an ecto-domain sheddase. Its expression level is upregulated when the SARS-CoV-2 S-protein binds to ACE-2. Whereas TMPRSS2 cleaves the cytoplasmic tail, ADAM17 cleaves the ectodomain of ACE-2 thus mediating viral entry [72]. Besides directly contributing to viral pathology, the release of ACE-2 by ADAM 17 into the extracellular environment raises the concern of co-morbidity, such as promoting vascular diseases as a "collateral" of the infection. Alpha-anti trypsin has been identified as a potential inhibitor for ADAM17 against SARS-CoV-2 infection [73]. Many other inhibitors against ADAM17 have been described for other diseases [74], however, not many of them have been tested against SARS-CoV-2.

Cathepsins are proteases that function to recycle/degrade cellular proteins. There are 11 types of cathepsins that are usually found within the endosomes/lysosomes (see Figure 10.2). They exist mainly as precursor enzymes, which require acidic pH for activation. Cathepsin L, a serine protease seems to be highly associated with the SARS-CoV-2 S protein. Once inside endosomes, cathepsin L further cleaves the SARS-Cov-2 S protein. This allows the membrane fusion of the viral envelope and endosomes, a critical step for the release of the viral genome into the cytoplasm [75]. The anti-Ebola cysteine protease inhibitor K11777, which specifically targets cathepsin, has been shown also to have some positive effects on SARS-CoV-2 [77]. As mentioned earlier, the Mpro inhibitor GC-376, also seems to exert cross reactivity with Cathepsin-L [45]. Furthermore, some evidence suggests that cathepsins work in cohort with TMPRSS2 to fully achieve effectiveness for SARS-CoV-2 entry [75]. This implies that combining drugs such as camostat with K11777 may optimize the therapy.

Cathepsins are also produced and stored in granules by neutrophils and are critical components of host innate immunity. In the case of viral infections, such as SARS-CoV-2, neutrophils are usually activated, thus leading to degranulation [76], allowing the release of cathepsins to the extracellular environment [77]. Although host cathepsins play a role in slowing down viral infections, they can also have detrimental effects on surrounding tissues, leading to severe inflammatory damage as seen in the lungs of many SARS-CoV-2 patients.

Therefore inhibiting cathepsin not only may control SARS-CoV-2 but it might also potentially attenuate host-inflammation, an apparent "win–win" therapy. However, the dichotomy is that since neutrophil cathepsin is important for host response, this can potentially lead to compromised innate immune responses, resulting in the host being susceptible to other infections, particularly those pathogens that require neutrophil degranulation. This is especially true since cathepsin inhibitors may also inhibit other neutrophil defensive enzymes such as elastase [78]. Therefore, more work needs to be done to optimize the targeting of cathepsins as therapeutics for SARS-CoV-2 infection. The proteases and potential inhibitors discussed above are summarized in Table 10.1.

Table 10.1 Key host and pathogen-specific drug targets involved in SARS-CoV-2 infection

Target	Origin	Major Function	Known Inhibitors
Mpro (3CLpro)	SARS-CoV-2, NSP5	Cleavage of NSP 7-10, required for formation of viral transcription-replication complex	GRL-1720 AT1001 N3, ebselen, VR23 nafamostat
PLpro	SARS-CoV-2, NSP3	Cleavage of NSPs1-5 to release Mpro, coordinates with Mpro in cleavage of NSP7-10, deubitinating agent of ISG15 (host antiviral)	GRL0617 VR23n nafamostat
TMPRSS2	Host cell surface membrane, endosomes, extracellular	Cleaves ACE2 cytoplasmic tail domain upon viral binding, facilitates viral entry. Can also directly cleave S protein	Camostat nafamostat
ADAM17	Host cell surface membrane	Cleaves ACE2 Ectodomain, releases ACE2 from cell surface, facilitates viral entry	TAPI-2
Cathepsin	Host cell surface, endosome/lysosome Extracellular by neutrophils (C/G)	Viral entry, cleavage of S-protein and allow viral envelope fusion w/endosome	K11777 GC-376
Furin	Host Golgi/endosome	Facilitate viral S-protein cleavage and fusion with endosome	D6R
Heparan sulfate proteoglycans (HSPGs)	Host cell surface membrane, extracellular matrix		Heparin
ACE-2	Viral receptor on host cell	Carboxypeptidase in RAAS	Recombinant ACE-2 (decoy receptor)
Neuropilin-1 (NRP-1)	Host cell surface membrane		
C-type lectin receptors (CLRs)	Host cell surface membrane		
Sialic acids	Host cell surface membrane glycoproteins and glycolipids	Bind receptors	Chloroquine (CLQ), hydroxychloroquine (HCQ), DAS-181
RNA-dependent RNA polymerase (RdRp)	SARS-COV-2	Catalyzes replication of viral RNA into genomic and nested RNAs	Remdesivir (Rmd), molnupiravir, favipiravir, sofosbuvir, daclatasvir, ribavirin

10.6 FURIN AND SARS-CoV-2 ENTRY INTO HOST CELLS

SARS-CoV and SARS-CoV-2 S proteins share 76.2% amino acid sequence homology and both use ACE-2 as a receptor [79]. Because of four amino acids (PRRA) insertion at the S1/S2 junction, a furin cleavage site (^{681}PRRAR|SV^{687}) has evolved for SARS-CoV-2 that is not present in SARS-CoV or its closest bat ancestor viruses [80]. Furin is a type-I transmembrane, trypsin-type, serine protease that belongs to the pro-protein convertase (PC: gene PCSK) family, which cleaves precursor proteins within the motif (R/K)–(X–X)n–(R/K)| (n = 0, 1, 2, or 3) [81]. PCs activate a wide variety of host secretory proteins and viral surface glycoproteins. PCs are abundant in multiple tissues including the respiratory tract and acquisition of a furin site has led to generation of highly pathogenic avian H5 and H7 influenza viruses [82]. In fact, the furin cleavage site exists in a number of human coronaviruses (CoVs) including MERS-CoV, HKU1-CoV, and OC43-CoV [82], suggesting that the existence of a furin site does not necessarily correlate with hyper-transmissibility and pathogenesis. However, the furin site greatly enhances SARS-CoV-2 transmission and pathogenesis in animal models [83]. Thus, it is highly likely that a gain of furin cleavage site has enabled SARS-CoV-2 to jump into humans and begin its current pandemic spread [84].

The hallmarks of advanced SARS-CoV-2 pathology are pneumocyte syncytia and thrombosis [85]. In autopsies of COVID-19 victims, many multinucleated giant cells resulting from syncytia of pneumocytes have been found in the lungs, which is the consequence of the fusogenic S protein activity of SARS-CoV-2 that promotes cell-to-cell spread of viral infection. Cell-to-cell infection is not only more efficient than virus-to-cell infection but can also evade host immunity. Thus many viruses, including HIV-1, herpes simplex virus, measles virus, and human hepatitis C virus, drive their dissemination via cell-to-cell infection [86]. Introduction of a furin cleavage site into the SARS-CoV S protein selectively enhanced its cell-to-cell fusion but not virus-to-cell infection [87]. Conversely, abolishing the furin cleavage site in SARS-CoV-2 S protein strongly inhibited its cell-to-cell fusion but not its virus-to-cell infection [88]. Thus the furin cleavage site may contribute to SARS-CoV-2 transmission and disease progression by promoting the cell-to-cell infection *in vivo*.

In addition to furin, CoV S proteins are processed by three other types of proteases [89]. Two of them are serine proteases, including secreted trypsin and cell surface trypsin-like proteases. The cell surface proteases include TMPRSS2 and the human airway trypsin-like protease (HAT, TMPRSS11D). The third type protease is a lumenal cysteine protease cathepsin L (CTSL) that is expressed in late endosomes and lysosomes. SARS-CoV-2 entry requires two sequential conformational changes in S proteins that are mediated by receptor-binding or proteolysis. The ACE-2-binding causes a conformational change that exposes two protease cleavage sites, and upon cleavage, these S proteins are further refolded into fusion-competent conformation. Depending on the abundance of these proteases during infection, CoVs enter cells by early or late pathways. In the presence of TMPRSS2 and HAT, S proteins are cleaved on the cell surface at neutral pH that triggers direct fusion with the plasma membrane. However, in the absence of these trypsin-like proteases, absorbed virions are delivered into late endosomes and cleaved by CSTL at high pH for membrane fusion. The furin-mediated cleavage at the S1/S2 boundary occurs during S protein biosynthesis in viral producer cells. This cleavage exposes the S2' site, which is required for the second cleavage by TMPRSS2 on the target cell membrane and promote cell-to-cell fusion. In contrast, furin-cleavage does not promote the CSTL-mediated late viral entry because of the instability of cleaved S1/S2 in the late endosomes.

Collectively, furin is an attractive therapeutic target for the development of novel antivirals that may be broadly effective to various infectious diseases. Peptide-based and small molecule inhibitors targeting furin/PCs have already been found to inhibit the syncytia formation effectively by blocking the SARS-CoV-2 S protein cleavage [90]. Thus these inhibitors may provide another tool to combat COVID-19 after further development.

10.7 TARGETING THE VIRAL REPLICATION MACHINERY

Immediately after entry into a host cell, CoVs translate their genomic RNA into polyprotein products that are subsequently processed to different non-structural proteins (NSPs). Some of these proteins assemble to give rise to the replication machinery of the virus. As in other RNA viruses, the RNA-dependent RNA polymerase (RdRp) is a major component of this machinery. It catalyzes the replication of the viral RNA into genomic and nested RNAs. The critical role played by the RdRp in the replication cycle of CoVs makes it a target in the development of therapeutics against SARS-CoV-2 [91].

Remdesvir (Rmd) is an adenosine analogue prodrug that interferes with the activity of the RdRp, serving as a chain terminator of polynucleotide synthesis. A significant impact of the drug on viral replication is a reduction in viral RNA levels and titers. Rmd has a broad-spectrum antiviral activity against CoVs from highly divergent lineages [92, 94]. It is one of the few drugs approved for treatment of COVID-19 patients in some countries, though there are concerns about the rise of drug-resistant mutations in the viral RdRp [94]. This resistance has yet to be seen for SARS-CoV-2, but it has been demonstrated for mouse hepatitis virus (MHV) where increased passaging of the virus in the presence of Rmd led to the development of polymerase mutations, conferring resistance to the drug. Interestingly, when these resistance mutations were introduced into SARS-CoV, the resistance phenotype was recapitulated [93]. This possibility in the genetically similar SARS-CoV-2 calls for structure-based analysis to identify residues in the viral RdRp prone to Rmd resistance [92]. Also, combination therapy with Rmd and other drugs is applied to reduce the chances of treatment failure. Molnupiravir, a cytosine analogue prodrug, was effective against MERS-CoV, SARS-CoV, SARS-CoV-2, and a recombinant Rmd-resistant MHV [92]. Favipiravir, sofosbuvir, daclatasvir, and ribavirin are proposed for COVID-19 treatment because of their ability to target the RdRp and inhibit viral replication [96–98]. Agents designed to affect the replication apparatus are summarized in Table 10.1.

In addition to the RdRp, the replication machinery includes a helicase, a proof-reading exoribonuclease, and accessory proteins that associate with the RdRp [94, 99]. Consideration of these proteins in the development of anti-replicase drugs may be helpful [100]. The design of nucleoside analogue-based drugs should consider the proof-reading activity of the exonuclease as a barrier to inhibiting viral replication effectively [95].

10.8 CONCLUSIONS

At the time of writing, ongoing clinical trials have identified promising inhibitors of the viral replication machinery and host cell entry mechanisms. Other avenues to combating SARS-CoV-2 include blockers and/or inhibitors of alternate cell entry pathways and in particular, proteases expressed by the host and/or virus, which are critical for viral entry and/or pathogenesis. All drug targets discussed here, and agents that may act on them, are summarized in Table 10.1. In some cases, druggable protease inhibitors already exist, and in other cases are under intense study and development. Given the worldwide effort devoted to solving this global problem, safe and effective antivirals are on the near horizon.

REFERENCES

1. Shang, J., Ye, G., Shi, K., Wan, Y., Luo, C., Aihara, H., Geng, Q., Auerbach, A., Li, F. (2020). Structural basis of receptor recognition by SARS-CoV-2. *Nature* 581(7807), 221–224.

2. Lan, J., Ge, J., Yu, J. (2020). Structure of the SARS-CoV-2 spike receptor-binding domain bound to the ACE2 receptor. *Nature* 581, 215–220.

3. Hoffmann, M., Kleine-Weber, H., Schroeder, S., Krüger, N., Herrler, T., Erichsen, S., Schiergens, T.S., Herrler, G., Wu, N.H., Nitsche, A., Müller, M.A., Drosten, C., Pöhlmann, S. (2020). SARS-CoV-2 cell entry depends on ACE2 and TMPRSS2 and is blocked by a clinically proven protease inhibitor. *Cell* 181(2), 271–280.

4. Li, X., Molina-Molina, M., Abdul-Hafez, A., Uhal, V., Xaubet, A., Uhal, B. D. (2008). Angiotensin converting enzyme-2 is protective but down-regulated in human and experimental lung fibrosis. *Am. J. Physiol. Lung Cell. Mol. Physiol.* 295(1), L178–L185.

5. Samavati, L., Uhal, B. (2020). ACE-2, much more than just a receptor for SARS-CoV-2. *Front. Cell. Infect. Microbiol. Virus Host* 10, 317. doi:10.3389/fcimb.2020.00317. eCollection 2020. PMID: 32582574.

6. Seyran, M., Takayama, K., Uversky, V. N., Lundstrom, K., Palù, G., Sherchan, S.P., Attrish, D., Rezaei, N., Aljabali, A., Ghosh, S., Pizzol, D., Chauhan, G., Adadi, P., Mohamed Abd El-Aziz, T., Soares, A.G., Kandimalla, R., Tambuwala, M., Hassan, S.S., Azad, G.K., Pal Choudhury, P., Uhal, B.D. (2020). The structural basis of accelerated host cell entry by SARS-CoV-2†. *FEBS J.* doi:10.1111/febs.15651.

7. Waidha, K., Saxena, A., Kumar, P., Sharma, S., Ray, D., Saha, B. (2021). Design and identification of novel Annomontine analogues against SARS-CoV-2: an in-silico approach. *Heliyon* 7(4), e06657. doi:10.1016/j.heliyon.2021.e06657. PMID: 33824915.

8. He, M., Wang, Y., Huang, S., Zhao, N., Cheng, M., Zhang, X. (2021). Computational exploration of natural peptides targeting ACE2. *J. Biomol. Struct. Dyn.* 1–12. doi:10.1080/07391102.2021.1905555. PMID: 33826484.

9. Sarwar, Z., Ahmad, T., Kakar, S. (2020). Potential approaches to combat COVID-19: A mini-review. *Mol. Biol. Rep.* 47(12), 9939–9949. doi:10.1007/s11033-020-05988-1. Epub 2020 Nov 13. PMID: 33185828.

10. Ou, X., Liu, Y., Lei, X., Li, P., Mi, D., Ren, L., Guo, L., Guo, R., Chen, T., Hu, J., Xiang, Z., Mu, Z., Chen, X., Chen, J., Hu, K., Jin, Q., Wang, J., Qian, Z. (2020). Characterization of spike glycoprotein of SARS-CoV-2 on virus entry and its immune cross-reactivity with SARS-CoV. *Nat. Commun.* 11(1), 1620. doi:10.1038/s41467-020-15562-9.

11. Lambert, D. W., Yarski, M., Warner, F. J. (2005). Tumor necrosis factor convertase (ADAM17)

mediates regulated ectodomain shedding of the severe-acute respiratory syndrome-coronavirus (SARS-CoV) receptor, angiotensin-converting enzyme-2 (ACE2). *J. Biol. Chem.* 280(34), 30113–30119.

12. McMillan, P., Dexhiemer, T., Neubig, R., Uhal, B. D. (2021). COVID-19: A theory of autoimmunity against ACE-2 explained. *Front. Immunol.* 12, 582166. doi:10.3389/fimmu.2021.582166.

13. Epelman, S., Tang, W. H. W., Chen, S. Y., Van Lente, F., Francis, G. S., Sen, S. (2008). Detection of soluble angiotensin-converting enzyme 2 in heart failure: Insights into the endogenous counter-regulatory pathway of the renin angiotensin-aldosterone system. *J. Am. Coll. Cardiol.* 52, 750–754. doi:10.1016/j.jacc.2008.02.088.

14. Yeung, M.L., Lee Teng, J.L., Jia, L., Zhang, C., Huang, C., Cai, J.-P., Zhou, R., Chan, K.-H., Zhao, H., Zhu, L., Siu, K.-L., Fung, S.-Y., Yung, S., Chan, T.M., Kai-Wang To, K., Fuk-Woo Chan, J., Cai, Z., Pui Lau, S. K., Chen, Z., Jin, D.-Y., Yat Woo, P. C., Yuen, K.-Y. (2021). Soluble ACE2- mediated cell entry of SARS-CoV-2 via interaction with proteins related to the renin-angiotensin system. *Cell* 184(8), 2212–2228.e12.

15. Clausen, T.M., Sandoval, D.R., Spliid, C.B., Pihl, J., Perrett, H.R., Painter, C.D., Narayanan, A., Majowicz, S.A., Kwong, E.M., McVicar, R.N. (2020). SARS-CoV-2 infection depends on cellular heparan sulfate and ACE2. *Cell* 183, 1043–1057.

16. Kim, S.Y., Jin, W., Sood, A., Montgomery, D.W., Grant, O.C., Fuster, M.M., Fu, L., Dordick, J.S., Woods, R.J., Zhang, F. (2020). Characterization of heparin and severe acute respiratory syndrome-related coronavirus 2 (SARSCoV-2) spike glycoprotein binding interactions. *Antiv. Res.* 181, 104873.

17. Cantuti-Castelvetri, L., Ojha, R., Pedro, L.D., Djannatian, M., Franz, J., Kuivanen, S., van der Meer, F., Kallio, K., Kaya, T., Anastasina, M. (2020). Neuropilin-1 facilitates SARS-CoV-2 cell entry and infectivity. *Science* 370, 856–860.

18. Li, F. (2015). Receptor recognition mechanisms of coronaviruses: A decade of structural studies. *J. Virol.* 89, 1954–1964.

19. Bermejo-Jambrina, M., Eder, J., Helgers, L.C., Hertoghs, N., Nijmeijer, B.M., Stunnenberg, M. Geijtenbeek, T.B. (2018). C-type lectin receptors in antiviral immunity and viral escape. *Front. Immunol.* 9, 590.

20. Matrosovich, M., Herrler, G., Klenk, H.D. (2015). Sialic acid receptors of viruses. *Top Curr. Chem.* 367, 1–28.

21. Qing, E. (2020). Distinct roles for sialoside and protein receptors in coronavirus infection. *MBio* 11(1), e02764.

22. Milanetti, E., Miotto, M., Di Rienzo, L., Monti, M. (2021). In-silico evidence for two receptors based strategy of SARS-CoV-2. *bioRxiv*. Preprint at doi:10.1101/2020.03,2020.24.

23. Liu, J. (2020). Hydroxychloroquine, a less toxic derivative of chloroquine, is effective in inhibiting SARS-CoV-2 infection in vitro. *Cell Discov.* 6(1), 1–4.

24. Fantini, J, Di Scala, C., Chahinian, H., Yahi, N. (2020). Structural and molecular modelling studies reveal a new mechanism of action of chloroquine and hydroxychloroquine against SARS-CoV-2 infection. *Int. J. Antimicrob. Agents* 55(5), 105960.

25. Singh, H., Chauhan, P., Kakkar, A.K. 2021. Hydroxychloroquine for the treatment and prophylaxis of COVID-19: The journey so far and the road ahead. *Eur. J. Pharmacol.*, 890, 173717.

26. Elavarasi, A., Prasad, M., Seth, T., Sahoo, R.K., Madan, K., Nischal, N., Soneja, M., Sharma, A., Maulik, S.K., Shalimar, G.P. (2020). Chloroquine and hydroxychloroquine for the treatment of COVID-19: A systematic review and meta-analysis. *J. Gen. Intern. Med.* 35(11), 3308–3314. doi:10.1007/s11606-020-06146-w. Epub 2020 Sep 3. PMID: 32885373; PMCID: PMC7471562.

27. Chan, R.W., Chan, M.C., Wong, A.C., Karamanska, R., Dell, A., Haslam, S.M., Sihoe, A.D., Chui, W.H., Triana-Baltzer, G., Li, Q., Peiris, J.S., Fang, F., Nicholls, J.M. (2009). DAS181 inhibits H5N1 influenza virus infection of human lung tissues. *Antimicrob. Agents Chemother.*, 53(9), 3935–3941.

28. Ho, J.H.-C., Zhao, Y, Liu, Z, Zhou, X., Chen, X, Xianyu, Y, Lewis, S, Fan, L, Tian, Y, Chang, N, Gong, Z, Hu, K. et al. (2019). Resolution of coronavirus disease Infection and pulmonary pathology with nebulized DAS181: A pilot study. *Crit. Care Explor.* 2(10): e0263.

29. Veldhuizen, R.A., Zuo, Y.Y., Petersen, N.O., Lewis, J.F., Possmayer, F. (2021). The COVID-19 pandemic: a target for surfactant therapy? *Expert Rev. Respir. Med.* 15(5), 597–608.

30. Devasena, T. (2021). The nanotechnology-COVID-19 interface. In *Nanotechnology-COVID-19 Interface*. Springer, pp. 31–58.

31. Seth, S., Batra, J., Srinivasan, S. (2020). COVID-19: Targeting proteases in viral invasion and host immune response. *Front. Mol. Biosci.*, 7, 215.

32. Li, H., Wang, Y., Xu, J., Cao, B. (2020). Potential antiviral therapeutics for 2019 Novel Coronavirus. *Chin. J. Tuberc. Respir. Dis.* 43, E002–E002.

33. Roe, M.K., Junod, N.A., Young, A.R., Beachboard, D.C., Stobart, C.C. (2021). Targeting novel structural and functional features of coronavirus protease nsp5 (3CL(pro), M(pro)) in the age of COVID-19. *J. Gen. Virol.* 102 (3), 001558.

34. Goyal, B., Goyal, D. (2020). Targeting the dimerization of the main protease of coronaviruses: A potential broad-spectrum therapeutic strategy. *ACS Combinat. Sci.* 22, 297–305.

35. Amin, S.A., Banerjee, S., Ghosh, K., Gayen, S., Jha, T. (2020). Protease targeted COVID-19 drug disCoVery and its challenges: Insight into viral main

protease (Mpro) and papain-like protease (PLpro) inhibitors. *Bioorg. Med. Chem.* 29, 115860.

36. Krichel, B., Falke, S., Hilgenfeld, R., Redecke, L., Uetrecht, C. (2020). Processing of the SARS-CoV pp1a/ab nsp7-10 region. *Biochem. J.* 477, 1009–1019.

37. Jin, X., Du, X., Xu, Y., Deng, Y., Liu, M., Zhao, Y., Zhang, B., Li, X., Zhang, L., Peng, C., Duan, Y., Yu, J., Wang, L., Yang, K., Liu, F., Jiang, R., Yang, X., You, T., Liu, X., Yang, X., Bai, F., Liu, H., Liu, X., Guddat, L.W., Xu, W., Xiao, G., Qin, C., Shi, Z., Jiang, H., Rao, Z., Yang, H. (2020). Structure of M^pro from SARS-CoV.2 and discovery of its inhibitors. *Nature* 582(7811), 289–293.

38. Zhang, L., Lin, D., Kusov, Y., Nian, Y., Ma, Q., Wang, J., Von Brunn, A., Leyssen, P., Lanko, K., Neyts, J. (2020). a-Ketoamides as broad-spectrum inhibitors of coronavirus and enterovirus replication: Structure-based design, synthesis, and activity assessment. *J. Med. Chem.* 63, 4562–4578.

39. Kumar, B.K., Sekhar, K.V.G.C., Kunjiappan, S., Jamalis, J., Balaña-Fouce, R., Tekwani, B.L., Sankaranarayanan, M. (2020). Druggable targets of SARS-CoV-2 and treatment opportunities for COVID-19. *Bioorg. Chem.* 104, 104269.

40. Zhang, L., Lin, D., Sun, X., Curth, U., Drosten, C., Sauerhering, L., Becker, S., Rox, K., Hilgenfeld, R. (2020). Crystal structure of SARS-CoV-2 main protease provides a basis for design of improved alpha-ketoamide inhibitors. *Science* 368, 409–412.

41. Daoud, S., Alabed, S.J., Dahabiyeh, L.A. (2021). Identification of potential COVID-19 main protease inhibitors using structure-based pharmacophore approach, molecular docking and repurposing studies. *Acta Pharm.* 71, 163–174.

42. Hattori, S.I., Higashi-Kuwata, N., Hayashi, H., Allu, S.R., Raghavaiah, J., Bulut, H., Das, D., Anson, B.J., Lendy, E.K., Takamatsu, Y., Takamune, N., Kishimoto, N., Murayama, K., Hasegawa, K., Li, M., Davis, D.A., Kodama, E.N., Yarchoan, R., Wlodawer, A., Misumi, S., Mesecar, A.D., Ghosh, A.K., Mitsuya, H. (2021). A small molecule compound with an indole moiety inhibits the main protease of SARS-CoV-2 and blocks virus replication. *Nat. Commun.* 12, 668.

43. Di Micco, S., Musella, S., Scala, M.C., Sala, M., Campiglia, P., Bifulco, G., Fasano, A. (2020). In silico analysis revealed potential anti-SARS-CoV-2 main protease activity by the Zonulin inhibitor Larazotide acetate. *Front. Chem.* 8, 628609.

44. Di Pierro, M., Lu, R., Uzzau, S., Wang, W., Margaretten, K., Pazzani, C., Maimone, F., Fasano, A. (2001). Zonula occludens toxin structure-function analysis: Identification of the fragment biologically active on tight junctions and of the zonulin receptor binding domain. *J. Biol. Chem.* 276, 19160–19165.

45. Sacco, M.D., Ma, C., Lagarias, P., Gao, A., Townsend, J.A., Meng, X., Dube, P., Zhang, X.,

Hu, Y., Kitamura, N., Hurst, B., Tarbet, B., Marty, M.T., Kolocouris, A., Xiang, Y., Chen, Y., Wang, J. (2020). Structure and inhibition of the SARS-CoV-2 main protease reveal strategy for developing dual inhibitors against M(pro) and cathepsin L. *Sci. Adv.* 6, eabe0751.

46. Yang, H., Xie, W., Xue, X., Yang, K., Ma, J., Liang, W., Zhao, Q., Zhou, Z., Pei, D., Ziebuhr, J., Hilgenfeld, R., Yuen, K.Y., Wong, L., Gao, G., Chen, S., Chen, Z., Ma, D., Bartlam, M., Rao, Z. (2005). Design of wide-spectrum inhibitors targeting coronavirus main proteases. *PLoS Biol.* 3, e324.

47. Ma, C., Hu, Y., Townsend, J. A., Lagarias, P.I., Marty, M.T., Kolocouris, A., Wang, J. (2020). Ebselen, disulfiram, carmofur, PX-12, tideglusib, and shikonin are nonspecific promiscuous SARS-CoV-2 main protease inhibitors. *ACS Pharmacol. Transl. Sci.* 3, 1265–1277.

48. Jin, Z., Du, X., Xu, Y., Deng, Y., Liu, M., Zhao, Y., Zhang, B., Li, X., Zhang, L., Peng, C. (2020). Structure of M pro from SARS-CoV-2 and disCoVery of its inhibitors. *Nature*, 582, 289–293.

49. Majumder, R., Mandal, M. (2020). Screening of plant-based natural compounds as a potential COVID-19 main protease inhibitor: An in silico docking and molecular dynamics simulation approach. *J. Biomol. Struct. Dyn.* 1–16. doi:10.1080/07391102.2020.1817787.

50. Teli, D.M., Shah, M.B., Chhabria, M.T. (2020). In silico screening of natural compounds as potential inhibitors of SARS-CoV-2 main protease and spike RBD: Targets for COVID-19. *Front. Mol. Biosci.* 7, 599079.

51. Neupane, N.P., Karn, A.K., Mukeri, I.H., Pathak, P., Kumar, P., Singh, S., Qureshi, I.A., Jha, T., Verma, A. (2021). Molecular dynamics analysis of phytochemicals from Ageratina adenophora against COVID-19 main protease (M(pro)) and human angiotensin-converting enzyme 2 (ACE2). *Biocatal. Agric. Biotechnol.* 32, 101924.

52. Mielech, A.M., Chen, Y., Mesecar, A.D., Baker, S.C. (2014). Nidovirus papain-like proteases: Multifunctional enzymes with protease, deubiquitinating and deISGylating activities. *Virus Res.* 194, 184–190.

53. Liu, J., Zhai, Y., Liang, L., Zhu, D., Zhao, Q., Qiu, Y. (2021). Molecular modeling evaluation of the binding effect of five protease inhibitors to COVID-19 main protease. *Chem. Phys.* 542, 111080. doi:10.1016/j.chemphys.2020.111080.

54. Kouznetsova, V.L., Zhang, A., Tatineni, M., Miller, M.A., Tsigelny, I.F., 2020. Potential COVID-19 papain-like protease PL(pro) inhibitors: repurposing FDA-approved drugs. *Peer J.* 8, e9965. doi:10.7717/peerj.9965.

55. Fu, Z., Huang, B., Tang, J., Liu, S., Liu, M., Ye, Y., Liu, Z., Xiong, Y., Zhu, W., Cao, D., Li, J., Niu, X., Zhou, H., Zhao, Y. J., Zhang, G., Huang, H. (2021). The complex structure of GRL0617 and

SARS-CoV-2 PLpro reveals a hot spot for antiviral drug disCoVery. *Nat. Commun.* 12, 488.

56. Bhowmik, D., Sharma, R. D., Prakash, A., Kumar, D. (2021). Identification of Nafamostat and VR23 as COVID-19 drug candidates by targeting 3CL(pro) and PL(pro). *J. Mol. Struct.* 1233, 130094.

57. Mirza, M.U., Ahmad, S., Abdullah, I., Froeyen, M. (2020). Identification of novel human USP2 inhibitor and its putative role in treatment of COVID-19 by inhibiting SARS-CoV-2 papain-like (PLpro) protease. *Comput. Biol. Chem.* 89, 107376.

58. Perng, Y.C., Lenschow, D.J. (2018). ISG15 in antiviral immunity and beyond. *Nat. Rev. Microbiol.*, 16, 423–439.

59. Villarroya-Beltri, C., Guerra, S., Sánchez-Madrid, F. (2017). ISGylation–a key to lock the cell gates for preventing the spread of threats. *J. Cell Sci.* 130, 2961–2969.

60. Liu, G., Lee, J.-H., Parker, Z. M., Acharya, D., Chiang, J.J., van Gent, M., Riedl, W., Davis-Gardner, M.E., Wies, E., Chiang, C. (2020). ISG15-dependent activation of the RNA sensor MDA5 and its antagonism by the SARS-CoV-2 papain-like protease. *bioRxiv.* doi:10.1101/2020.10.26.356048.

61. Freitas, B.T., Durie, I.A., Murray, J., Longo, J.E., Miller, H.C., Crich, D., Hogan, R.J., Tripp, R.A., Pegan, S.D. (2020). Characterization and NonCoValent inhibition of the deubiquitinase and deISGylase activity of SARS-CoV-2 papain-like protease. *ACS Infect. Dis.* 6, 2099–2109.

62. McClain, C.B., Vabret, N. (2020). SARS-CoV-2: The many pros of targeting PLpro. *Signal Transduct. Target. Ther.* 5, 223.

63. Shin, D., Mukherjee, R., Grewe, D., Bojkova, D., Baek, K., Bhattacharya, A., Schulz, L., Widera, M., Mehdipour, A.R., Tascher, G., Geurink, P.P., Wilhelm, A., van der Heden van Noort, G.J., Ovaa, H., Muller, S., Knobeloch, K.P., Rajalingam, K., Schulman, B.A., Cinatl, J., Hummer, G., Ciesek, S., Dikic, I. (2020). Papain-like protease regulates SARS-CoV-2 viral spread and innate immunity. *Nature* 587, 657–662.

64. Gupta, V., Murthy, M.K., Patil, S. (2020). Can host cell proteins like ACE2, ADAM17, TMPRSS2, androgen receptor be the efficient targets in SARS-CoV-2 infection? *Curr. Drug Targets* 22(10), 1149–1157.

65. Iwata-Yoshikawa, N., Okamura, T., Shimizu, Y., Hasegawa, H., Takeda, M., Nagata, N. (2019). TMPRSS2 contributes to virus spread and immunopathology in the airways of murine models after coronavirus infection. *J. Virol.* 93, e01815.

66. Shen, L.W., Mao, H.J., Wu, Y.L., Tanaka, Y., Zhang, W. (2017). TMPRSS2: A potential target for treatment of influenza virus and coronavirus infections. *Biochimie* 142, 1–10.

67. De Toma, I., Dierssen, M. (2021). Network analysis of down syndrome and SARS-CoV-2 identifies risk and protective factors for COVID-19. *Sci. Rep.* 11, 1–12.

68. Matsuyama, S., Nagata, N., Shirato, K., Kawase, M., Takeda, M., Taguchi, F. (2010). Efficient activation of the severe acute respiratory syndrome coronavirus spike protein by the transmembrane protease TMPRSS2. *J. Virol.* 84, 12658–12664.

69. Zhirnov, O., Klenk, H., Wright, P. (2011). Aprotinin and similar protease inhibitors as drugs against influenza. *Antiv. Res.* 92, 27–36.

70. Hoffmann, M., Schroeder, S., Kleine-Weber, H., Müller, M.A., Drosten, C., Pöhlmann, S. (2020). Nafamostat mesylate blocks activation of SARS-CoV-2: New treatment option for COVID-19. *Antimicrob. Agents Chemother.* 64, e00754.

71. Glowacka, I., Bertram, S., Müller, M.A., Allen, P., Soilleux, E., Pfefferle, S., Steffen, I., Tsegaye, T.S., He, Y., Gnirss, K. (2011). Evidence that TMPRSS2 activates the severe acute respiratory syndrome coronavirus spike protein for membrane fusion and reduces viral control by the humoral immune response. *J. Virol.* 85, 4122–4134.

72. Zipeto, D., da Fonseca Palmeira, J., Argañaraz, G.A., Argañaraz, E.R. (2020). ACE2/ADAM17/TMPRSS2 interplay may be the main risk factor for COVID-19. *Front. Immunol.* 11, 2642.

73. Yang, C., Keshavjee, S., Liu, M. (2020). Alpha-1 antitrypsin for COVID-19 treatment: Dual role in antiviral infection and anti-inflammation. *Front. Pharmacol.* 11, 615398.

74. Bae, E.H., Kim, I.J., Choi, H.S., Kim, H.Y., Kim, C.S., Ma, S.K., Kim, I.S., Kim, S.W. (2018). Tumor necrosis factor a-converting enzyme inhibitor attenuates lipopolysaccharide-induced reactive oxygen species and mitogen-activated protein kinase expression in human renal proximal tubule epithelial cells. *Korean J. Physiol. Pharmacol.* 22, 135.

75. Zhou, Y., Vedantham, P., Lu, K., Agudelo, J., Simmon, G. (2015). Protease inhibitors targeting coronavirus and filovirus entry. *Antiv. Res.* 116, 76–84.

76. Liu, T., Luo, S., Libby, P., Shi, G.-P. (2020). Cathepsin L-selective inhibitors: A potentially promising treatment for COVID-19 patients. *Pharmacol. Ther.* 213, 107587.

77. Akgun, E., Tuzuner, M.B., Sahin, B., Kilercik, M., Kulah, C., Cakiroglu, H.N., Serteser, M., Unsal, I., Baykal, A.T. (2020). Proteins associated with neutrophil degranulation are upregulated in nasopharyngeal swabs from SARS-CoV-2 patients. *PLoS One* 15, e0240012.

78. Methot, N., Rubin, J., Guay, D., Beaulieu, C., Ethier, D., Reddy, T.J., Riendeau, D., Percival, M.D. (2007). Inhibition of the activation of multiple serine proteases with a cathepsin C inhibitor requires sustained exposure to prevent pro-enzyme processing. *J. Biol. Chem.* 282, 20836–20846.

79. Lu, R., Zhao, X., Li, J., Niu, P., Yang, B., Wu, H., Wang, W., Song, H., Huang, B., Zhu, N., et al. (2020). Genomic characterisation and epidemiology of 2019 novel coronavirus: Implications for virus origins and receptor binding. *Lancet* 395, 565–574, doi:10.1016/S0140-6736(20)30251-8.

80. Andersen, K.G., Rambaut, A., Lipkin, W.I., Holmes, E.C., Garry, R.F. (2020). The proximal origin of SARS-CoV-2. *Nat. Med.* 26, 450–452, doi:10.1038/s41591-020-0820-9.

81. Seidah, N.G., Sadr, M.S., Chretien, M., Mbikay, M. (2013). The multifaceted proprotein convertases: Their unique, redundant, complementary, and opposite functions. *J. Biol. Chem.* 288, 21473–21481, doi:10.1074/jbc.R113.481549.

82. Izaguirre, G. (2019). The proteolytic regulation of virus cell entry by Furin and other proprotein convertases. *Viruses* 11, doi:10.3390/v11090837.

83. Millet, J.K., Whittaker, G.R. (2015). Host cell proteases: Critical determinants of coronavirus tropism and pathogenesis. *Virus Res.* 202, 120–134, doi:10.1016/j.virusres.2014.11.021.

84. Johnson, B.A., Xie, X., Bailey, A.L., Kalveram, B., Lokugamage, K.G., Muruato, A., Zou, J., Zhang, X., Juelich, T., Smith, J.K., et al. (2021).Loss of furin cleavage site attenuates SARS-CoV-2 pathogenesis. *Nature* 591, 293–299, doi:10.1038/s41586-021-03237-4.

85. Bussani, R., Schneider, E., Zentilin, L., Collesi, C., Ali, H., Braga, L., Volpe, M.C., Colliva, A., Zanconati, F., Berlot, G., et al. (2020). Persistence of viral RNA, pneumocyte syncytia and thrombosis are hallmarks of advanced COVID-19 pathology. *EBioMedicine* 61, 103104, doi:10.1016/j.ebiom.2020.103104.

86. Cheng, C.C., Yang, C.F., Lo, Y.P., Chiang, Y.H., Sofiyatun, E., Wang, L.C., Chen, W.J. (2020). Cell-to-cell spread of dengue viral RNA in mosquito cells. *BioMed Res. Int.* 2020, 2452409, doi:10.1155/2020/2452409.

87. Follis, K.E., York, J., Nunberg, J.H. (2006). Furin cleavage of the SARS coronavirus spike glycoprotein enhances cell-cell fusion but does not affect virion entry. *Virology* 350, 358–369. doi:10.1016/j.virol.2006.02.003.

88. Hoffmann, M., Kleine-Weber, H., Pohlmann, S. (2020). A Multibasic cleavage site in the spike protein of SARS-CoV-2 is essential for infection of human lung cells. *Mol. Cell* 78, 779–784. doi:10.1016/j.molcel.2020.04.022.

89. Hoffmann, M., Kleine-Weber, H., Schroeder, S., Kruger, N., Herrler, T., Erichsen, S., Schiergens, T.S., Herrler, G., Wu, N.H., Nitsche, A., et al. (2020). SARS-CoV-2 cell entry depends on ACE2 and TMPRSS2 and is blocked by a clinically proven protease inhibitor. *Cell* 181, 271–280.e278. doi:10.1016/j.cell.2020.02.052.

90. Cheng, Y.W., Chao, T.L., Li, C.L., Chiu, M.F., Kao, H.C., Wang, S.H., Pang, Y.H., Lin, C.H., Tsai, Y.M., Lee, W.H., et al. (2020). Furin inhibitors block SARS-CoV-2 spike protein cleavage to suppress virus production and cytopathic effects. *Cell Rep.* 33, 108254, doi:10.1016/j.celrep.2020.108254.

91. Aftab, S.O. et al. (2020). Analysis of SARS-CoV-2 RNA-dependent RNA polymerase as a potential therapeutic drug target using a computational approach. *J. Transl. Med.* 18, 275.

92. Sheahan, T.P. et al. (2017). Broad-spectrum antiviral GS-5734 inhibits both epidemic and zoonotic coronaviruses. *Sci. Transl. Med.* 9, eaal3653.

93. Pruijssers, A.J. et al. (2020). Remdesivir inhibits SARS-CoV-2 in human lung cells and chimeric SARS-CoV expressing the SARS-CoV-2 RNA polymerase in mice. *Cell Rep.* 32, 107940.

94. Padhi, A.K., Shukla, R., Saudagar, P., Tripathi, T. (2021). High-throughput rational design of the remdesivir binding site in the RdRp of SARS-CoV-2: Implications for potential resistance. *iScience* 24, 101992.

95. Agostini, M.L. et al. (2018). Coronavirus susceptibility to the antiviral remdesivir (GS-5734) is mediated by the viral polymerase and the proofreading exoribonuclease. *mBio* 9, e00221-18.

96. Dabbous, H.M. et al. (2021). Efficacy of favipiravir in COVID-19 treatment: a multi-center randomized study. *Arch. Virol.* 166, 949–954.

97. Sadeghi, A. et al. (2020). Sofosbuvir and daclatasvir compared with standard of care in the treatment of patients admitted to hospital with moderate or severe coronavirus infection (COVID-19): A randomized controlled trial. *J. Antimicrob. Chemother.* 75, 3379–3385.

98. Ko, W.-C. et al. (2020). Arguments in favour of remdesivir for treating SARS-CoV-2. *Int. J. Antimicrob. Agents* 55, 105933.

99. Hillen, H.S., Kokic, G., Farnung, L., Dienemann, C., Tegunov, D., Cramer, P. (2020). Structure of replicating SARS-CoV-2 polymerase. *Nature* 584, 154.

100. Stertz, S. et al. (2007). The intracellular sites of early replication and budding of SARS-coronavirus. *Virology* 361, 304–315.

Chapter 11 Computational Biology and Bioinformatics in Anti-SARS-CoV-2 Drug Development

Vladimir N. Uversky

11.1 CHALLENGES ASSOCIATED WITH COVID-19 TREATMENT

Notwithstanding obvious problems associated with the fast and massive spread of the severe acute respiratory syndrome coronavirus 2 (SARS-CoV-2) infection around the globe causing the global coronavirus disease 2019 (COVID-19) pandemic, treatment options for COVID-19 remain scarce. As it was rightly pointed out by James Pandarakalam: "Medical profession was unprepared to face the coronavirus pandemic, and the pharmaceutical armamentarium is currently not robust enough to combat with SARS-CoV-2" (https://www.sciencerepository.org/the-clinical-and-treatment-challenges-posed-by-covid-19_JCMCR-2020-2-105).

What makes SARS-CoV-2 infection so special? COVID-19 is a very complex illness characterized by high transmission potential and unpredictability of disease progression [1], with senior citizens and people with compromised immunity or some comorbidities being more vulnerable to infection. Since entry of SARS-CoV-2 to the host cells depends on the presence of the specific receptor, ACE2 (angiotensin-converting enzyme 2), on the cell surface, and since cells of many tissues and organs have these receptors, SARS-CoV-2 infection often represents a multi-hit pathology affecting different organs and causing multiple health issues. Though initial symptoms of SARS-CoV-2 infection are typical for the respiratory disease and include persistent dry cough, sore throat, and fever, COVID-19 may progress to breathlessness and pneumonia, fatigue, headache, aches and pains. Many patients show olfactory and gustatory dysfunctions, such as the loss of the sense of smell (anosmia) and of taste (ageusia). In some patients, SARS-CoV-2 infection can initiate a "cytokine storm", generating massive production of chemokines and cytokines such as IL1-β, IL1RA, IL7, IL8, IL9, IL10, basic FGF2, GCSF, GMCSF, IFNγ, IP10, MCP1, MIP1α, MIP1β, PDGFB, TNFα, and VEGFA [2]. Increased severity of disease, especially in the patients admitted to intensive care units (ICUs), is associated with the increased levels of pro-inflammatory cytokines such as IL2, IL7, IL10, GCSF, IP10, MCP1, MIP1α, and TNFα [3]. SARS-CoV-2 can access the central nervous system via multiple pathways [4], causing both ischaemic and haemorrhagic strokes, encephalitis, Guillain-Barré syndrome, confusion, disorientation, and other neurological symptoms [5], and may lead to an amplification of existing mental health issues and result in a surge of cases of post-traumatic stress disorder (PTSD; the incidence of PTSD during the pandemic COVID-19 outbreak is 18%, whereas the prevalence of PTSD-related symptoms in coronavirus survivors is 29% [6]) and increase in depression, anxiety, and insomnia [7]. This virus can also cause venous thrombosis leading to pulmonary embolism [8], and, more generally, it affects the heart and vascular system directly or indirectly [9]. Many patients show renal, liver, and gastrointestinal pathologies [10], and adverse effects of SARS-CoV-2 on male fertility potential are also reported [11]. Furthermore, COVID-19 can be associated with visual impairments manifested in dacryoadenitis, conjunctivitis, tonic pupils, vitritis, central retinal artery/venous occlusion, retinitis, retinal bleeding, panuveitis, anterior ischemic optic neuropathy, optic nerve stroke, optic neuritis, optic perineuritis, or occipital ischemic stroke [12]. Such a multi-hit potential not only defines the unpredictability of disease progression, but also represents a very serious challenge to the development of anti-COVID-19 therapies. Another most serious challenge is given by the rather fast mutation rate of this RNA virus. In fact, the currently reported rate of the acquisition of new mutations by SARS-CoV-2 is 0.9×10^{-3} during the substitutions/site/year [13], which corresponds to 26 substitutions per year [14], or more than two changes per month [15]. Therefore, SARS-CoV-2 is not only a difficult multi-hit pathogen, but is also a rapidly moving target that requires the development of promptly amendable and swiftly adaptable preventive and treatment strategies. It is likely that bioinformatics and computational biology might represent important means for fulfilling these goals.

11.2 SARS-CoV-2 SEQUENCING, DATA STORAGE, RETRIEVAL, AND ANALYSIS

Whole genome sequencing represents an important means for tracing the origin, spread, and transmission chains of SARS-CoV-2, and is crucial for monitoring the evolution of this virus

DOI: 10.1201/9781003190394-11

and the emergence of reinfections. The first complete genomic sequences of SARS-CoV-2 were reported in late December 2019 [16–18]. The reference genome assembly was achieved through metatranscriptomic approaches augmented by PCR and Sanger sequencing [16–18]. This information was crucial as it provided vital means for the development of diagnostic tests based on real-time PCR [19]. This success in the identification of SARS-CoV-2 was a result of the use of next-generation sequencing (NGS) and readily available bioinformatics pipelines, which can be assembled into an NGS data analysis workflow consisting of several essential steps, such as quality control of the NGS data, removal of host/rRNA data, reads assembly, taxonomic classification, and virus genome verification [20]. A recent review describes numerous bioinformatics tools, which are currently available for every step of the NGS data analysis, and discusses the advantages and disadvantages of these bioinformatics resources [20]. Importantly, these same NGS technologies and bioinformatics resources can be used efficiently for the ongoing genomic surveillance of SARS-CoV-2 worldwide, tracking its spread, evolution, and patterns of variation on a global scale [20]. Another comprehensive review introduces currently available platforms and methodological approaches for the sequencing of SARS-CoV-2 genomes, and outlines some of the repositories and databases delivering access to SARS-CoV-2 genomic data and associated metadata [21].

The unmatched efforts to develop effective surveillance strategies based on real-time sequencing of the SARS-CoV-2 genome were triggered by the COVID-19 pandemic [15, 22–26], and the results of these efforts are truly astonishing. For example, the Centers for Disease Control and Prevention (CDC) established the SARS-CoV-2 Sequencing for Public Health Emergency Response, Epidemiology and Surveillance (SPHERES) program to coordinate SARS-CoV-2 sequencing (https://www.cdc.gov/coronavirus/2019-ncov/covid-data/spheres.html). SeqCOVID, a consortium in Spain focusing on genomic epidemiology of SARS-CoV-2, received 28,132 SARS-CoV-2 samples, 14,797 of which were sequences (http://seqcovid.csic.es/). The EpiCov repository, which is a part of the GISAID (Global Initiative on Sharing All Influenza Data) initiative [27, 28], included 1,670,279 submissions of SARS-CoV-2 sequences as of May 22, 2021 (https://www.gisaid.org/). The major centralized depository of SARS-CoV-2–related information, the NCBI SARS-CoV-2 Resources (https://www.ncbi.nlm.nih.gov/sars-cov-2/), contains massive SARS-CoV-2 data that include 608,864 Sequence Read Archive (SRA) runs, 498,354 nucleotide records, 3,591,571 viral protein records, 136,701 PubMed publications on this virus, and 5,761 records on SARS-CoV-2-related clinical trials. One can find a regularly updated SARS-CoV-2 phylogeny on an open-source platform to harness the scientific and public health potential of pathogen genome data at Nextstrain [29], which, has provided information on 3,921 SARS-CoV-2 genomes sampled between December 2019 and May 2021 (as of May 22, 2021) (https://nextstrain.org/) (see Figure 11.1).

With all the advantages of having massive amounts of information of SARS-CoV-2 sequences in different countries on different continents, and the related publicly available epidemiological, biological, and clinical data, there is an obvious issue pertaining to these big data (i.e., large and diverse data sets that require computational analysis): the need to be able analyze them in a meaningful way. To address this issue, numerous web tools and online methods were developed by bioinformaticians to give non-computational users an opportunity to conduct SARS-CoV-2- and COVID-19–related research and analyses. Therefore, among the crucial roles of bioinformatics in addressing various aspects related to COVID-19 research and providing solutions to different SARS-CoV-2–related questions are the capability to reduce the vaccine development time, to discover potential clinical interventions, and to deal with the big data via the development of well-ordered information hubs and web resources, and efficient information retrieval from the current massive information sources about SARS-CoV-2 [30]. A detailed description of a set of web platforms designed to visualize and mine data from four major branches: epidemiology, genomics, interactomics, and pharmacology/clinical studies, is provided in a recent comprehensive review containing information on web links, sources, and architectures of at least 30 such COVID-19 web platforms [31]. An important review by Hufsky et al. can serve as a detailed manual describing a large set of bioinformatics workflows and tools for multi-level COVID-19 research, starting from the routine detection of SARS-CoV-2 infection, to the trustworthy analysis of sequencing data, to pursuing the COVID-19 pandemic and assessment of containment measures, to the study of coronavirus (CoV) evolution, to the discovery of potential drug targets and development of therapeutic strategies [32]. To facilitate clinical research on COVID-19, a web portal OverCOVID (http://bis.zju.edu.cn/overcovid/) was created,

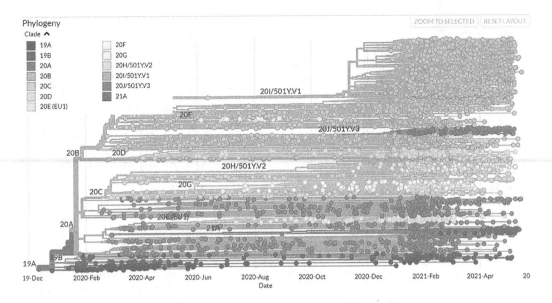

Figure 11.1 SARS-CoV-2 phylogeny on an open-source platform Nextstrain [29], which, as of May 22, 2021, provides information on 3,921 SARS-CoV-2 genomes sampled between December 2019 and May 2021 (https://nextstrain.org/).

where a detailed interpretation of SARS-CoV-2 basics is provided, and a collection of resources that may contribute to therapeutic advances is introduced [33].

11.3 EVOLUTION OF SARS-CoV-2

The genomic sequence of viruses (especially in the case of viruses with RNA genomes) is prone to mutations caused either by random replication errors or introduced by RNA editing, which is a defense mechanism of the host [34, 35]. Synonymous (when there is no change in the encoded amino acid because of nucleotide substitutions) and non-synonymous (nucleotide substitutions that cause amino acid changes) mutations occur on a regular basis in the viral genome, with the reported rate of acquired new mutations for SARS-CoV-2 being approximately two changes per month [15] (or approximately 26 substitutions per year [14]), and as of September 2020, the SARS-CoV-2 was shown to have a mutation rate of 0.9×10^{-3} substitution/site/year [13]. This evolutionary rate is similar to those of other human CoVs: $0.80 - 2.38 \times 10^{-3}$, $0.63 - 1.12 \times 10^{-3}$, and 0.43×10^{-3} substitutions/site/year for SARS-CoV [36], MERS-CoV [37–39], and HCoV OC43 [40], respectively.

Furthermore, the evolution of CoVs occurs not only by nucleotide mutations but also by recombination [14]. Therefore, information on sequence variability can be used for the phylogenetic analysis of various human CoVs (SARS-CoV, MERS-CoV, and SARS-CoV-2) in order

to get a glimpse at their evolutionary correlations. Such phylogenetic analysis, for example, demonstrated that SARS-CoV and SARS-CoV-2 are relatively distantly related, and suggested that their spill-over into humans were distinct events [41]. This conclusion was further supported by an integrated semi-alignment based computational technique used to compare 340, 291, and 2,391 SARS-CoV, MERS-CoV, and SARS-CoV-2 genome sequences, respectively, which were shown to form three non-overlapping clusters [42]. This analysis showed that the SARS-CoV-2 genomic sequences were ~77% similar to those of SARS-CoV, whereas there was only ~36% sequence similarity between the SARS-CoV-2 and MERS-CoV genomes [42].

Phylogenetic analysis of different SARS-CoV-2 isolates allows researchers to look at the in-host evolution of this virus and to find clades – clusters of related genomes grouped according to common mutations. For example, such analysis conducted for over 5,000 SARS-CoV-2 genomes isolated from Indian COVID-19 patients produced a phylogeny with 6,888 mutation events [15]. Here, the presence of a prominent clade I/A3i, which was characterized by a set of 4 mutations and likely arose from a single outbreak, was noticed in samples retrieved during the early spread of infection. Importantly, while originally 42% of all genomes sequenced in India belonged to this clade, it evolved quickly via changes in the Nucleocapsid (N) and Membrane (M) genes, and has become almost non-existent in recent samples [15]. An integrated semi-alignment–based computational technique was utilized to analyze 2,391 genomic SARS-CoV-2 sequences to look at the SARS-CoV-2 sequence variability in human hosts from 54 different countries and to analyze sequence variability between the CoV family and country-specific SARS-CoV-2 sequences in human hosts [42].

While one would expect that the presence of multiple genome sequences from various SARS-CoV-2 isolates would represent a solid ground for reliable phylogenetic analysis, it was pointed out that inferring reliable phylogenies are associated with multiple difficulties rooted in the large number of closely related sequences with a low number of mutations [43]. This study used a quality-filtered subset of 8,736 out of 16,453 virus sequences from GISAID (gisaid.org) and showed that one cannot reliably root the inferred SARS-CoV-2 phylogeny either via the bat and pangolin outgroups or by applying the novel computational methods on the ingroup phylogeny, and that an automatic classification of the current sequences into subclasses is also challenging [43]. These observations indicated that while some insight into the evolution and spread on COVID-19 can be provided by phylogenetic analyses, the results of such analyses should be considered and interpreted with extreme caution [43].

Another important notion is that not all SARS-CoV-2 mutants are equal, with some of them being classified as Variants of Concern/Interest (VOC/I) because of their greater health risks associated with enhanced transmissibility and/or severity, immune escape, diagnostic and/or treatment failure, and reduced vaccine efficacy (https://www.who.int/publications/m/item/covid-19-weekly-epidemiological-update). These variants can be considered as pandemics within the pandemic [44]. Obviously, bioinformatics approaches, including literature mining, are required to acquire information on emerging VOC/Is. Recent analysis showed that the frequency of VOC/Is is increasing globally, thereby reflecting the continuous adaptation of this virus to transmission in humans. These variants represent a serious challenge to pandemic management achieved through a herd immunity approach, and their prevalent existence indicates the need for updates of existing vaccines [44].

11.4 COVID-19 AND A MULTI-OMICS APPROACH: SOME GENERAL CONSIDERATIONS

COVID-19 is a complex pandemic, and there is no single research tool that would allow one

to disentangle the transmission mode of viral pathogens, decipher specific alterations of the biological pathways needed for viral survival, and understand all the intricacies of the host immune response to the virus. Solving all COVID-19–related mysteries and understanding the pathobiology of SARS-CoV-2 in humans require a complex multi-omics approach, where various high-throughput "omics" technologies, such as protein microarrays, genomics, proteomics, metabolomics, and microbiomics play a central role. In fact, integration of machine learning (ML), i.e., complex computer algorithms capable of self-improvement following the input of relevant data; artificial intelligence (AI), i.e., computer systems that are able to perform tasks generally needing humans, such as decision-making; and big data into "omics" opens new, fast, practical, and efficient ways to collect, integrate, and process massive volumes of information [45].

These approaches constitute the next-generation computational tools and technological resources for unraveling the mechanistic pathways of viral infection [46]. Such multi-omics tools and studies can be used to prepare and guide lab-based investigations. Illustrative examples are given by the in-depth proteome analysis using mass spectrometry (MS)-based proteomics and the MS-based metabolomics [46], as various diseases are associated with distorted metabolomics, and viral infection can alter host metabolism for viral survival and reproduction [47]. The success of this combined proteomics–metabolomics approach is based on the premises that an altered biomolecule profile promotes a better understanding of the altered biological pathways, which leads to a better comprehension of the complex COVID-19 pathogenesis [48]. Among the omics-based technological platforms that can be used for finding proteome biomarkers with disease diagnosis or prognosis value are plasma/serum proteomics, nasopharyngeal swab/gargle proteomics, postmortem sample proteomics, urine proteomics, and cell line model proteomics [48].

On the other hand, metabolomics studies on plasma and serum biospecimens can provide useful information on SARS-CoV-2-promoted alterations of various metabolites that can be used as specific metabolite biomarkers [48]. Further, proteomics tools can provide information on novel biomarkers of the innate and adaptive immune response [48]. Obviously, an integrated view of perturbations in host responses at both the proteome and metabolome levels can be generated by meta-analysis of all available information and integration of all these proteomics and metabolomics data into a common picture [48]. An illustrative example of the successful use of such meta-analysis is given by a recent study, where bioinformatics tools were used to decipher alterations in the immune response, fatty acid, and amino acid metabolism and other pathways associated with SARS-CoV-2 infection [48].

An interesting recent development comprises the emergence of the computational immune proteomics, immunoinformatics, that "makes use of tailored bioinformatics tools and data repositories to facilitate the analysis of data from a plurality of disciplines and helps drive novel research hypotheses and *in silico* screening investigations in a fast, reliable, and cost-effective manner" [49]. Immunoinformatics was used to target the most promiscuous antigenic epitopes from the SARS-CoV-2 proteome for acceleration of the vaccine development process [46].

Stukalov et al. used a multi-omics approach in a concurrent study of SARS-CoV-2 and SARS-CoV in order to obtain a holistic view of virus–host interactions and to define the pathogenic properties of these viruses [50]. This multilevel proteomics analysis not only generated the interactomes of both viruses, but also characterized their effects on the proteome, transcriptome, ubiquitinome, and phosphoproteome [50]. Subsequent projection of these data on to the global network of cellular interactions discovered the presence of crosstalk between the infection-induced perturbations at different levels, identified specific and common features in the molecular mechanisms of these CoVs, and discovered multiple hotspots that could be targeted by existing drugs or be utilized for guiding rational design of virus- and host-directed therapies [50].

In their multi-omics analysis of hospitalized COVID-19 patients, Sullivan et al. integrated the outputs of the whole blood transcriptome, plasma proteomics with two complementary platforms, cytokine profiling, plasma and red blood cell metabolomics, deep immune cell phenotyping by mass cytometry, and clinical data annotation in the multi-dimensional computational online researcher portal, COVIDome Explorer [51]. This portal represents a useful tool for multi-omics analysis and visualization of the data in real time, which can accelerate data sharing, hypothesis testing, and discoveries in the COVID-19 field [51].

Willforss et al. elaborated the OmicLoupe software for visual data exploration across multiple omics datasets that provides more than 15 interactive cross-dataset visualizations for omics data [52]. The utility of this tool for SARS-CoV-2 research was demonstrated by the identification of gene products with consistent expression changes across datasets at both the transcript and protein levels [52].

Stephenson et al. reported the results of their single-cell multi-omics analysis of the immune response in COVID-19 [53]. This study integrated the outputs of single-cell transcriptome, surface proteome, and T and B lymphocyte antigen receptor analyses of peripheral blood mononuclear cells from patients with varying severities of COVID-19. It showed that the coordinated immune response contributes to the COVID-19 pathogenesis, and those discrete cellular components potentially serving as targeted for therapy can be identified [53].

11.5 DEEP LEARNING AND ARTIFICIAL INTELLIGENCE IN COVID-19 RESEARCH

Artificial Intelligence (AI) has found a number of great applications in tackling scientific problems from different angles and in many aspects. AI is an evidence-based tool that can deal with multi-dimensional data-rich frameworks, help to build models used in prediction–validation workflows, and improve drug discovery and repositioning [54, 55]. Important components of AI are machine learning (ML), a method of data analysis where analytical model building is automated, based on the idea that systems can learn from data, identify patterns, and make decisions with minimal human intervention; and deep learning (DL), a part of ML based on artificial neural networks with representation learning, where the AI neural networks with multiple hidden layers are capable of learning unsupervised from data that are unstructured or unlabeled. The more DL platforms learn, the better they perform. An important advantage of DL is its exceptional adaptability in the design of neural systems it can utilize. In fact, DL can use repetitive neural networks (RNNs), convolutional neural networks (CNNs), deep belief networks (DBNs), and completely associated feed-forward systems [54].

Handling massive SARS-CoV-2- and COVID-19–related data generated since the beginning of the pandemic (e.g., as of May 24, 2021, there were almost 140,000 PubMed publications dealing with SARS-CoV-2 or COVID-19), clearly requires AI help [54–56]. For example, based on many similarities between the SARS-CoV-2 and SARS-CoV viruses and the existing data that caused SARS, AI models can be created to predict drug structures that could potentially be used to treat COVID-19 patients [57]. Zhu et al. developed an integrative, antiviral drug repurposing methodology that implemented a systems pharmacology-based network medicine platform and was able to quantify the interplay between the human CoV-host interactome and drug targets in the human protein–protein interaction network [58]. Various aspects of AI, ML, and DL applications in SARS-CoV-2 and COVID-19 research are presented in a recent comprehensive review by Tayarani [56].

11.6 DRUG DISCOVERY

A rigorous search for potential drugs to treat and prevent SARS-CoV-2 infection was conducted by many researchers utilizing both computational methods and experimental techniques, and enormous efforts have been made to identify potent drugs for COVID-19 based on drug repurposing and finding potential novel compounds from ligand libraries, natural products, short peptides, and RNAseq analysis [59]. In general, various entities with different levels of structural and organizational complexity can serve as drugs [60]. These entities could be small chemical compounds and (stapled) peptides [61–69], various therapeutic proteins such as antibodies or nanobodies [70–81], vaccines [82, 83], and even entire cells [84–86]. Computer-aided drug discovery represents an important means of enabling cost- and time-efficient development of new drugs and target-specific drugs to combat any disease, including COVID-19. Computational approaches in drug discovery are traditionally focused on finding targets for drug design and on identifying lead compounds. In application to viral infections, the search for drug design targets can be further subdivided into identification of viral and host targets. The sections below briefly introduce some of the computational methods used in these endeavors. It is worth noting, however, that most of the computer-aided drug discovery tools require knowledge of the structure of various target proteins present in SARS-CoV-2, or the structures of target host proteins.

11.6.1 Search for Potential Drug Targets

11.6.1.1 Viral Targets

Obviously, efficiency of a drug as a potent anti-viral agent capable of specific elimination of a pathogen can be ensured by targeting viral proteins. Therefore, the discovery of novel viral targets for anti-COVID-19 drugs using computer-aided drug discovery tools requires knowledge of the structure of the virus, structure of viral proteins, and an understanding of the functions of these proteins and their roles in the viral life cycle, where drugs might act at different stages of the infection (for example, viral attachment, entry, replication, assembly, and dissemination) [60, 63, 87–93]. It is clear that in the search for therapeutic options for COVID-19, any SARS-CoV-2 enzymes and proteins involved in viral replication and the control of host cellular machineries should be considered as potential drug targets [60, 87].

All structural SARS-CoV-2 proteins, i.e., the spike (S) glycoprotein, envelope (E) protein, membrane (M) protein, and the nucleocapsid (N) protein, can be targeted by drugs. This is because in addition to their obvious role in the formation of the viral particle, all of them have a multitude of functions at different stages of the viral life cycle. For example, S is crucial for virus pathogenesis and organ tropism, as it is involved in attachment and viral entry through receptor recognition and membrane fusion [94]. Despite being the smallest of the CoV structural proteins, E is crucial for virus assembly, budding, envelope formation, and virulence [95]. The capability of M to bend membranes defines the role of this protein in the promotion of viral assembly [96]. Finally, because of the capability of N to interact with genomic RNA and viral M protein during virion assembly, this structural CoV protein is responsible for packaging of the RNA into nucleocapsids, a ribonucleoprotein complex required for genome protection, and plays a critical role in enhancing the efficiency of virus transcription and assembly [97].

Among the 16 SARS-CoV-2 non-structural proteins (NSPs), the primary drug targets are the main protease (3CLpro, NSP5), the papain-like protease (PLpro, NSP3), and the RNA-dependent RNA polymerase (RdRp, NSP12), in complex with cofactors NSP7 and NSP8, the methyltransferase-stimulatory factor NSP16-NSP10 complex, the NSP9-binding protein, the endoribonuclease NSP15, for which crystal structures are known, and the NSP13 helicase, because of its crucial role in the replication-transcription complex of CoVs that catalyzes the separation of duplex oligonucleotides into single strands in a nucleotide triphosphate (NTP) hydrolysis-dependent manner [87].

Based on the presumption that the extremely highly conserved regions of SARS-CoV-2 proteins (i.e., regions recognizable across many viruses and organisms) may serve as important targets, being related to crucial functions and less likely to exhibit escape mutations that would make them resistant to vaccines and therapeutic agents, Robson et al. conducted a comprehensive search for such regions in all open reading frames of SARS-CoV-2 [98]. This analysis revealed the presence of such an extremely highly conserved motif in the SARS-CoV-2 NSP3. This motif is related to the highly conserved structural module known as the macro domain, which is broadly distributed across various organisms, including humans [98]. The authors also pointed to the presence of three especially conserved subsequences,

VVVNAANVYLKHGGGVAGALNK,PLLSAGIFG, and LHVVGPNVNKG, in NSP3 [98].

Another interesting set of viral drug targets comprises viroporins, viral proteins capable of ion-channel formation. In SARS-CoV-2, such viroporins are the envelope protein E (ORF4a, which, being smallest of CoV structural proteins, is an integral membrane protein embedded in the envelope bilayer membrane), ORF3a (a 274-amino acid–long viral ion-channel protein involved in viral release, inflammasome activation, and cell death), and ORF8 (a cysteine-rich 29-amino acid single-passage transmembrane peptide), which are utilized by the virus to take control of the endoplasmic reticulum–Golgi complex intermediate compartment (ERGIC) [99]. Furthermore, the E and ORF3a proteins are highly promiscuous binders that can interact with more than 400 target proteins in infected host cells because of the presence of a PDZ-binding domain [99].

An important notion was recently voiced by Grenga and Armengaud who, based on the analysis of numerous proteomics studies of SARS-CoV-2, indicated that the "molecular machinery of SARS-CoV-2 is much more complex than initially believed, as many post-translational modifications can occur, leading to a myriad of proteoforms and a broad heterogeneity of viral particles" [100]. Obviously, such structural heterogeneity should be taken into account not only in the detection of SARS-CoV-2, but also in the development of new antiviral drugs.

11.6.1.2 Search for Potential Host Targets of Viral Proteins

Selection of host proteins as drug targets and/or the discovery of drug candidates depends on the knowledge of the SARS-CoV-2/human interactome [101–103]. MS-assisted proteomics represents an important means for a better understanding of the roles of viral and host proteins during SARS-CoV-2 infection, their protein–protein interactions, and post-translational modifications. Bittremieux et al. describe freely available data and computational resources that can be used to facilitate mass spectrometry-based analysis of SARS-CoV-2 [104]. Important information on the potentially druggable host proteins and the molecular mechanisms at play during infection can also be retrieved from the comparisons of SARS-CoV-2 with other viruses [105].

Obviously, the host receptor(s) responsible for virus binding should be considered as primary target(s) for drug development, since blocking or disturbing virus-receptor interactions should reduce or prevent virus entry. In COVID-19, the main virus receptor is angiotensin-converting enzyme 2 (ACE2), whose activity is related to the renin–angiotensin system (RAS) involved in the maintenance of blood pressure homeostasis, and fluid and salt balance [106]. Another important host target is transmembrane serine protease 2 (TMPRSS2), as following receptor interaction, specific cleavage of viral S protein at the S1/S2 site by this protease can activate the virus–host cell membrane fusion for subsequent genome delivery [107]. The S protein of SARS-CoV-2 contains a specific multi-basic furin-like cleavage site [108, 109], which is not found in other CoVs [110]. Furin, which is a type 1 membrane-bound protease from the subtilisin-like proprotein convertase family expressed in multiple tissues, serves as another attractive drug target [87]. It was pointed out that while the furin-like enzymes play a pleiotropic role in a large number of cellular processes, drugs targeting this protein might show noticeable side effects [111].

Cathepsin L, which is involved in SARS-CoV-2 endocytosis entry [112], serves as one more potential therapeutic option for COVID-19 [113]. The main entry pathway for SARS-CoVs is receptor-mediated endocytosis, in which adaptor-associated kinase 1 (AAK1) and cyclin G-associated kinase (GAK) play key roles in receptor-mediated endocytosis and clathrin-mediated trafficking, respectively. Since AAK1 and GAK regulate intracellular viral trafficking during entry, assembly, and release of RNA viruses, inhibition of their activity represents a promising therapy for COVID-19 [87]. Phosphatidylinositol-3,5-bisphosphate (PI(3,5) P2) synthesized in late endosomes by the phosphatidylinositol 3-phosphate 5-kinase (PIKfyve) regulates the dynamic process of endosome maturation [114, 115]. Therefore, inhibition of PIKfyve represents a useful strategy to modulate infection by SARS-CoV-2 and viruses that enter through endocytosis [116].

Novel host proteins that can serve as potential targets for the anti-SARS-CoV-2 drugs can be found based on careful analysis of currently available literature. For example, Parkinson et al. conducted a dynamic ranking of host genes implicated in the infection by human betacoronavirus (MERS-CoV, SARS-CoV, SARS-CoV-2, and seasonal CoVs) using Meta-Analysis by Information Content (MAIC) [117]. This analysis generated a comprehensive ranked list of host genes implicated in COVID-19, where one can find PPIA encoding druggable cyclophilin A, as well as several prognostic factors (CD3E, CD4, and CXCL10) and investigational therapeutic targets (for example, IL1A) [117].

Jaiswal et al. emphasized the importance of using systems biology approaches and integration of multiple omics (transcriptomics, proteomics, genomics, lipidomics, immunomics, and in silico computational modeling) while dealing with analysis of host–virus interactions in search of potential therapeutic targets against the COVID-19 [118].

Finally, the utility of the Eukaryotic Linear Motif (ELM) resource (http://elm.eu.org/), which is capable of finding short linear motif (SLiM) candidates in intrinsically disordered regions of host target proteins such as ACE2 and integrins, was emphasized by Meszaros et al. [119]. This analysis revealed the presence of a multitude of such motifs with potential roles in endocytosis, membrane dynamics, autophagy, cytoskeleton, and cell signaling, and indicated that such motifs can be used for establishing molecular links and generating testable hypotheses pertaining to the molecular mechanisms of SARS-CoV-2 attachment, entry, and replication [119].

11.6.2 Structure-Based Drug Design

11.6.2.1 Structural Bioinformatics

The major role of structural biology and structural bioinformatics is defined by the ability of the corresponding techniques to provide key information on the 3D structures, define critical residues/mutations in SARS-CoV-2, and host proteins that can be implicated in infectivity, molecular recognition, and the capability of target proteins to be engaged in a broad range of interactions [120]. A structure-guided drug design relies on the detailed understanding of viral proteins and their complexes with host receptors and candidate epitope/lead compounds. In addition to the experimental determination of structures of several SARS-CoV-2 proteins, multiple specialized structural bioinformatics tools, and resources have been elaborated for building theoretical models, analysis of structural dynamics by computer simulations, and evaluation of the impact of variants/mutations and molecular therapeutics on target structure and dynamics [120].

One can find information pertaining to experimentally determined structures of SARS-CoV-2 proteins in the PDB [121] that assembled all COVID-19/SARS-CoV-2 related resources to the dedicated platform RCSB.org/covid19, containing over 1,220 structures of SARS-CoV-2 proteins. Figure 11.2 shows the architecture of the SARS-CoV-2 genome and proteome and represents illustrative examples of experimentally determined 3D structures of SARS-CoV-2 proteins. Predicted 3D structures of SARS-CoV-2 proteins are presented in various repositories, such as Coronavirus3D [122], SWISS-Model [123], Aquaria [124], the Krokin lab repository [125], and Kiharalab (http://www.kiharalab.org/covid19/index.html). Additional SARS-CoV-2-related sources, such as CASP_Commons (https://predictioncenter.org/caspcommons/) and CAPRI COVID-19 open science initiative, were started by CASP (Critical Assessment of protein Structure Prediction) and CAPRI (Critical Assessment of Predicted Interactions), respectively.

Multiple repositories for storage of the molecular trajectories generated by simulations involving SARS-CoV-2 proteins have been developed [120]. Some of these resources are CHARMM COVID library of Wonpil Im (http://www.charmm-gui.org/?doc=archive&lib=covid19), the SIRAH-CoV-2 initiative by Sergio Pantano (https://www.cluster.uy/web-covid/), the COVID-19 molecular structure and therapeutic hub by MOLSSI, BioExcel (https://covid.molssi.org/), and the long simulation trajectories generated by D.E. Shaw Research using Anton-2 supercomputers (https://www.deshawresearch.com/downloads/download_trajectory_sarscov2.cgi/).

11.6.3 Search for Potential Drug Leads

11.6.3.1 Docking and Virtual Screening

Traditional structure-based drug discovery applies the computational ligand-receptor-binding modeling and virtual screening, whereas the stability of the resulting ligand-protein complexes is confirmed by molecular dynamics simulation. All potentially druggable SARS-CoV-2 proteins were subjected to these analyses, and the number of computational studies dedicated to finding potential drugs targeting these proteins is mounting. For example, Hosseini et al. conducted molecular docking and virtual screening of 1,615 FDA-approved drugs on the binding pocket of SARS-CoV-2 MPro, PLPro, and RdRp proteins [127]. The authors used AutoDock Vina, Glide, and rDock followed by MD simulation using GROMACS on the top inhibitors and identified six novel ligands as potential inhibitors against SARS-CoV-2, such as antiemetics rolapitant and ondansetron for M^{pro}; labetalol and levomefolic acid for PLpro; and leucal and antifungal natamycin for RdRp [127]. Chourasia et al. investigated in silico binding of epigallocatechin gallate (EGCG), and other catechins to SARS-CoV-2 proteins and identified papain-like protease protein (PLPro) as a binding partner [128].

11.6.3.2 Computational Drug Repurposing

Drug repurposing or repositioning represents one of the more efficient approaches for finding potential therapeutics via identification of new applications for existing drugs at a lower cost and in a shorter time [129–139]. In applications to SARS-CoV-2, computational drug-repositioning approaches can be grouped into network-based

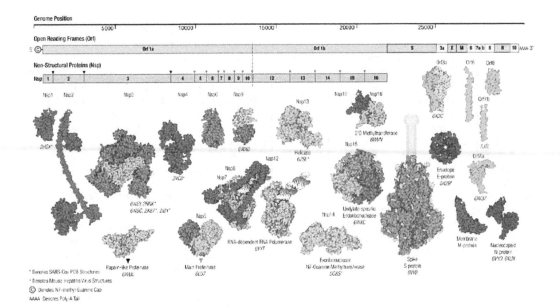

Figure 11.2   Architecture of the SARS-CoV-2 genome and proteome, including non-structural proteins derived from Pp1a and Pp1ab (NSPs, shades of blue), virion structural proteins (pink/purple), and open reading frame proteins (ORFs, shades of green). Polyprotein cleavage sites are indicated by inverted triangles for papain-like proteinase (PL^Pro, black) and the main protease (NSP5, blue). The double-stranded RNA substrate-product complex of the RNA-dependent RNA polymerase (shown as the NSP7-NSP82-NSP12 heterotetramer, and separately with only NSP12) is color coded (yellow: product strand; red: template strand). Transmembrane portions of the S protein are shown in cartoon form (pink).

Source: Reproduced from [126].

models, structure-based approaches, signature-based approaches, molecular docking, genome-wide association studies (GWAS), and AI approaches [130, 140]. In signature-based drug repositioning, high-throughput omics data (transcriptomic, proteomic, or metabolomic), as well as molecular structures, and adverse effect profiles are used to compare the pattern of gene expression profiles of a drug against gene expression profiles of another drug (i.e., drug–drug comparison), disease (i.e., drug-disease comparison), or clinical phenotype [141]. In molecular docking, which is an important component of the structure-based drug repurposing (SBDR) techniques [142], unknown interactions between receptor target and leads are discovered by screening of compound libraries against targets to discover candidates for drug repurposing processes [143]. The network-based and pathway-based drug repurposing relies on the construction of biological networks by using different data types, such as disease pathology, gene expression patterns, and protein interactions [144]. The differences in genetic material related to common diseases that can be found

by GWAS generate an important knowledge that can give rise to repurposing of drugs [145].

Since earlier studies of viruses from the Coronaviridae family established several viral proteins, such as RdRp, M^pro (also called 3CL^pro), and PL^pro as candidate drug targets, the homologue proteins from SARS-CoV-2 were utilized in drug repurposing studies [140]. A few illustrative examples of successful use of computational drug repurposing for COVID-19 are given below. Efliky reported that RdRp of SARS-CoV-2 can be targeted efficiently by several FDA-approved drugs, such as IDX-184, remdesivir, ribavirin, and sofosbuvir [146]. According to Krishnan et al., SARS-CoV-2 endoribonuclease NSP15 can be potentially inhibited by eight compounds from a set of 3,978 compounds with antiviral properties retrieved from the Enamine database [147]. Mark et al. docked 970,000 chemical compounds obtained from the ZINC database and Enamine library to SARS-CoV-2 helicase NSP13 and found that lumacaftor and cepharanthine can serve as inhibitors of this protein [148].

Tomazou et al. elaborated a network-based platform integrating multi-omics and multi-source

137

publicly available data from patients, cell lines, and databases to prioritize the most important COVID-19–related genes [149]. This multiplex drug repurposing approach generated a highly informed integrated drug shortlist, which, in addition to the known potential drugs such as dexamethasone and remdesivir, included inhibitors of Src tyrosine kinase (bosutinib, dasatinib, cytarabine and saracatinib), specific immunomodulators and anti-inflammatory drugs, such as dactolisib and methotrexate, as well as inhibitors of histone deacetylase: for example, hydroquinone and vorinostat [149]. In another multi-target SBDR study, Wu et al. identified 21 viral and host proteins, such as NSP1, NSP3b, NSP3c, PLpro, NSP3e, 3CLpro, NSP7-NSP8 complex, NSP9, NSP10, NSP12/RdRp, NSP13/helicase, NSP14, NSP15, NSP16, ORF7a, Spike, NNRBD, NCRBD, Envelope, ACE2, and TMPRSS2 as potential drug targets [150]. Docking compounds from the ZINC database to these proteins revealed that several drugs from different groups, such as anti-asthmatic, antibacterial, and antiviral classes can serve as candidate medicines for treating COVID-19 [150].

11.6.3.3 Phytochemicals and Natural Products

An immense supply of products is provided by nature, and many of these natural products and their derivatives have been used for the control and prevention of various diseases, including viral infections [151–160]. It has been pointed out that various herbal-based compounds can potentially inhibit SARS-CoV-2 infectivity by blocking the host ACE2 receptor or interrupting the activity of various viral proteins, such as the S protein, 3CL^{pro}, PL^{pro}, helicase, and RdRp [151]. Swain et al. conducted an exhaustive literature search for studies on phytochemicals with reported anti-CoV activity and used the ChemMine tool (https://chemminetools. ucr.edu/) to perform hierarchical clustering analysis of all selected phytochemicals [161]. As a result, 78 phytochemicals with reported CoV activity were found and classified into six clusters. At the next stage, these compounds were docked to 3CL^{pro}. This analysis revealed that the most potent compound from each cluster (abietane, epigallocatechin gallate/EGCG, homoharringtonine, tomentine E, papyriflavonol A, and scutellarein) showed similar binding affinity to 3CL^{pro} as two existing repurposed FDA-approved drugs, lopinavir and ritonavir [161]. Raimundo et al. emphasized the importance of ethnopharmacology in drug discovery by conducting a search for articles addressing plant-based natural products, plant extracts, and essential oils as potential anti-SARS-CoV-2 agents, followed by the principal component

analysis (PCA) of their Chemometrics descriptors [162]. The study revealed that 29 medicinal plant species and more than 300 isolated substances can serve as potential anti-CoV agents [162]. It is important to keep in mind that most studies on plant-based drugs typically rely on empirical and anecdotal experiences and not on thorough clinical evaluation. Further, one should remember that despite the enormous potential of computational and bioinformatics approaches, the "real deal" is to test plant-based drugs in vitro and in vivo.

11.6.3.4 Dietary Supplements and Functional Foods

Li et al. suggested that the prevention and management of COVID-19 can be enhanced via the development of specific dietary supplements and functional foods [163]. This is based on the idea that there is a great variety of edible and medicinal plants and/or natural compounds that show potential benefits in managing the SARS-CoV (and potentially SARS-CoV-2) infection, with many plants and natural compounds being proposed to be protective against COVID-19 [163]. Since this information is based on data-driven approaches and computational chemical biology techniques, bioinformatics plays a crucial role in finding promising candidates of edible and medicinal plants for the prevention and management of COVID-19 [163]. The authors also indicated that some of these natural compounds (such as acetoside, glyasperin, isorhamnetin, and several flavonoid compounds) can represent bioactive dietary components, which, being used either alone or in combination, can serve as the foundation for the development of dietary supplements or functional foods for managing COVID-19 [163].

11.6.4 Computational Polypharmacology

It is now recognized that the desired effects of most therapeutics are exerted via modulation of multiple targets and pathways [164–167], whereas severe side effects can sometimes be associated with the excessive selectivity of a drug for a single target [168]. Moreover, it deals with pharmaceutical agents characterized by the promiscuous binding to multiple targets and acting on multiple disease pathways, thereby generating different phenotypic or pharmacological effects [167]. Polypharmacology deals with multi-target binding, drug off targeting, and molecular promiscuity, and thereby opposes the "single drug, single target" approach. Therefore, polypharmacology has emerged as a powerful alternative paradigm for development of versatile therapeutic agents capable of modulating multiple biological targets simultaneously, often displaying higher efficacy, less resistance, and an improved safety profile [169]. It is important to emphasize that, while in the past the identification of multi-targeting agents has largely been fortuitous and serendipitous, recent advances in computational sciences enable rational design of drug poly-pharmacology (reviewed in [167, 170, 171]). Since a single therapeutic can act on multiple targets and a single target can be affected by multiple therapeutics, one can differentiate ligand-based and target-based polypharmacology, whereas network pharmacology integrates multi-omics technologies and systems biology for drug dis-covery and development [172].

In applications for COVID-19, several studies reported a polypharmacology nature of action of analyzed leads. For example, Omotuyi et al. showed that several secondary metabolites from *Aframomum melegueta* can bind efficiently to host furin and several SARS-CoV-2 pro-teins in a polypharmacological manner [173]. Molecular docking analysis of 688 phase III, and 1,702 phase IV clinical trial drugs binding to the SARS-CoV-2 PL^{pro}, found a set of covalent and non-covalent inhibitors showing potential multi-target activities and possessing desir-able polypharmacology profiles [174]. Similarly, Pinzi et al. conducted in silico screening (dock-ing) of 13,227 compounds from the DrugBank database and identified 22 candidates showing putative SARS-CoV-2 M^{pro} inhibitory activity, with some candidates possessing a polyphar-macology profile [175]. Kumar et al. conducted a bioinformatics-based screen of FDA approved drugs against nine SARS-CoV-2 proteins and human proteins, whose expression in the lung changed during SARS-CoV-2 infection and identified 74 molecules that can bind to various SARS-CoV-2 and human host proteins [176].

11.6.5 Target Prioritization

Several aspects can be considered when one is dealing with target prioritization. In fact, drug leads can be prioritized based on their goals, such as whether they should hit one target or several targets in a pathway [60, 177–184], whereas prioritization of targets often involves the identification of druggable or ligand-binding pockets, such as binding cavities, hot-spots, and cryptic sites [185–191].

11.7 MICROBIOME ANALYSIS

The human microbiome represents an impor-tant type of omics that has gained exponen-tially increased attention since the year 2000. This is because of its vast size (in comparison with 20,000–25,000 protein coding genes in the human genome, the microbiome found in the human gut is estimated to contain many millions of microbial genes), highly dynamic and changeable genetic diversity [38], and the very important roles that microbiota play in food digestion, regulating the immune system, protecting against potentially pathogenic bac-teria, and producing various vitamins such as vitamin B$_{12}$, thiamine, riboflavin, and vitamin K. Therefore, the microbiome is a crucial compo-nent of human well-being and illness in general [192] and may play an important role in SARS-CoV-2 infections (e.g., a proper gut microbiota may influence disease severity [193]).

Since the human microbiome biodiversity, which is studied by metagenomics and asso-ciated bioinformatics methods and tools, can change in response to illness, analysis of the gut microbiome in COVID-19 patients can provide useful information for fighting SARS-CoV-2 infections and disparity. These studies aim at understanding how the gut microbiome is influ-enced by or affects the SARS-CoV-2 and utilizes various metagenomics bioinformatics platforms and tools [192]. Based on a comprehensive review of the available information on the gut microbiome of COVID-19 patients it was pointed out that the microbiota of COVID-19 patients is enriched in opportunistic microorganisms, sug-gesting that microbiome profiling can be used for diagnosis [192]. It was also pointed out that in COVID-19 patients, an altered gut microbiota and its associated leaky gut may contribute to the onset of gastrointestinal symptoms and occasionally to additional multi-organ com-plications that may lead to severe illness by allowing leakage of the causative CoV into the circulatory system [193].

11.8 VACCINE DEVELOPMENT

Although vaccine development has traditionally used the "trial-and-error" approach, computa-tional vaccinology constitutes a promising devel-opment that can facilitate vaccine design and speed up this long and costly process. Russo et al. indicated that a combination of AI and systems biology represents a very promising direction for the intelligent anti-COVID-19 vaccine design [194], whereas Hwang et al. emphasized that computational tools have been applied success-fully as a part of the reverse vaccinology approach for SARS-CoV-2 vaccine development, where they were used for antigen selection, and epitope, toxicity and allergenicity predictions [195].

Structure-based reverse vaccinology [196, 197] represents an important constituent of ratio-nal vaccine design, which attempts to pro-duce a vaccine using information from the observed crystallographic structure of neutral-izing monoclonal antibodies (mAbs) bound to their complementary epitopes. Such structural vaccinology represents a way to facilitate rational design of better antigens able to act as vaccine immunogens. The reverse computer-based vaccine engineering methodology utilizes the available structures of pathogenic proteins and antigen-antibody complexes and uses docking and modeling studies to predict epitopes to reconstruct an epitope capable of mAb binding. The structure of mAb is used as a template in a process similar to rational drug design, where the 3D structure of a biological target is used for designing molecules capable of selective binding to and specific inhibition of the biological activity of a target molecule [198].

Furthermore, successful epitope identifications can be achieved as a result of the recent advancements in B cell and T cell epitope predictions by bioinformatics analysis [199]. This computational approach represents an important complement to the experimental search for immunodominant epitopes that relies on the evaluation of peptides representing the epitopes from overlapping peptide libraries, which can be costly and labor-intensive. The importance of this field of study is further illustrated by the steady increase in the interest in the linear B-cell epitope (BCE) predictions, which is reflected in the development of several B-cell epitope prediction methods [200].

Recently, Galanis *et al.* analyzed the performance of several most widely used linear B-cell epitope predictors, such as BcePred, BepiPred, ABCpred, COBEpro, SVMTriP, LBtope, and LBEEP, and developed a consensus classifier, BepiPred-2.0, which accelerates the epitope-based vaccine design by combining the separate predictions of these methods into a single output [200]. Yang et al. used DL in designing their DeepVacPred predictor containing BepiPred-2.0, SVMtrip, ABCPred, and BCPREDS for successful linear BCE prediction of the SARS-CoV-2 S protein [82]. Crooke et al. developed a computational workflow using a series of open-source algorithms and webtools to identify putative T cell and B cell epitopes in the SARS-CoV-2 proteome [201]. Application of this tool to all structural, non-structural, and accessory proteins from SARS-CoV-2 revealed the presence of 41 T cell epitopes (5 HLA class I, 36 HLA class II) and 6 B cell epitopes that could serve as potential targets for peptide-based anti-COVID-19 vaccine development [201]. Noorimotlagh et al. used bio-immunoinformatics to screen the SARS-CoV-2-derived B-cell and T-cell epitopes within the basic immunogenic regions of the SARS-CoV-2 proteins, and found a set of inferred B cell and T cell epitopes in the S and N proteins with high antigenicity and without allergenic properties or toxic effects [202].

In contrast to the frequently employed structure-based reverse vaccinology, Goh et al. focused their attention on the computational evaluation of the correlation between the intrinsic disorder status of the N and M proteins forming the viral shell and the transmission mode [203]. Based on the detected correlations, it was proposed that, by influencing the intrinsic disorder status of their N and M proteins, a novel strategy for vaccine development could be developed [203].

11.9 SEARCH FOR BIOMARKERS

While detection of SARS-CoV-2 relies on the search for SARS-CoV-2 RNA (RT-PCR) and specific host immunoglobulins, and proteins associated with blood coagulation (D-dimer), cell damage (lactate dehydrogenase), and inflammatory responses (for example, C-reactive protein) have already been identified as possible predictors of COVID-19 severity or mortality, more biomarkers are needed to better understand various aspects of this complex disease, including its severity or complications [204, 205], as well as the presence of long COVID or post-COVID-19 syndromes [206]. Proteomics approaches that are used for biomarker discovery should use techniques for comprehensive data acquisition (such as MS) combined with informatics approaches (for example, AI) to extract information from large data sets [204]. Griffin and Downard emphasized the versatility of MS-based proteomics analysis for identifying host cell responses to SARS-CoV-2 infection, identification of abundant peptides in clinical specimens, and the analysis of viral protein glycoforms [207]. Fröberg and Diavatopoulos indicated that identification of mucosal biomarkers associated with viral clearance is needed, since such biomarkers will allow monitoring the SARS-CoV-2 infection-induced immunity [208].

Dos Santos et al. indicated that because of the potential link between the severity of SARS-CoV-2 infections and genetic polymorphisms in the population, one should look for specific biomarkers indicating the presence of such genetic polymorphisms in several host proteins, such as HLA, ACE1, OAS-1, MxA, PKR, MBL, E-CR1, FcγRIIA, MBL2, L-SIGN (CLEC4M), IFN-γ, CD14, ICAM3, RANTES, IL-12 RB1, TNF-α, CXCL10/IP-10, CD209 (DC-SIGN), AHSG, CYP4F3, and CCL2 [209]. Genetic polymorphisms in several cytokine encoding genes (such as IFNAR2, TNF, INF-γ, INF-β, IL-4, IL-1RN, IL-6, IL-10, IL-12, IL-17, CXCL10, and CCL7) can be related to the cytokine storm, emphasizing the need for using inflammatory cytokines and chemokines as biomarkers that can provide guidelines for decision-making and appropriate clinical management of COVID-19 [210]. Since cardiovascular disease (CVD) and cardiac injury represent risk factors for severe COVID-19, corresponding biomarkers of cardiac injury should be taken into consideration during hospital stays of COVID-19 patients [211].

The list of similar studies on various biomarkers reflecting different aspects of SARS-CoV-2 infection and COVID-19 is rapidly increasing. This is a result of the very complex nature of COVID-19, which is not a simple localized respiratory infection, but a multi-system disease caused by a diffuse systemic process involving a complex interplay of the coagulative, immunological, and inflammatory pathways and cascades [212]. It seems that almost all organs can be affected by this infection, indicating the need for finding multiple specific biomarkers that can reflect development of COVID-19–associated pathologies in at least major organs, such as lungs and the respiratory system, heart, brain, central nervous system, liver, kidneys, eyes, and reproductive systems.

11.10 CONCLUSIONS

It is clear that modern science is at loss without the systematic use of various computational tools. There are also no doubts about the defining roles of bioinformatics and computational biology in the successful development of various branches of biology, such as biochemistry, biophysics, biomedicine, and pharmacology. This is especially evident in the present days of havoc generated world-wide by the COVID-19 pandemic. To a large degree, success in the research on SARS-CoV-2 and COVID-19 is heavily dependent on the utilization of various computational platforms, tools, and databases. New computational means for COVID-19–related research are developed on a daily basis. New massive data sets are systematically generated based on the routine sequencing of samples from COVID-19 patients. One can find almost endless evidence of the validity that bioinformatics and computational biology are at the heart of COVID-19 research. Figure 11.3 presents some of the roles that bioinformatics and computational biology can contribute to SARS-CoV-2 and COVID-19 research. This chapter describes only the tip of the iceberg. In fact, analysis of PubMed using "SARS-CoV-2 OR COVID-19" AND "bioinformatics OR computational biology" as search terms generated 2,544 hits, which represent 1.8% of the 141,057 publications on SARS-CoV-2 or COVID-19. While it is clear that many more important discoveries will be made through bioinformatics and computational biology, and their novel tools and resources that help in generating

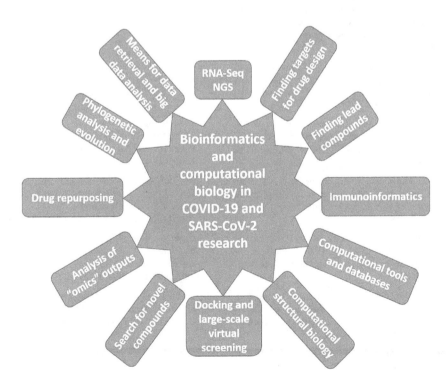

Figure 11.3 Some of the roles of bioinformatics and computational biology in SARS-CoV-2 and COVID-19 research.

and analyzing vital pieces of information, one should keep in mind that computational studies do not give rise to the final truth, and all in silico data, indications and observations require careful in vitro and in vivo validation.

REFERENCES

1. Lee, P.I., Hsueh, P.R. (2020). Emerging threats from zoonotic coronaviruses-from SARS and MERS to 2019-nCoV. *J. Microbiol. Immunol. Infect.* 53(3), 365–367.

2. Huang, C., Wang, Y., Li, X., et al. (2020). Clinical features of patients infected with 2019 novel coronavirus in Wuhan, China. *Lancet* 395(10223), 497–506.

3. Rothan, H.A., Byrareddy, S.N. (2020). The epidemiology and pathogenesis of coronavirus disease (COVID-19) outbreak. *J. Autoimmun.* 109, 102433.

4. Uversky, V.N., Elrashdy, F., Aljadawi, A., et al. (2021). Severe acute respiratory syndrome coronavirus 2 infection reaches the human nervous system: How? *J. Neurosci. Res.* 99(3), 750–777.

5. Severo Bem Junior, L., do Rego Aquino, P.L., Nunes Rabelo, N., et al. (2020). SARS-CoV-2 and nervous system – Neurological manifestations in patients with COVID-19: A systematic review. *J. Neurol. Res.* 10(4), 113–121.

6. Salehi, M., Amanat, M., Mohammadi, M., et al. (2021). The prevalence of post-traumatic stress disorder related symptoms in Coronavirus outbreaks: A systematic-review and meta-analysis. *J. Affect. Disord.* 282, 527–538.

7. Liu, C., Pan, W., Li, L., et al. (2021). Prevalence of depression, anxiety, and insomnia symptoms among patients with COVID-19: A meta-analysis of quality effects model. *J. Psychosom. Res.* 147, 110516.

8. Zhang, Y., Xiao, M., Zhang, S., et al. (2020). Coagulopathy and Antiphospholipid antibodies in patients with COVID-19. *N. Engl. J. Med.* 382(17), e38.

9. Ding, Y., Wang, H., Shen, H., et al. (2003). The clinical pathology of severe acute respiratory syndrome (SARS): A report from China. *J. Pathol.* 200(3), 282–289.

10. Xu, Z., Shi, L., Wang, Y., et al. (2020). Pathological findings of COVID-19 associated with acute respiratory distress syndrome. *Lancet Respir. Med.* 8(4), 420–422.

11. Moshrefi, M., Ghasemi-Esmailabad, S., Ali, J., et al. (2021). The probable destructive mechanisms behind COVID-19 on male reproduction system and fertility. *J. Assist. Reprod. Genet.*

12. Finsterer, J., Scorza, F.A., Scorza, C.A., et al. (2021). SARS-CoV-2 impairs vision. *J. Neuroophthalmol.* 41(2), 166–169.

13. Rahimi, A., Mirzazadeh, A., Tavakolpour, S. (2021). Genetics and genomics of SARS-CoV-2: A review of the literature with the special focus on genetic diversity and SARS-CoV-2 genome detection. *Genomics* 113(1 Pt 2), 1221–1232.

14. Nakagawa, S., Miyazawa, T. (2020). Genome evolution of SARS-CoV-2 and its virological characteristics. *Inflamm. Regen.* 40, 17.

15. Srivastava, S., Banu, S., Singh, P., et al. (2021). SARS-CoV-2 genomics: An Indian perspective on sequencing viral variants. *J. Biosci.* 46, 22.

16. Wu, F., Zhao, S., Yu, B., et al. (2020). A new coronavirus associated with human respiratory disease in China. *Nature* 579(7798), 265–269.

17. Zhou, P., Yang, X.L., Wang, X.G., et al. (2020). A pneumonia outbreak associated with a new coronavirus of probable bat origin. *Nature* 579(7798), 270–273.

18. Lu, R., Zhao, X., Li, J., et al. (2020). Genomic characterisation and epidemiology of 2019 novel coronavirus: Implications for virus origins and receptor binding. *Lancet* 395(10224), 565–574.

19. Corman, V.M., Landt, O., Kaiser, M., et al. (2020). Detection of 2019 novel coronavirus (2019-nCoV) by real-time RT-PCR. *Eur. Surveill.* 25(3), 2000045.

20. Hu, T., Li, J., Zhou, H., et al. (2021). Bioinformatics resources for SARS-CoV-2 discovery and surveillance. *Brief Bioinform.* 22(2), 631–641.

21. Chiara, M., D'Erchia, A.M., Gissi, C., et al. (2021). Next generation sequencing of SARS-CoV-2 genomes: Challenges, applications and opportunities. *Brief Bioinform.* 22(2), 616–630.

22. Maurano, M.T., Ramaswami, S., Zappile, P., et al. (2020). Sequencing identifies multiple early introductions of SARS-CoV-2 to the New York City region. *Genome Res.* 30(12), 1781–1788.

23. Meredith, L.W., Hamilton, W.L., Warne, B., et al. (2020). Rapid implementation of SARS-CoV-2 sequencing to investigate cases of health-care associated COVID-19: A prospective genomic surveillance study. *Lancet Infect. Dis.* 20(11), 1263–1271.

24. Rockett, R.J., Arnott, A., Lam, C., et al. (2020). Revealing COVID-19 transmission in Australia by SARS-CoV-2 genome sequencing and agent-based modeling. *Nat. Med.* 26(9), 1398–1404.

25. Gonzalez-Reiche, A.S., Hernandez, M.M., Sullivan, M.J., et al. (2020). Introductions and early spread of SARS-CoV-2 in the New York City area. *Science* 369(6501), 297–301.

26. Gudbjartsson, D.F., Helgason, A., Jonsson, H., et al. (2020). Spread of SARS-CoV-2 in the Icelandic population. *N. Engl. J. Med.* 382(24), 2302–2315.

27. Kamil, J.P. (2021). Virus variants: GISAID policies incentivize surveillance in global south. *Nature* 593(7859), 341.

28. Shu, Y., McCauley, J. (2017). GISAID: Global initiative on sharing all influenza data – from vision to reality. *Eur. Surveill.* 22(13), 30494.

29. Hadfield, J., Megill, C., Bell, S.M., et al. (2018). Nextstrain: Real-time tracking of pathogen evolution. *Bioinformatics* 34(23), 4121–4123.

30. Fahmi, M., Kharisma, V.D., Ansori, A.N.M., et al. (2021). Retrieval and investigation of data on SARS-CoV-2 and COVID-19 using bioinformatics approach. *Adv. Exp. Med. Biol.* 1318, 839–857.

31. Mercatelli, D., Holding, A.N., Giorgi, F.M. (2021). Web tools to fight pandemics: The COVID-19 experience. *Brief Bioinform.* 22(2), 690–700.

32. Hufsky, F., Lamkiewicz, K., Almeida, A., et al. (2021). Computational strategies to combat COVID-19: Useful tools to accelerate SARS-CoV-2 and coronavirus research. *Brief Bioinform.* 22(2), 642–663.

33. Ahsan, M.A., Liu, Y., Feng, C., et al. (2021). Bioinformatics resources facilitate understanding and harnessing clinical research of SARS-CoV-2. *Brief Bioinform.* 22(2), 714–725.

34. van Dorp, L., Richard, D., Tan, C.C.S., et al. (2020). No evidence for increased transmissibility from recurrent mutations in SARS-CoV-2. *Nat. Commun.* 11(1), 5986.

35. van Dorp, L., Tan, C.C., Lam, S.D., et al. (2020). Recurrent mutations in SARS-CoV-2 genomes isolated from mink point to rapid host-adaptation. *bioRxiv.* doi:10.1101/2020.11.16.384743.

36. Zhao, Z., Li, H., Wu, X., et al. (2004). Moderate mutation rate in the SARS coronavirus genome and its implications. *BMC Evol. Biol.* 4, 21.

37. Cotten, M., Watson, S.J., Kellam, P., et al. (2013). Transmission and evolution of the Middle East respiratory syndrome coronavirus in Saudi Arabia: A descriptive genomic study. *Lancet* 382(9909), 1993–2002.

38. Dudas, G., Carvalho, L.M., Rambaut, A., et al. (2018). MERS-CoV spillover at the camel–human interface. *Elife* 7, e31257.

39. Cotten, M., Watson, S.J., Zumla, A.I., et al. (2014). Spread, circulation, and evolution of the Middle East respiratory syndrome coronavirus. *mBio* 5(1), e01062.

40. Vijgen, L., Keyaerts, E., Moes, E., et al. (2005). Complete genomic sequence of human coronavirus OC43: Molecular clock analysis suggests a relatively recent zoonotic coronavirus transmission event. *J. Virol.* 79(3), 1595–1604.

41. Andersen, K.G., Rambaut, A., Lipkin, W.I., et al. (2020). The proximal origin of SARS-CoV-2. *Nat. Med.* 26(4), 450–452.

42. Sarkar, J.P., Saha, I., Seal, A., et al. (2021). Topological analysis for sequence variability: Case study on more than 2K SARS-CoV-2 sequences of COVID-19 infected 54 countries in comparison with SARS-CoV-1 and MERS-CoV. *Infect. Genet. Evol.* 88, 104708.

43. Morel, B., Barbera, P., Czech, L., et al. (2021). Phylogenetic analysis of SARS-CoV-2 data is difficult. *Mol. Biol. Evol.* 38(5), 1777–1791.

44. Boehm, E., Kronig, I., Neher, R.A., et al. (2021).Novel SARS-CoV-2 variants: The pandemics within the pandemic. *Clin. Microbiol. Infect.* 27(8), 1109–1117.

45. D'Adamo, G.L., Widdop, J.T., Giles, E.M. (2021). The future is now? Clinical and translational aspects of "Omics" technologies. *Immunol. Cell Biol.* 99(2), 168–176.

46. Kangabam, R., Sahoo, S., Ghosh, A., et al. (2021). Next-generation computational tools and resources for coronavirus research: From detection to vaccine discovery. *Comput. Biol. Med.* 128,104158.

47. Song, J.W., Lam, S.M., Fan, X., et al. (2020). Omics-driven systems interrogation of metabolic dysregulation in COVID-19 pathogenesis. *Cell Metab.* 32(2), 188–202 e5.

48. Aggarwal, S., Acharjee, A., Mukherjee, A., et al. (2021). Role of multiomics data to understand host–pathogen interactions in COVID-19 pathogenesis. *J. Proteome Res.* 20(2), 1107–1132.

49. Tilocca, B., Britti, D., Urbani, A., et al. (2020). Computational immune proteomics approach to target COVID-19. *J. Proteome Res.*19(11), 4233–4241.

50. Stukalov, A., Girault, V., Grass, V., et al. (2021). Multilevel proteomics reveals host perturbations by SARS-CoV-2 and SARS-CoV. *Nature* 594(7862), 246–252.

51. Sullivan, K.D., Galbraith, M.D., Kinning, K.T., et al. (2021). The COVIDome explorer researcher portal. *medRxiv.* doi:10.1101/2021.03.04.21252945.

52. Willforss, J., Siino, V., Levander, F. (2021). OmicLoupe: Facilitating biological discovery by interactive exploration of multiple omic datasets and statistical comparisons. *BMC Bioinformatics* 22(1), 107.

53. Stephenson, E., Reynolds, G., Botting, R.A., et al. (2021). Single-cell multi-omics analysis of the immune response in COVID-19. *Nat. Med.* 27(5), 904–916.

54. Mohanty, S., Harun Ai Rashid, M., Mridul, M., et al. (2020). Application of Artificial Intelligence in COVID-19 drug repurposing. *Diabetes Metab. Syndr.* 14(5), 1027–1031.

55. Aishwarya, T., Ravi Kumar, V. (2021). Machine learning and deep learning approaches to analyze and detect COVID-19: A review. *SN Comput. Sci.* 2(3), 226.

56. Tayarani, N.M. (2021). Applications of artificial intelligence in battling against COVID-19: A literature review. *Chaos Solitons Fractals* 142, 110338.

57. Gns, H.S., Gr, S., Murahari, M., et al. (2019). An update on drug repurposing: Re-written saga of the drug's fate. *Biomed. Pharmacother.* 110, 700–716.

58. Zhou, Y., Hou, Y., Shen, J., et al. (2020). Network-based drug repurposing for novel coronavirus 2019-nCoV/SARS-CoV-2. *Cell Discov.* 6(1), 14.

59. Shanmugam, A., Muralidharan, N., Velmurugan, D., et al. (2020). Therapeutic targets and computational approaches on drug development for COVID-19. *Curr. Top. Med. Chem.* 20(24), 2210–2220.

60. Singh, N., Villoutreix, B.O. (2021). Resources and computational strategies to advance small molecule SARS-CoV-2 discovery: Lessons from the pandemic and preparing for future health crises. *Comput. Struct. Biotechnol. J.* 19, 2537–2548.

61. Maas, M.N., Hintzen, J.C.J., Loffler, P.M.G., et al. (2021). Targeting SARS-CoV-2 spike protein by stapled hACE2 peptides. *Chem. Commun.* 57(26), 3283–3286.

62. Ojha, P.K., Kar, S., Krishna, J.G., et al. (2021). Therapeutics for COVID-19: From computation to practices – where we are, where we are heading to. *Mol. Divers.* 25(1), 625–659.

63. Su, H., Zhou, F., Huang, Z., et al. (2021). Molecular insights into small-molecule drug discovery for SARS-CoV-2. *Angew. Chem. Int. Ed. Engl.* 60(18), 9789–9802.

64. Yan, X.C., Sanders, J.M., Gao, Y.D., et al. (2020). Augmenting hit identification by virtual screening techniques in small molecule drug discovery. *J. Chem. Inf. Model.* 60(9), 4144–4152.

65. Wang, P., Zhou, J. (2018). Proteolysis Targeting Chimera (PROTAC): A paradigm-shifting approach in small molecule drug discovery. *Curr. Top. Med. Chem.* 18(16), 1354–1356.

66. Acar, H., Ting, J.M., Srivastava, S., et al. (2017). Molecular engineering solutions for therapeutic peptide delivery. *Chem. Soc. Rev.* 46(21), 6553–6569.

67. Henninot, A., Collins, J.C., Nuss, J.M. (2018). The current state of peptide drug discovery: Back to the Future? *J. Med. Chem.* 61(4), 1382–1414.

68. Fosgerau, K., Hoffmann, T. (2015). Peptide therapeutics: Current status and future directions. *Drug Discov. Today* 20(1), 122–128.

69. Di, L. (2015). Strategic approaches to optimizing peptide ADME properties. *AAPS J.* 17(1), 134–143.

70. Carter, P.J., Lazar, G.A. (2018). Next generation antibody drugs: Pursuit of the 'high-hanging fruit'. *Nat. Rev. Drug Discov.* 17(3), 197–223.

71. Sauna, Z.E., Lagasse, D., Pedras-Vasconcelos, J., et al. (2018). Evaluating and mitigating the immunogenicity of therapeutic proteins. *Trends Biotechnol.* 36(10), 1068–1084.

72. Jing, X., Hou, Y., Hallett, W., et al. (2019). Key physicochemical characteristics influencing adme properties of therapeutic proteins. *Adv. Exp. Med. Biol.* 1148, 115–129.

73. Krause, M.E., Sahin, E. (2019). Chemical and physical instabilities in manufacturing and storage of therapeutic proteins. *Curr. Opin. Biotechnol.* 60, 159–167.

74. Bojkova, D., Bechtel, M., McLaughlin, K.M., et al. (2020). Aprotinin inhibits SARS-CoV-2 replication. *Cells* 9(11), 2377.

75. Glasgow, A., Glasgow, J., Limonta, D., et al. (2020). Engineered ACE2 receptor traps potently neutralize SARS-CoV-2. *Proc. Natl. Acad. Sci. U.S.A.* 117(45), 28046–28055.

76. Ji, P., Chen, J., Golding, A., et al. (2020). Immunomodulatory therapeutic proteins in COVID-19: Current clinical development and clinical pharmacology considerations. *J. Clin. Pharmacol.* 60(10), 1275–1293.

77. Papageorgiou, A.C., Mohsin, I. (2020). The SARS-CoV-2 spike glycoprotein as a drug and vaccine target: Structural insights into its complexes with ACE2 and antibodies. *Cells* 9(11), 2343

78. Pecetta, S., Finco, O., Seubert, A. (2020). Quantum leap of monoclonal antibody (mAb) discovery and development in the COVID-19 era. *Semin. Immunol.* 50, 101427.

79. Schuster, J., Koulov, A., Mahler, H.C., et al. (2020). In vivo stability of therapeutic proteins. *Pharm. Res.* 37(2), 23.

80. Butreddy, A., Janga, K.Y., Ajjarapu, S., et al. (2021). Instability of therapeutic proteins: An overview of stresses, stabilization mechanisms and analytical techniques involved in lyophilized proteins. *Int. J. Biol. Macromol.* 167, 309–325.

81. Khodabakhsh, F., Salimian, M., Hedayati, M.H., et al. (2021). Challenges and advancements in the pharmacokinetic enhancement of therapeutic proteins. *Prep. Biochem. Biotechnol.* 1–11.

82. Yang, Z., Bogdan, P., Nazarian, S. (2021). An in silico deep learning approach to multi-epitope vaccine design: A SARS-CoV-2 case study. *Sci. Rep.* 11(1), 3238.

83. He, L., Zhu, J. (2015). Computational tools for epitope vaccine design and evaluation. *Curr. Opin. Virol.* 11, 103–112.

84. Frohlich, E. (2021). Therapeutic potential of mesenchymal stem cells and their products in lung diseases – intravenous administration versus inhalation. *Pharmaceutics* 13(2), 232.

85. Mahendiratta, S., Bansal, S., Sarma, P., et al. (2021). Stem cell therapy in COVID-19: Pooled evidence from SARS-CoV-2, SARS-CoV, MERS-CoV and ARDS: A systematic review. *Biomed. Pharmacother.* 137, 111300.

86. Lanzoni, G., Linetsky, E., Correa, D., et al. (2021). Umbilical cord mesenchymal stem cells for COVID-19 acute respiratory distress syndrome: A double-blind, phase 1/2a, randomized controlled trial. *Stem Cells Transl. Med.* 10(5), 660–673.

87. Gil, C., Ginex, T., Maestro, I., et al. (2020). COVID-19: Drug targets and potential treatments. *J. Med. Chem.* 63(21), 12359–12386.

88. Jomah, S., Asdaq, S.M.B., Al-Yamani, M.J. (2020). Clinical efficacy of antivirals against novel

coronavirus (COVID-19): A review. *J. Infect. Public Health* 13(9), 1187–1195.

89. Martinez-Ortiz, W., Zhou, M.M. (2020). Could PROTACs protect us from COVID-19? *Drug Discov. Today* 25(11), 1894–1896.

90. Singh, R.K., Yadav, B.S., Mohapatra, T.M. (2020). Molecular targets and system biology approaches for drug repurposing against SARS-CoV-2. *Bull. Natl. Res. Cent.* 44(1), 193.

91. Khalil, B.A., Elemam, N.M., Maghazachi, A.A. (2021). Chemokines and chemokine receptors during COVID-19 infection. *Comput. Struct. Biotechnol. J.* 19, 976–988.

92. Muus, C., Luecken, M.D., Eraslan, G., et al. (2021). Single-cell meta-analysis of SARS-CoV-2 entry genes across tissues and demographics. *Nat. Med.* 27(3), 546–559.

93. Wong, N.A., Saier, Jr. M.H. (2021). The SARS–coronavirus infection cycle: A survey of viral membrane proteins, their functional interactions and pathogenesis. *Int. J. Mol. Sci.* 22(3), 1308.

94. Gallagher, T.M., Buchmeier, M.J. (2001). Coronavirus spike proteins in viral entry and pathogenesis. *Virology* 279(2), 371–374.

95. Castano-Rodriguez, C., Honrubia, J.M., Gutierrez-Alvarez, J., et al. (2018). Role of severe acute respiratory syndrome coronavirus viroporins E, 3a, and 8a in replication and pathogenesis. *mBio* 9(3), e02325.

96. Neuman, B.W., Kiss, G., Kunding, A.H., et al. (2011). A structural analysis of M protein in coronavirus assembly and morphology. *J. Struct. Biol.* 174(1), 11–22.

97. McBride, R., van Zyl, M., Fielding, B.C. (2014). The coronavirus nucleocapsid is a multifunctional protein. *Viruses* 6(8), 2991–3018.

98. Robson, B. (2020). The use of knowledge management tools in viroinformatics. Example study of a highly conserved sequence motif in Nsp3 of SARS-CoV-2 as a therapeutic target. *Comput. Biol. Med.* 125, 103963.

99. Barrantes, F.J. (2021). Structural biology of coronavirus ion channels. *Acta Crystallogr. D. Struct. Biol.* 77(Pt 4), 391–402.

100. Grenga, L., Armengaud, J. (2021). Proteomics in the COVID-19 battlefield: First semester check-up. *Proteomics* 21(1), e2000198.

101. Zhou, N., Bao, J., Ning, Y. (2021). H2V: A database of human genes and proteins that respond to SARS-CoV-2, SARS-CoV, and MERS-CoV infection. *BMC Bioinformatics* 22(1), 18.

102. Gordon, D.E., Hiatt, J., Bouhaddou, M., et al. (2020). Comparative host-coronavirus protein interaction networks reveal pan-viral disease mechanisms. *Science* 370(6521), eabe9403.

103. Gordon, D.E., Jang, G.M., Bouhaddou, M., et al. (2020). A SARS-CoV-2 protein interaction map reveals targets for drug repurposing. *Nature* 583(7816), 459–468.

104. Bittremieux, W., Adams, C., Laukens, K., et al. (2021). Open science resources for the mass spectrometry-based analysis of SARS-CoV-2. *J. Proteome. Res.* 20(3), 1464–1475.

105. Ekins, S., Mottin, M., Ramos, P., et al. (2020). Deja vu: Stimulating open drug discovery for SARS-CoV-2. *Drug Discov. Today* 25(5), 928–941.

106. Kuba, K., Imai, Y., Ohto-Nakanishi, T., et al. (2010). Trilogy of ACE2: A peptidase in the renin-angiotensin system, a SARS receptor, and a partner for amino acid transporters. *Pharmacol. Ther.* 128(1), 119–128.

107. Iwata-Yoshikawa, N., Okamura, T., Shimizu, Y., et al. (2019). TMPRSS2 contributes to virus spread and immunopathology in the airways of murine models after coronavirus infection. *J. Virol.* 93(6), e01815.

108. Walls, A.C., Park, Y.J., Tortorici, M.A., et al. (2020). Structure, function, and antigenicity of the SARS-CoV-2 spike glycoprotein. *Cell* 181(2), 281–292 e6.

109. Coutard, B., Valle, C., de Lamballerie, X., et al. (2020). The spike glycoprotein of the new coronavirus 2019-nCoV contains a furin-like cleavage site absent in CoV of the same clade. *Antiviral Res.* 176, 104742.

110. Hoffmann, M., Kleine-Weber, H., Pohlmann, S. (2020). A multibasic cleavage site in the spike protein of SARS-CoV-2 is essential for infection of human lung cells. *Mol. Cell* 78(4), 779–784 e5.

111. Ivanova, T., Hardes, K., Kallis, S., et al. (2017). Optimization of substrate-analogue furin inhibitors. *ChemMedChem* 12(23), 1953–1968.

112. Ou, X., Liu, Y., Lei, X., et al. (2020). Characterization of spike glycoprotein of SARS-CoV-2 on virus entry and its immune cross-reactivity with SARS-CoV. *Nat. Commun.* 11(1), 1620.

113. Adedeji, A.O., Severson, W., Jonsson, C., et al. (2013). Novel inhibitors of severe acute respiratory syndrome coronavirus entry that act by three distinct mechanisms. *J. Virol.* 87(14), 8017–8028.

114. He, K., Marsland III, R., Upadhyayula, S., et al. (2017). Dynamics of phosphoinositide conversion in clathrin-mediated endocytic traffic. *Nature* 552(7685), 410–414.

115. Shisheva, A. (2008). PIKfyve: Partners, significance, debates and paradoxes. *Cell Biol. Int.* 32(6), 591–604.

116. Kang, Y.L., Chou, Y.Y., Rothlauf, P.W., et al. (2020). Inhibition of PIKfyve kinase prevents infection by Zaire Ebolavirus and SARS-CoV-2. *Proc. Natl. Acad. Sci. U.S.A.* 117(34), 20803–20813.

117. Parkinson, N., Rodgers, N., Head Fourman, M., et al. (2020). Dynamic data-driven meta-analysis for prioritisation of host genes implicated in COVID-19. *Sci. Rep.* 10(1), 22303.

118. Jaiswal, S., Kumar, M., Dixit, M., et al. (2020). Systems biology approaches for therapeutics development against COVID-19. *Front. Cell Infect. Microbiol.* 10, 560240.

119. Meszaros, B., Samano-Sanchez, H., Alvarado-Valverde, J., et al. (2021). Short linear motif candidates in the cell entry system used by SARS-CoV-2 and their potential therapeutic implications. *Sci. Signal.* 14(665).

120. Waman, V.P., Sen, N., Varadi, M., et al. (2021). The impact of structural bioinformatics tools and resources on SARS-CoV-2 research and therapeutic strategies. *Brief Bioinform.* 22(2), 742–768.

121. ww, P.D.B.c. (2019). Protein Data Bank: The single global archive for 3D macromolecular structure data. *Nucleic Acids Res.* 47(D1), D520–D528.

122. Sedova, M., Jaroszewski, L., Alisoltani, A., et al. (2020). Coronavirus3D: 3D structural visualization of COVID-19 genomic divergence. *Bioinformatics* 36(15), 4360–4362.

123. Bienert, S., Waterhouse, A., de Beer, T.A., et al. (2017). The SWISS-MODEL repository-new features and functionality. *Nucleic Acids Res.* 45(D1), D313–D319.

124. O'Donoghue, S.I., Sabir, K.S., Kalemanov, M., et al. (2015). Aquaria: Simplifying discovery and insight from protein structures. *Nat. Methods* 12(2), 98–99.

125. Srinivasan, S., Cui, H., Gao, Z., et al. (2020). Structural genomics of SARS-CoV-2 indicates evolutionary conserved functional regions of viral proteins. *Viruses* 12(4), 360.

126. Lubin, J.H., Zardecki, C., Dolan, E.M., et al. (2020). Evolution of the SARS-CoV-2 proteome in three dimensions (3D) during the first six months of the COVID-19 pandemic. *bioRxiv.* doi:10.1101/2020.12.01.406637.

127. Hosseini, M., Chen, W., Xiao, D., et al. (2021). Computational molecular docking and virtual screening revealed promising SARS-CoV-2 drugs. *Precis. Clin. Med.* 4(1), 1–16.

128. Chourasia, M., Koppula, P.R., Battu, A., et al. (2021). EGCG, a green tea catechin, as a potential therapeutic agent for symptomatic and asymptomatic SARS-CoV-2 infection. *Molecules* 26(5), 1200.

129. Vela, J.M. (2020). Repurposing Sigma-1 receptor ligands for COVID-19 therapy? *Front. Pharmacol.* 11, 582310.

130. Dotolo, S., Marabotti, A., Facchiano, A., et al. (2021). A review on drug repurposing applicable to COVID-19. *Brief Bioinform.* 22(2), 726–741.

131. Zhou, Y., Wang, F., Tang, J., et al. (2020). Artificial intelligence in COVID-19 drug repurposing. *Lancet. Digit. Health* 2(12), e667–e676.

132. Edwards, A. (2020). What are the odds of finding a COVID-19 drug from a lab repurposing screen? *J. Chem. Inf. Model.* 60(12), 5727–5729.

133. Wang, X., Guan, Y. (2021). COVID-19 drug repurposing: A review of computational screening methods, clinical trials, and protein interaction assays. *Med. Res. Rev.* 41(1), 5–28.

134. Abdulla, A., Wang, B., Qian, F. F., et al. (2020). Project IDentif.AI: Harnessing artificial intelligence to rapidly optimize combination therapy development for infectious disease intervention. *Adv. Ther.* 2000034.

135. Touret, F., Gilles, M., Barral, K., et al. (2020). In vitro screening of a FDA approved chemical library reveals potential inhibitors of SARS-CoV-2 replication. *Sci. Rep.* 10(1), 13093.

136. Riva, L., Yuan, S., Yin, X., et al. (2020). Discovery of SARS-CoV-2 antiviral drugs through large-scale compound repurposing. *Nature* 586(7827), 113–119.

137. Ke, Y.Y., Peng, T.T., Yeh, T.K., et al. (2020). Artificial intelligence approach fighting COVID-19 with repurposing drugs. *Biomed. J.* 43(4), 355–362.

138. Wang, J. (2020). Fast identification of possible drug treatment of coronavirus disease-19 (COVID-19) through computational drug repurposing study. *J. Chem. Inf. Model.* 60(6), 3277–3286.

139. Brimacombe, K.R., Zhao, T., Eastman, R.T., et al. (2020). An OpenData portal to share COVID-19 drug repurposing data in real time. *bioRxiv* doi:10.1101/2020.06.04.135046.

140. Altay, O., Mohammadi, E., Lam, S., et al. (2020). Current status of COVID-19 therapies and drug repositioning applications. *iScience* 23(7), 101303.

141. Keiser, M.J., Setola, V., Irwin, J.J., et al. (2009). Predicting new molecular targets for known drugs. *Nature* 462(7270), 175–181.

142. Masoudi-Sobhanzadeh, Y., Salemi, A., Pourseif, M.M., et al. (2021). Structure-based drug repurposing against COVID-19 and emerging infectious diseases: Methods, resources and discoveries. *Brief Bioinform.*, bbab113. doi:10.1093/bib/bbab113.

143. Kitchen, D.B., Decornez, H., Furr, J.R., et al. (2004). Docking and scoring in virtual screening for drug discovery: Methods and applications. *Nat. Rev. Drug Discov.* 3(11), 935–949.

144. Greene, C.S., Voight, B.F. (2016). Pathway and network-based strategies to translate genetic discoveries into effective therapies. *Hum. Mol. Genet.* 25(R2), R94–R98.

145. Sanseau, P., Agarwal, P., Barnes, M.R., et al. (2012). Use of genome-wide association studies for drug repositioning. *Nat. Biotechnol.* 30(4), 317–320.

146. Elfiky, A.A. (2020). Anti-HCV, nucleotide inhibitors, repurposing against COVID-19. *Life Sci.* 248, 117477.

147. Krishnan, D.A., Sangeetha, G., Vajravijayan, S., et al. (2020). Structure-based drug designing towards the identification of potential anti-viral for COVID-19 by targeting endoribonuclease NSP15. *Inform. Med. Unlocked* 20, 100392.

148. White, M.A., Lin, W., Cheng, X. (2020). Discovery of COVID-19 inhibitors targeting the SARS-CoV-2 Nsp13 helicase. *J. Phys. Chem. Lett.* 11(21), 9144–9151.

149. Tomazou, M., Bourdakou, M.M., Minadakis, G., et al. (2021). Multi-omics data integration and network-based analysis drives a multiplex drug repurposing approach to a shortlist of candidate drugs against COVID-19. *Brief Bioinform.* bbab114. doi:10.1093/bib/bbab114.

150. Wu, C., Liu, Y., Yang, Y., et al. (2020). Analysis of therapeutic targets for SARS-CoV-2 and discovery of potential drugs by computational methods. *Acta Pharm. Sin. B* 10(5), 766–788.

151. Khare, P., Sahu, U., Pandey, S.C., et al. (2020). Current approaches for target-specific drug discovery using natural compounds against SARS-CoV-2 infection. *Virus Res.* 290, 198169.

152. Sardanelli, A.M., Isgro, C., Palese, L.L. (2021). SARS-CoV-2 main protease active site ligands in the human metabolome. *Molecules* 26(5), 1409.

153. Saakre, M., Mathew, D., Ravisankar, V. (2021). Perspectives on plant flavonoid quercetin-based drugs for novel SARS-CoV-2. *Beni Suef Univ. J. Basic Appl. Sci.* 10(1), 21.

154. Liskova, A., Samec, M., Koklesova, L., et al. (2021). Flavonoids against the SARS-CoV-2 induced inflammatory storm. *Biomed. Pharmacother.* 138, 111430.

155. Grigore, A., Cord, D., Tanase, C., et al. (2020). Herbal medicine, a reliable support in COVID therapy. *J. Immunoassay Immunochem.* 41(6), 976–999.

156. Zheng, C., Pei, T., Huang, C., et al. (2016). A novel systems pharmacology platform to dissect action mechanisms of traditional Chinese medicines for bovine viral diarrhea disease. *Eur. J. Pharm. Sci.* 94, 33–45.

157. Ganjhu, R.K., Mudgal, P.P., Maity, H., et al. (2015). Herbal plants and plant preparations as remedial approach for viral diseases. *Virusdisease* 26(4), 225–236.

158. Lin, L.T., Hsu, W.C., Lin, C.C. (2014). Antiviral natural products and herbal medicines. *J. Tradit. Complement. Med.* 4(1), 24–35.

159. Wang, S.X., Zhang, X.S., Guan, H.S., et al. (2014). Potential anti-HPV and related cancer agents from marine resources: An overview. *Mar. Drugs* 12(4), 2019–2035.

160. Ajaiyeoba, E.O., Ogbole, O.O. (2006). A phytotherapeutic approach to Nigerian anti-HIV and immunomodulatory drug discovery. *Afr. J. Med. Med. Sci.* 35 Suppl, 71–76.

161. Swain, S.S., Panda, S.K., Luyten, W. (2021). Phytochemicals against SARS-CoV as potential drug leads. *Biomed. J.* 44(1), 74–85.

162. Raimundo, E.S.J.P., Acevedo, C.A.H., de Souza, T.A., et al. (2021). Natural products as potential agents against SARS-CoV and SARS-CoV-2. *Curr. Med. Chem.*, 28(27), 5498–5526.

163. Li, S., Cheng, C.S., Zhang, C., et al. (2021). Edible and herbal plants for the prevention and management of COVID-19. *Front. Pharmacol.* 12, 656103.

164. Ramsay, R.R., Popovic-Nikolic, M.R., Nikolic, K., et al. (2018). A perspective on multi-target drug discovery and design for complex diseases. *Clin. Transl. Med.* 7(1), 3.

165. Klaeger, S., Heinzlmeir, S., Wilhelm, M., et al. (2017). The target landscape of clinical kinase drugs. *Science* 358(6367), eaan4368.

166. Saginc, G., Voellmy, F., Linding, R. (2017). Cancer systems biology: Harnessing off-target effects. *Nat. Chem. Biol.* 13(12), 1204–1205.

167. Chaudhari, R., Fong, L.W., Tan, Z., et al. (2020). An up-to-date overview of computational polypharmacology in modern drug discovery. *Expert Opin. Drug Discov.* 15(9), 1025–1044.

168. Kroschinsky, F., Stolzel, F., von Bonin, S., et al. (2017). New drugs, new toxicities: Severe side effects of modern targeted and immunotherapy of cancer and their management. *Crit. Care* 21(1), 89.

169. Anighoro, A., Bajorath, J., Rastelli, G. (2014). Polypharmacology: Challenges and opportunities in drug discovery. *J. Med. Chem.* 57(19), 7874–7887.

170. Chaudhari, R., Tan, Z., Huang, B., et al. (2017). Computational polypharmacology: A new paradigm for drug discovery. *Expert Opin. Drug Discov.* 12(3), 279–291.

171. Tan, Z., Chaudhai, R., Zhang, S. (2016). Polypharmacology in drug development: A mini-review of current technologies. *ChemMedChem* 11(12), 1211–1218.

172. Lim, H., Xie, L. (2019). Omics data integration and analysis for systems pharmacology. *Methods Mol. Biol.* 1939, 199–214.

173. Omotuyi, I.O., Nash, O., Ajiboye, B.O., et al. (2021). Aframomum melegueta secondary metabolites exhibit polypharmacology against SARS-CoV-2 drug targets: In vitro validation of furin inhibition. *Phytother. Res.* 35(2), 908–919.

174. Delre, P., Caporuscio, F., Saviano, M., et al. (2020). Repurposing known drugs as covalent and non-covalent inhibitors of the SARS-CoV-2 papain-like protease. *Front. Chem.* 8, 594009.

175. Pinzi, L., Tinivella, A., Caporuscio, F., et al. (2021). Drug repurposing and polypharmacology to fight SARS-CoV-2 through inhibition of the main protease. *Front. Pharmacol.* 12, 636989.

176. Kumar, S., Singh, B., Kumari, P., et al. (2021). Identification of multipotent drugs for COVID-19 therapeutics with the evaluation of their SARS-CoV2 inhibitory activity. *Comput. Struct. Biotechnol. J.* 19, 1998–2017.

177. Bergstrom, F., Lindmark, B. (2019). Accelerated drug discovery by rapid candidate drug identification. *Drug Discov. Today* 24(6), 1237–1241.

178. Canning, P., Birchall, K., Kettleborough, C.A., et al. (2020). Fragment-based target screening as an empirical approach to prioritising targets: A case study on antibacterials. *Drug Discov. Today*, S1359-6446(20)30339-1.

179. Duarte, Y., Marquez-Miranda, V., Miossec, M.J., et al. (2019). Integration of target discovery, drug discovery and drug delivery: A review on computational strategies. *Wiley Interdiscip. Rev. Nanomed. Nanobiotechnol.* 11(4), e1554.

180. Emmerich, C.H., Gamboa, L.M., Hofmann, M.C.J., et al. (2021). Improving target assessment in biomedical research: The GOT-IT recommendations. *Nat. Rev. Drug Discov.* 20(1), 64–81.

181. Siramshetty, V.B., Preissner, R. (2018). Drugs as habitable planets in the space of dark chemical matter. *Drug Discov. Today* 23(3), 481–486.

182. Sosa, E.J., Burguener, G., Lanzarotti, E., et al. (2018). Target-pathogen: A structural bioinformatic approach to prioritize drug targets in pathogens. *Nucleic Acids Res.* 46(D1), D413–D418.

183. Sydow, D., Burggraaff, L., Szengel, A., et al. (2019). Advances and challenges in computational target prediction. *J. Chem. Inf. Model.* 59(5), 1728–1742.

184. Wilkinson, I.V.L., Terstappen, G.C., Russell, A.J. (2020). Combining experimental strategies for successful target deconvolution. *Drug Discov. Today*, S1359-6446(20)30373-1.

185. Cavasotto, C.N., Lamas, M.S., Maggini, J. (2021). Functional and druggability analysis of the SARS-CoV-2 proteome. *Eur. J. Pharmacol.* 890, 173705.

186. Abrusan, G., Marsh, J.A. (2019). Ligands and receptors with broad binding capabilities have common structural characteristics: An antibiotic design perspective. *J. Med. Chem.* 62(21), 9357–9374.

187. Vajda, S., Beglov, D., Wakefield, A.E., et al. (2018). Cryptic binding sites on proteins: Definition, detection, and druggability. *Curr. Opin. Chem. Biol.* 44, 1–8.

188. Stank, A., Kokh, D.B., Fuller, J.C., et al. (2016). Protein binding pocket dynamics. *Acc. Chem. Res.* 49(5), 809–815.

189. Surade, S., Blundell, T.L. (2012). Structural biology and drug discovery of difficult targets: The limits of ligandability. *Chem. Biol.* 19(1), 42–50.

190. Kufareva, I., Ilatovskiy, A.V., and Abagyan, R. (2012). Pocketome: An encyclopedia of small-molecule binding sites in 4D. *Nucleic Acids Res.* 40(Database issue), D535–D540.

191. Perot, S., Sperandio, O., Miteva, M.A., et al. (2010). Druggable pockets and binding site centric chemical space: A paradigm shift in drug discovery. *Drug Discov. Today* 15(15–16), 656–667.

192. Sehli, S., Allali, I., Chahboune, R., et al. (2021). Metagenomics approaches to investigate the gut microbiome of COVID-19 patients. *Bioinform. Biol. Insights* 15, 1177932221999428.

193. Kim, H.S. (2021). Do an altered gut microbiota and an associated leaky gut affect COVID-19 severity? *mBio* 12(1), E03022-20.

194. Russo, G., Reche, P., Pennisi, M., et al. (2020). The combination of artificial intelligence and systems biology for intelligent vaccine design. *Expert Opin. Drug Discov.* 15(11), 1267–1281.

195. Hwang, W., Lei, W., Katritsis, N.M., et al. (2021). Current and prospective computational approaches and challenges for developing COVID-19 vaccines. *Adv. Drug Deliv. Rev.* 172, 249–274.

196. Masignani, V., Rappuoli, R., Pizza, M. (2002). Reverse vaccinology: A genome-based approach for vaccine development. *Expert Opin. Biol. Ther.* 2(8), 895–905.

197. Rappuoli, R. (2001). Reverse vaccinology, a genome-based approach to vaccine development. *Vaccine* 19(17–19), 2688–2691.

198. Burton, D.R. (2002). Antibodies, viruses and vaccines. *Nat. Rev. Immunol.* 2(9), 706–713.

199. Lim, H.X., Lim, J., Jazayeri, S.D., et al. (2021). Development of multi-epitope peptide-based vaccines against SARS-CoV-2. *Biomed. J* 44(1), 18–30.

200. Galanis, K.A., Nastou, K.C., Papandreou, N.C., et al. (2021). Linear B-cell epitope prediction for in silico vaccine design: A performance review of methods available via command-line interface. *Int. J. Mol. Sci.* 22(6), 3210.

201. Crooke, S.N., Ovsyannikova, I.G., Kennedy, R.B., et al. (2020). Immunoinformatic identification of B cell and T cell epitopes in the SARS-CoV-2 proteome. *Sci. Rep.* 10(1), 14179.

202. Noorimotlagh, Z., Karami, C., Mirzaee, S.A., et al. (2020). Immune and bioinformatics identification of T cell and B cell epitopes in the protein structure of SARS-CoV-2: A systematic review. *Int. Immunopharmacol.* 86, 106738.

203. Goh, G.K., Dunker, A.K., Foster, J.A., et al. (2020). A novel strategy for the development of vaccines for SARS-CoV-2 (COVID-19) and other viruses using AI and viral shell disorder. *J. Proteome Res.* 19(11), 4355–4363.

204. Whetton, A.D., Preston, G.W., Abubeker, S., et al. (2020). Proteomics and informatics for understanding phases and identifying biomarkers in COVID-19 disease. *J. Proteome. Res.* 19(11), 4219–4232.

205. Safiabadi Tali, S.H., LeBlanc, J.J., Sadiq, Z., et al. (2021). Tools and techniques for severe acute respiratory syndrome coronavirus 2 (SARS-CoV-2)/COVID-19 detection. *Clin. Microbiol. Rev.* 34(3), E00228-20.

206. Yong, S.J. (2021). Long COVID or post-COVID-19 syndrome: Putative pathophysiology, risk factors, and treatments. *Infect. Dis.* 53(10), 737–754.

207. Griffin, J.H., Downard, K.M. (2021). Mass spectrometry analytical responses to the SARS-CoV2 coronavirus in review. *Trends Analyt. Chem.* 142, 116328.

208. Froberg, J., Diavatopoulos, D.A. (2021). Mucosal immunity to severe acute respiratory syndrome coronavirus 2 infection. *Curr. Opin. Infect. Dis.* 34(3), 181–186.

209. Dos Santos, A.C.M., Dos Santos, B.R.C., Dos Santos, B.B., et al. (2021). Genetic polymorphisms as multi-biomarkers in severe acute respiratory syndrome (SARS) by coronavirus infection: A systematic review of candidate gene association studies. *Infect. Genet. Evol.* 93, 104846.

210. Paim, A.A.O., Lopes-Ribeiro, A., Daian, E.S.D.S.O., et al. (2021. Will a little change do you good? A putative role of polymorphisms in COVID-19. *Immunol. Lett.* 235, 9–14.

211. Long, J., Luo, Y., Wei, Y., et al. (2021). The effect of cardiovascular disease and acute cardiac injury on fatal COVID-19: A meta-analysis. *Am. J. Emerg. Med.* 48, 128–139.

212. Samprathi, M., Jayashree, M. (2020). Biomarkers in COVID-19: An up-to-date review. *Front. Pediatr.* 8, 607647.

Chapter 12 Nanomaterials in COVID-19 Drug Development

Alaa A. A. Aljabali, Ángel Serrano-Aroca, Kenneth Lundstrom, and Murtaza M. Tambuwala

12.1 INTRODUCTION

The current pandemic was first reported in Wuhan, China, in December 2019 and is now the deadliest outbreak ever since World War II, with more than 243 million infections as a significant part is asymptomatic, and five million casualties by October 2021 [1]. It is concerning that the global effect of this pandemic is as yet not quite at the peak. Mainly because of the compulsory isolation and shutdowns, the human population is experiencing a crisis. The financial system is now in danger, and if the spread is not restricted, the situation will worsen [2]. SARS-CoV-2, which is the cause of the novel coronavirus disease (COVID-19), is a threat to global health that is urgently in need of advanced alternative treatments. In this context, nanotechnology can play an important role. In this chapter, the role of nanomaterials to counter the shortcomings of current antiviral and biotherapeutic drugs will be addressed. Thus nanomaterials in the form of engineered nanocarriers provide alternative robust and reliable drug delivery strategies.

Furthermore, a broad range of nanomaterial types has exhibited the ability to block initial interactions between the viral spike glycoprotein and host cell surface receptors and interrupts virion formation. On the other hand, nanotechnology provides a safe and effective alternative for COVID-19 vaccinations. Thus the first two approved COVID-19 vaccines for human use are based on nanoparticle-encapsulated mRNA.

12.1.1 Nanotechnology versus Coronavirus

In the absence of selective and effective treatment, it is necessary to search for alternative, nontoxic treatments. While nanotechnology-based techniques are used to construct vaccine delivery vectors, few other nanotechnology methods are being developed to address the current pandemic. Throughout the context of therapies and vaccines, attempts should systematically present the nanotechnology application's actual state. The illness caused by SARS-CoV-2 is not very distinct from many other serious diseases, regarding interventional science, clinical progress, and challenges. We also need to study these closely related therapeutic/vaccination techniques and related nanotechnology to rapidly follow up on the latest studies employing reused nanotechnology [3, 4]. The nano-carrier-based treatment provides different approaches to overcome the shortcomings of existing antiviral therapy. Nanoprotein-based vaccines, the alteration of their pharmacokinetic/pharmacodynamic features and dosage reduction, reduction of toxicity and increased drug bioavailability, and the preservation of suppressed viral spread are significant problems as are weak aqueous solubility and low bioavailability. Effective, targeted nanostructures could cross biological barriers in reasonable viral reservoirs and reach sufficient therapeutic concentrations. Unique tissue, cell, and intercellular positions engaged in SARS-CoV-2 pathogenesis may also be targeted, such as ACE2 expressing cells, viral S protein domains, cathepsin-binding sites, and various other sites [5].

Several nanomaterials have been evaluated against coronaviruses, including nanotubes, nanowires, nanocrystals, nanosheets, nanocapsules, lipid-based nanocarriers, carboxy terminated quantum dots, silver nanoparticles, gold nanoparticles, polymeric nanoparticles (chitosan, poly lactic-co-glycolic acid (PLGA), and poly(hydroxyethyl) methacrylate) and carbon-based nanomaterials [6, 7]. Iron oxide nanoparticles (IONPs), previously approved by the US Food and Drug Administration (FDA) for anemia treatment, showed in docking experiments interaction with the receptor-binding domain (RBD) of the SARS-CoV-2 S protein, which is anticipated to lead to conformational changes and viral inactivation and therefore serves as a potential approach for drug repurposing [8]. Furthermore, inorganic polyphosphate (polyP), a physiological polymer released from blood platelets, can efficiently inhibit the binding of the S protein to the ACE2 receptor [9]. Soluble silica/polyP nanoparticles significantly inhibited the interaction of the S protein with ACE2 at a concentration of 1 µg/ml, potentially providing a novel strategy for the prevention and treatment of SARS-CoV-2 infections in the oropharyngeal cavity [9].

12.2 SCOPE OF NANOTECHNOLOGY APPROACHES

Nanotechnology may contribute to combating COVID-19 through different means, such as preventing viral contamination and spreading, by developing personal protective equipment [10] to improve the safety of health professionals,

DOI: 10.1201/9781003190394-12

and to develop effective antiviral disinfectant and surface coatings [11] capable of inactivating and preventing the spread of the virus, and developing highly selective designs and delivery systems to boost therapeutic effectiveness. Thus, for example, very recently, an antiviral face mask filter capable of inactivating SARS-CoV-2 in one minute of contact has been developed as a promising tool to combat the spread of the COVID-19 pandemic [12]. The mask filter also inactivated Gram-positive multidrug-resistant bacteria such as *Staphylococcus pneumoniae*, contributing to the SARS-CoV-2-mediated pneumonia disease complex. Moreover, antibiotic resistance in pneumonia therapeutics is rising at an alarming rate. Nanotechnology-based studies in the production of new materials open prospects for self-cleaning surfaces. These mechanisms may be antimicrobial, or slow-release chemicals which can extend their time of action. Additional properties including such receptive structures may contribute to the production of active substances in response to various stimuli, such as photothermal, photocatalytic, or other stimuli. According to the manufacturer, a disinfectant formulation for titanium dioxide and silver nanoparticles, by the Nanotech Surface Company enabled self-sterilization of surfaces and was recently used to clean buildings in Milan. Italy during the COVID-19 pandemic [13].

Many material moieties could be mounted and transported by nanocarriers, including antivirals, biologics, and nucleic acids. In the context of viruses, nanocarriers with negative amphiphilic structures display a full range of inhibitory activities against viruses. It has been demonstrated for herpes simplex virus (HSV), though it should also be applicable to other types of viruses [14]. This may be attributed to the rapid treatment of membrane damage by the mechanism of self-repair. Therefore it is considered that an excellent SARS-CoV-2 inhibitor can be established with the principle of envelope rupture.

To succeed against SARS-CoV-2 it is necessary to conjugate the right therapeutic candidate to the right nanocarrier, which is intended to treat a particular disease condition. This nanomedicine method must be used for all licensed reformulation and trial drug candidates, primarily by resolving drug molecule limits and mitigating toxicity or side effects, to boost the therapeutic index. The nanomedicine systems currently available for anticancer therapies should also be considered to support this strategy [15]. The critical decision is to research and choose basic and intelligent nanomedicine designs that adopt nanosystems techniques to optimize the effect of nanomedicines. Strategic recommendations

are of considerable significance, stressing the right spheres and straightforward methods to track COVID-19 nanomedicine science quickly. Several nanomaterial types such as carbon-based nanomaterials (CBNs), polymeric nanoparticles, dendrimers, and lipid-based nanomaterials have been proposed to combat COVID-19 [16] (Figure 12.1).

12.2.1 Antiviral Metallic Nanomaterials

Copper-based nanomaterials (CuNPs) have been used against SARS-CoV-2. The antiviral mechanism is based on virus inhibition by disrupting the activity of specific viral proteins using Cu^{2+} ion-generated hydroxyl radicals located on the surface of nanomaterials and in direct contact with the viral surface [17]. CuNPs or copper oxides (CuOs) are the most appropriate technique for destroying SARS-CoV-2 externally by coating the mask materials with CuNPs.

Alternatively, iron oxide NPs have proven to interact with the spike protein receptor-binding domain (S1-RBD) of SARS-CoV-2, essential for virus attachment to the host cell surface receptors [18]. Furthermore, the ability of iron oxide nanomaterials to generate reactive oxygen species (ROS) holds great potential in the inactivation of the viral particles outside the host cell and might have a role in preventing infections. Other metallic nanomaterials such as those based on silver, titanium, or zinc nanoparticles or composite nanomaterials such as SiO_2-Ag have also shown broad-spectrum solid antimicrobial properties, including antiviral activity against SARS-CoV-2 [19].

12.2.2 Carbon-Based Antiviral Nanomaterials

CBNs, such as fullerene, carbon dots, graphene, and derivatives, promise to combat COVID-19 because they possess unique properties, broad-spectrum antimicrobial properties, none or low cytotoxicity, low-risk of microbial resistance, and they are capable of inducing tissue regeneration. CBNs with low or no toxicity to humans have shown antiviral activity against 13 enveloped positive-sense single-stranded RNA viruses: human coronavirus (HCoV-229E), porcine reproductive and respiratory syndrome virus, porcine epidemic diarrhea virus, human immunodeficiency virus type 1 and type 2, feline coronavirus, Japanese encephalitis, simian immunodeficiency virus, Moloney murine leukemia virus, Zika virus, dengue virus, hepatitis C virus, and SARS-CoV-2. Furthermore, a very recent study has shown that graphene sheets can be used as nanoplatforms to carry alkyl chains capable of inhibiting the infection of enveloped viruses such as the SARS-CoV-2 [20].

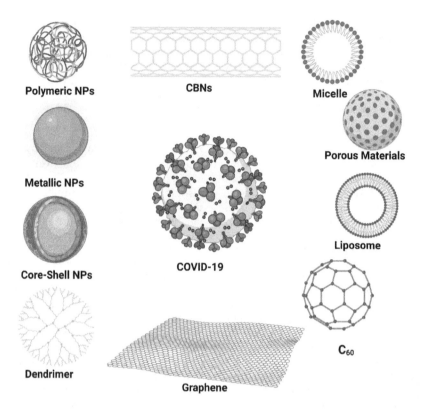

Figure 12.1 A schematic illustration of how various nanomaterial can combat the COVID-19 pandemic. Carbon-based nanomaterials (CNTs, buckyballs, graphene), polymeric dendrimers, and lipid-based nanomaterials are currently under investigation against COVID-19.

Source: Image created by Biorender.

The oxidized form of graphene, graphene oxide (GO), is also a 2D nanomaterial (see Figure 12.2B) with a high surface/volume ratio with hydrophilic properties from their hydroxyl, carbonyl, and epoxy groups located at the edges and basal planes [21], with wide-spectrum antimicrobial properties [22].

The functional groups present in GO can be crosslinked by coordination chemistry with divalent cations such as Ca^{2+} or antimicrobial cations such as Zn^{2+} or Mg^{2+} to produce novel filamentous micrometric materials (Figures 12.2C–12.2E) [24].

1D carbon nanomaterials such as carbon nanofibers are hydrophobic filamentous materials (see Figure 12.2A) with great potential to be used as nanoweapons against life-threatening multidrug-resistant bacteria such as methicillin-resistant *Staphylococcus epidermidis* (MRSE) [25]. Further, they can enhance the antiviral properties of antiviral biopolymers such as calcium alginate [26].

These types of 1D and 2D CBNs can also induce cell proliferation and enhance cell adhesion at non-cytotoxic concentrations in biomedical applications [27].

These results confirmed that the broad-spectrum antimicrobial properties of CBNs render them as very promising agents to inactivate viruses, bacteria, fungi, and multidrug-resistant microorganisms. Furthermore, CBNs possess immunostimulatory potential [28] and can be used in combination with stem cells as very promising therapeutics to treat COVID-19 [29]. CBNs can induce the production of angiogenic factors that can induce angiogenesis by promoting the proliferation and differentiation of endothelial cells or mesenchymal stem cells [30]. CBNs in combination with MSCs have the potential to target tissue inflammation, immune system damage (leukopenia, lymphopenia), respiratory microstructure and distal organs injury and secondary infections, and microvascular systems (see Figure 12.3).

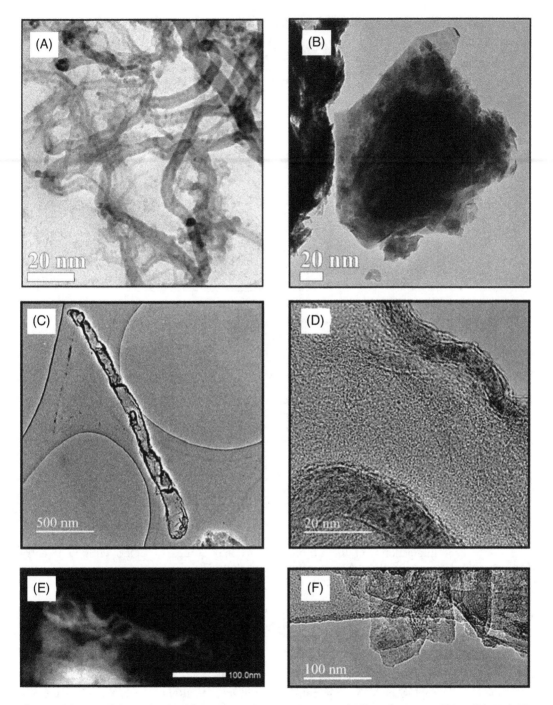

Figure 12.2   High-resolution electron microscopy images of 1D carbon nanofibers (A) and 2D graphene oxide nanosheets (B) reproduced from [23]. High-resolution transmission electron micrographs at two magnifications (C & D) with STEM dark field (E) of GO crosslinked with antimicrobial Zn^{2+} and the pristine GO nanosheets used in the crosslinking process (F) [24].

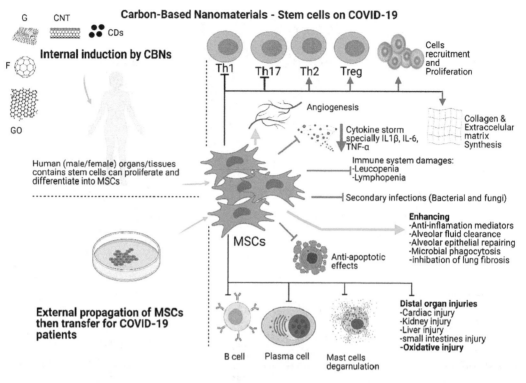

Figure 12.3 Carbon-based nanomaterials such as graphene (G), graphene oxide (GO), fullerene (F), carbon dots (CDs), or carbon nanotubes (CNT), and stem cells on COVID-19. Mesenchymal stem cells (MSCs) or MSCs from many tissues internally induced by CBNs (G: graphene, GO: graphene oxide, F: fullerene, CDs: carbon dots, or CNT: carbon nanotubes).

Source: Reprinted with permission from our peer-review ACS Nano publication: https://doi.org/10.1021/acsnano.1c00629. Copyright 2021 American Chemical Society.

CBNs have recently proved to be promising candidates for viral inhibition through permitting multivalent interactions on the virions. For example, because of their strong affinity to bacteria or viruses, modified graphene nanoplatforms have significantly increased various potential infections. While a challenging question is still the potential mechanics of the interactions between graphene derivatives and pathogens, numerous approaches have been developed to deter pathogens from acting against host cells. Graphene materials that are capable of trapping or wrapping pathogens by interaction with particular antibodies or ligands, electrostatic interactions are currently under evaluation as an alternative treatment approach [31]. Carbon dots conjugated with boric acid suppress human coronavirus HCoV-229E [32]. Antiviral activity was observed for seven different carbon quantum dots (CQDs). CQDs showed concentration-dependent virus inactivation of HCoV-229E. Second-generation anti-HCoV nanomaterials showed superior EC_{50} concentrations, and HCoV-229E inhibition was based on the interaction between functional groups of CQDs with viral entry receptors [32].

12.2.3 Small Interfering RNA

Large, hydrophilic, and anionic small interfering RNA (siRNA) delivery can be improved with nanoparticles, or conjugates that actively target ligands on the cell surface, or using natural interactions with the body (e.g., serum proteins) to passively target the cell of interest because it is not easy for siRNA to cross the cell membrane alone [34]: (Figure 12.4).

SiRNA also appears to be an excellent alternative technique for controlling SARS-CoV-2. The ability of siRNA to target the coding sequences for the SARS-CoV S protein was demonstrated to inhibit viral replication in the Vero E6 cell line [34]. Moreover, siRNA has been applied for SARS-CoV, whereby targeting the leader sequence, SARS-CoV replication in Vero E6 was inhibited [35].

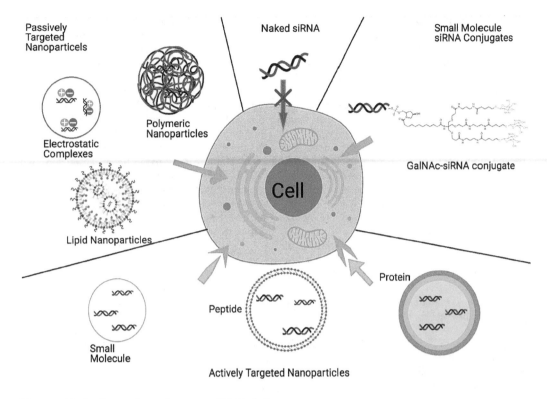

Figure 12.4 Strategies to improve siRNA delivery.

Source: Reproduced with permission from Elsevier [33].

12.2.4 CRISPR/Cas9

CRISPR-based technologies have also been emphasized as an option for the search for SARS-CoV-2 containment. The CRISPR-Cas13-based strategy was demonstrated to efficiently degrade SARS-CoV-2 RNA in human lung epithelial cells using the PAC-MAN (prophylactic antiviral CRISPR in human cells) system [36]. Application of bioinformatics indicated that six designed CRISPR RNAs (crRNAs) were able to target 90% of CoVs, providing an attractive pan-CoV inhibition strategy. The endonuclease of Cas13d RNA and the guide RNA (gRNA) are used for targeted inhibition and decomposition of the viral genome and the synthesis of mRNA. There have been promising findings with RNA degradation of the SARS-CoV-2 sequence [36]. The CRISPR/Cas13d method is also described by Nguyen et al. [37] as an option for SARS-CoV2 control. They designed 10,333 gRNAs to specifically target 10 peptide coding regions of SARS-CoV-2. Adeno-associated virus (AAV) has been proposed for the delivery of Cas13d effector, and utilization of tissue-specific promoters and a lung-specific AAV serotype supports precise delivery and expression in lung tissue. In another approach, the CRISPR-Cas9 system has been used to introduce point mutations into the human ACE2 receptor gene to decrease the interaction between the SARS-CoV-2 S protein and the ACE2 receptor [38].

12.2.5 Antiviral and Nanomaterial Delivery

As antiviral medication or vaccine delivery tools, specially engineered nanostructures, can also specifically combat viruses directly. In this regard, it is essential to engineer the appropriate antiviral approach to block viral replication.

The emergence of DNA origami innovation has further expanded the initial nanomaterial inventory, which is also in its initial antiviral research stages. DNA may be prevented by interference with a spatial pattern by designing the DNA nanoarchitecture to have a unique star shape. The nanoarchitecture was explicitly updated to identify ED3 clusters on the viral surface using ED3 targeting aptamers [39].

In addition, gold nanocomposites used as broad-spectrum viral inhibitors were engineered with heparan sulfate proteoglycan (HSPG). Except for previous HSPG compounds, newly synthesized mercaptoundecanoic sulfonic (MUS) acid-containing ligands were also reported to bind to the viral attachment ligands in very diluted concentrations, creating viral deforming effects. HSPG has also been used in nanogels with extra versatility to prevent the penetration of viruses. The broad spectrum of antiviral studies has included MUS acid-modified cyclodextrins, as altered MUS acid can emulate HSPG to create a virucidal response [39].

The formulation of nanoparticles made from poly(ethylene glycol)–poly(lactide) with an inhibitor of Aurora B demonstrated increased efficacy and decreased toxicity as contrasted to their free form, which in phase II clinical trials developed intolerable side effects [40]. Lipid-based siRNA nanoparticles are just an illustration of a nanotechnology tool (Onpattro) to prevent systemic breakdown and benefit liver targeting. For example, encapsulation of the ML336 antiviral compound in lipid-coated mesoporous silica nanoparticles resulted in extended circulation time and demonstrated inhibition of Venezuelan equine encephalitis virus (VEE) *in vivo* [41]. In the screening of LNPs that can bypass the liver and provide functional mRNA to cells in vivo, Dahlman et al. [33] reported a high-performance approach (called FIND). This approach can be used widely to elucidate the relations between nanoparticles' arrangement, and mRNA in vivo delivery targets. Nanocarriers are used for the prevention of protein-based systemic immunotoxicity and facilitate immuno-oncology treatment [42].

One of the major research areas in the current pandemic is nanomaterial delivery into the nasal cavity. Because SARS-CoV-2 enters mucosal surfaces, causing infections of both the eye and thoracic mucosa, the primary strategy for treating such infectious conditions is mucosal therapy. The NP is absorbed efficiently and instantly, attributable to the cavity's ample capillary plexus and extensive surface area, which is not only straightforward and inexpensive but also noninvasive. To improve the process of nasal cavity delivery, the properties of the NPs, such as surface charge, dimensions, and shape, should also be considered. The process of administration to the lungs by delivering NPs to the nasal cavity has been tested using small animals. There is no easy way to generalize the outcomes of these animal experiments for humans. To date, three types of NPs have been engineered with transmission capability (organic, inorganic, and virus-like NP), which are tailored to medicinal uses and can also be delivered intranasally successfully.

12.2.5.1 Chemical Engineering of Drug Delivery Systems

Drug molecules are changed to comply with various groups or nanocarriers more common for drug candidates with identical physico-chemical properties. Wei et al. documented the use of modified cholesterol hydroxychloroquine (HCQ) loaded liposomes, which reduced HCQ doses and toxicity, thereby reducing pulmonary fibroblasts inhibiting the proliferation of the rat lung fibroblast. COVID-19 patients with pulmonary fibrosis and viral load may benefit from this strategy. A hydrolyzable ester conjugate has been synthesized as anticancer drug conjugates irinotecan (hydrophilic) and chlorambucil (hydrophobic) [42]. The nanomaterials, which are synthesized with self-assemblies, display sustained structural persistence, aggregation of cellular tissue, and improved cellular absorption of the amphiphilic drug conjugate.

12.2.5.2 Nanomedicine for Combination Drug Therapeutics

Combined pharmaceutical therapy is also a way to treat COVID-19 that provides many benefits, such as reduced doses for specific medications that decrease the number and strength of side effects, and meet multiple treatment goals. A few other combinations are documented in the WHO landscape details for novel coronavirus therapy. Inherently, nanocomposites are also quite helpful in supplying several medicines with various physicochemical properties that guarantee the true potential of hybrid strategies. Nanomaterials can also be evaluated and supplied in conjunction with drug formulations. Besides, it is understood that pneumonia-related hypoxia suppresses antiviral drug efficacy in patients with extreme COVID-19. Nanomaterials will be used soon to co-providing causes for angiogenesis (or other medications for hypoxia relief) and antivirals to produce improved results. Another exciting way is when antiviral nanomaterials are administered via aerosol delivery [43].

12.2.6 Nano-Based Vaccine Delivery

Antigens from microbe/virus, toxins, or surface proteins are generally used as vaccine components. Antigens trigger the body's immune system to produce antibodies, which in case of microbial, toxin, or cancer cell invasion recognize the invasion and kill the relevant target. Antigen proteins, generally combined with adjuvants, are administered directly to induce immune responses. Nanomaterials can also function as antigen carriers and, in some cases as adjuvants Nanomaterial-based vaccines can protect anti-antigens from premature degradation, and guarantee controlled delivery, improved antigen stability and controlled immunogen distribution, and increase the time of antigenic exposure to antigen-presenting cells (APCs) [44].

The full-length or specific regions of the SARS-CoV-2 S protein have been targeted for vaccine development. For example, the receptor-binding domain (RBD) and the N-terminal sequence encoding a CD5 signal sequence, enhanced humoral and cellular immune response. In phase I/II clinical trials, Novavax NVX-CoV2373, the full-length SARS-CoV-2 S protein in combination with the saponin-based Matrix-M adjuvant, showed a good safety profile and elicited superior immune responses compared to levels detected in convalescent COVID-19 patients (NCT04368988) [45]. Furthermore, the NVX-CoV2373 vaccine demonstrated an efficacy of 86% against the SARS-CoV-2 B.1.1.7 UK variant and 60% against the B.1.351 South African variant in phase II trials [46]. Nanoparticles act in a similar way to viruses and can be used for delivery of cargo to a particular target. The application of nanoparticles can enhance immune responses of vaccines due to cell membrane penetration and subcellular targeting. Various materials such as lipids, polymers, and polysaccharides may be used for the formulation of nanocarriers. For example, lipid nanoparticle encapsulation can protect DNA or RNA from enzymatic degradation leading to an improved immune response to nanomaterial-based vaccines.

Nanomaterials have played a key role in DNA and RNA vaccine delivery confirmed by the two approved COVID-19 RNA vaccines based on liposome nanoparticle encapsulated mRNA [47, 48]. Additionally, innovative nanomaterials such as Nuvec have been formulated by conjugation of silica-based nanomaterials and polyethyleneimine (PEI) [49]. The surface traps nuclear acids from nuclease enzymes on their way through cells and protects them efficiently. Once within the cell, nucleic acids are released, and the foreign/target protein is expressed, contributing to cellular and humoral immune responses and stimulation of the immune system [49].

Although SARS-CoV-2 resembles other viruses concerning structure and life cycle, there are very few examples of conventional or repurposed drugs showing efficacy for treating COVID-19 patients. However, the strong similarity between SARS-CoV-2 and other viruses such as SARS-CoV and MERS-CoV can support vaccine development against COVID-19. We foresee that application of nanomaterials for the encapsulation of antivirals, particularly liposomes and PLGA nanomaterials, can provide prolonged distribution, continuous release of antivirals, and multiple drugs to enhance the antiviral potency. Surface modifications with antibodies directed against SARS-CoV-2 proteins will improve the pharmaceutical application range of nanomaterials and reduce adverse effects of treatment.

Crucially, it has recently been reported that virus-like particles (VLPs) are ideal for developing MERS-CoV vaccines [50]. VLPs have the characteristic features of virus particles for superior delivery compared to other alternative approaches. VLPs are naturally occurring nanomaterials, which can be used to deliver various antigenic epitopes to enhance the safety and efficacy of antigen-presenting cells. In the context of VLP-based COVID-19 vaccines, the trivalent pan-coronavirus vaccine candidate VBI-2901 was engineered to express the S protein of SARS-CoV. MERS-CoV and SARS-CoV-2 [50]. Moreover, the monovalent SARS-CoV-2 has shown strong immunogenicity in hamsters and has entered phase I/II clinical trials [51].

12.3 CONCLUSION AND OUTLOOK

Recent developments in nanotechnology have shown that they can contribute quickly to the manufacture of vaccines and targeted therapeutics. Also, nano-based formulations are characterized by a low risk of antiviral resistance, a common, life-threatening problem found in many currently available traditional antiviral medications. CBNs such as fullerene, carbon dots, graphene, and derivatives have shown antiviral activity against many enveloped RNA viruses, including SARS-CoV-2. Further, they can induce tissue regeneration, possess immunostimulatory potential, and be used in combination with stem cells. Nano-based formulations can also be engineered to target a particular tissue with controlled release properties, enhancing therapeutic efficacy and reducing the dose/care time for virus management. In all these approaches, the multidrug therapy currently employed may be simplified. The confirmation of the safe application of nanomaterial is of utmost importance as most of the research has focused on only *in vitro* biocompatibility so far. Since the interaction of nanomaterials with physiological processes *in vivo* is complicated, both preclinical studies in animal models and clinical trials in humans are needed. As this chapter shows, improvements in diagnostics and prophylactic and therapeutic interventions have been achieved for other viral diseases due to nanotechnology. The fight against COVID-19 (and other future outbreaks) will receive much-needed support from nanotechnology and nanomaterials.

REFERENCES

1. Cucinotta, D., Vanelli, M. (2020). WHO declares COVID-19 a pandemic. *Acta Biomed.* 91 (1), 157.

2. Mogaji, E. (2020). Financial vulnerability during a pandemic: Insights for coronavirus disease (COVID-19). *Res. Agenda Work. Pap.* 2020 (5), 57–63.

3. Aljabali, A.A., Bakshi, H.A., Satija, S., Metha, M., Prasher, P., Ennab, R.M., Chellappan, D.K., Gupta, G., Negi, P., Goyal, R. et al. (2020). COVID-19: Underpinning RESEARCH FOR Detection therapeutics, and vaccines development. *Pharm. Nanotechnol.* 8 (4), 323–353.

4. Amawi, H., Abu Deiab, G.A.I., Aljabali, A.A.A., Dua, K., Tambuwala, M.M. (2020). COVID-19 Pandemic: An overview of epidemiology, pathogenesis, diagnostics and potential vaccines and therapeutics. *Ther. Deliv.* 11 (4), 245–268.

5. Aljabali, A.A., Al Zoubi, M.S., Al-Batayneh, K.M., Pardhi, D.M., Dua, K., Pal, K., Tambuwala, M.M. (2020). Innovative applications of plant viruses in drug targeting and molecular imaging: A review. *Curr. Med. Imaging* 17 (4), 491–506.

6. Serrano-Aroca, Á., Takayama, K., Tuñón-Molina, A., Seyran, M., Hassan, S.S., Pal Choudhury, P., Uversky, V.N., Lundstrom, K., Adadi, P., Palù, G., Aljabali, A.A.A., Chauhan, G., Kandimalla, R., Tambuwala, M.M., Lal, A., Abd El-Aziz, T.M., Sherchan, S., Barh, D., Redwan, E.M., Bazan, N.G., Mishra, Y.K., Uhal, B.D., Brufsky, A. (2021). Carbon-based nanomaterials: Promising antiviral agents to combat COVID-19 in the microbial-resistant era. *ACS Nano* 15 (5), 8069–8086.

7. Wu, J., Wang, H., Li, B. (2020). Structure-aided ACEI-capped remdesivir-loaded novel PLGA nanoparticles: Toward a computational simulation design for anti-SARS-CoV-2 therapy. *Phys. Chem. Chem. Phys.* 22 (48), 28434–28439.

8. Abo-Zeid, Y., Ismail, N.S.M., McLean, G.R., Hamdy, N.M. (2020). A molecular docking study repurposes FDA approved iron oxide nanoparticles to treat and control COVID-19 infection. *Eur. J. Pharm. Sci.* 153, 105465.

9. Neufurth, M., Wang, X., Tolba, E., Lieberwirth, I., Wang, S., Schröder, H.C., Müller, W.E.G. (2020). The inorganic polymer, polyphosphate, blocks binding of SARS-CoV-2 spike protein to ACE2 receptor at physiological concentrations. *Biochem. Pharmacol.* 182, 114215.

10. De Maio, F., Palmieri, V., Babini, G., Augello, A., Palucci, I., Perini, G., Salustri, A., De Spirito, M., Sanguinetti, M., Delogu, G. et al. (2020). Graphene nanoplatelet and graphene oxide functionalization of face mask materials inhibits infectivity of trapped SARS-CoV-2. *medRxiv* 2020.09.16.20194316, doi:https://doi.org/10.1101/2020.09.16.20194316.

11. Hasan, J., Pyke, A., Nair, N., Yarlagadda, T., Will, G., Spann, K., Yarlagadda, P.K. (2020). Antiviral nanostructured surfaces reduce the viability of SARS-CoV-2. *ACS Biomater. Sci.* 6 (9), 4858–4861.

12. Martí, M., Tuñón-Molina, A., Aachmann, F.L., Muramoto, Y., Noda, T., Takayama, K., Serrano-Aroca, Á. (2021). Protective face mask filter capable of inactivating SARS-CoV-2, and methicillin-resistant *Staphylococcus aureus* and *Staphylococcus epidermidis*. *Polymers* 13 (2), 207.

13. Gopalan, D., Pandey, A., Nayak, U.Y., Mutalik, S.J. (2020). Role of nanotechnology in the management of COVID-19. *COVID-19: A Multidimensional Response* Vol. 17, 256256.

14. Takano, H. (2020). Pulmonary surfactant itself must be a strong defender against SARS-CoV-2. *Med. Hypoth.* 144, 110020.

15. van der Meel, R., Sulheim, E., Shi, Y., Kiessling, F., Mulder, W.J., Lammers, T. (2019). Smart cancer nanomedicine. *Nat. Nanotechnol.* 14 (11), 1007–1017.

16. Gurunathan, S., Qasim, M., Choi, Y., Do, J.T., Park, C., Hong, K., Kim, J.-H., Song, H., Antiviral potential of nanoparticles: Can nanoparticles fight against coronaviruses? *Nanomaterials* 2020, 10 (9), 1645.

17. Henry, R. (1943). The mode of action of sulfonamides. *Bacteriol. Rev.* 7 (4), 175.

18. Seyran, M., Takayama, K., Uversky, V.N., Lundstrom, K., Palù, G., Sherchan, S.P., Attrish, D., Rezaei, N., Aljabali, A.A., Ghosh, S. (2021). The structural basis of accelerated host cell entry by SARS-CoV-2. *FEBS J.* 288 (17), 5010–5020.

19. Assis, M., Simoes, L.G.P., Tremiliosi, G.C., Coelho, D., Minozzi, D.T., Santos, R.I., Vilela, D.C., Santos, J.R.D., Ribeiro, L.K., Rosa, I.L.V.J.N. (2021). SiO$_2$-Ag composite as a highly virucidal material: A roadmap that rapidly eliminates SARS-CoV-2. *Nanomaterials* 11 (3), 638.

20. Donskyi, I.S., Nie, C., Ludwig, K., Trimpert, J., Ahmed, R., Quaas, E., Achazi, K., Radnik, J., Adeli, M., Haag, R.J. (2021). Graphene sheets with defined dual functionalities for the strong SARS-CoV-2 interactions. *Small* 17 (11) 2007091.

21. Zhao, J., Liu, L., Li, F., Fabrication and reduction. In *Graphene Oxide: Physics and Applications*, Heidelberg: Springer, 2015, pp. 1–13.

22. Innocenzi, P., Stagi, L.J. (2020). Carbon-based antiviral nanomaterials: Graphene, C-dots, and Fullerenes. A perspective. *Chem. Sci.* 11 (26), 6606–6622.

23. Salesa, B., Llorens-Gámez, M., Serrano-Aroca, Á. (2020). Study of 1D and 2D carbon nanomaterial in alginate films. *Nanomaterials* 10 (2), 206.

24. Serrano-Aroca, A., Deb, S.J. (2017). Synthesis of irregular graphene oxide tubes using green chemistry and their potential use as reinforcement materials for biomedical applications. *PLoS One* 12 (9), e0185235.

25. Salesa, B., Martí, M., Frígols, B., Serrano-Aroca, Á. (2019). Carbon nanofibers in pure form and in calcium alginate composites films: new cost-effective antibacterial biomaterials against the life-threatening multidrug-resistant Staphylococcus epidermidis. *Polymers* 11 (3), 453.

26. Nouri, A., Yaraki, M.T., Ghorbanpour, M., Agarwal, S., Gupta, V.K. (2018). Enhanced antibacterial effect of chitosan film using Montmorillonite/CuO nanocomposite. *Int. J. Biol. Macromol.* 109, 1219–1231.

27. Rivera-Briso, A.L., Aachmann, F.L., Moreno-Manzano, V., Serrano-Aroca, Á.J. (2020). Graphene oxide nanosheets versus carbon nanofibers: Enhancement of physical and biological properties of poly (3-Hydroxybutyrate-co-3-Hydroxyvalerate) films for biomedical applications. *Int. J. Biol. Macromol.* 143, 1000–1008.

28. Maiti, D., Tong, X., Mou, X., Yang, K.J. (2019). Carbon-based nanomaterials for biomedical applications: A recent study. *Front. Pharmacol.* 9, 1401.

29. Sahu, K.K., Siddiqui, A.D., Cerny, J.J. (2021). Mesenchymal stem cells in COVID-19: A journey from bench to bedside. *Lab. Med.* 52 (1), 24–35.

30. Shao, D., Lu, M., Xu, D., Zheng, X., Pan, Y., Song, Y., Xu, J., Li, M., Zhang, M., Li, J.J. (2017). Carbon dots for tracking and promoting the osteogenic differentiation of mesenchymal stem cells. *Biomater. Sci. 5* (9), 1820–1827.

31. Donskyi, I.S., Nie, C., Ludwig, K., Trimpert, J., Ahmed, R., Quaas, E., Achazi, K., Radnik, J., Adeli, M., Haag, R., Osterrieder, K., (2021). Graphene sheets with defined dual functionalities for the strong SARS-CoV-2 interactions. *Small* 17 (11), 2007091.

32. Łoczechin, A., Séron, K., Barras, A., Giovanelli, E., Belouzard, S., Chen, Y.-T., Metzler-Nolte, N., Boukherroub, R., Dubuisson, J., Szunerits, S.J. (2019). Functional carbon quantum dots as medical countermeasures to human coronavirus. *ACS Appl. Mater. Interf.* 11 (46), 42964–42974.

33. Dahlman, J.E., Kauffman, K.J., Langer, R., Anderson, D.G. (2014). Nanotechnology for in vivo targeted siRNA delivery. *Adv. Genet.* 88, 37–69.

34. Wu, C.-J., Huang, H.-W., Liu, C.-Y., Hong, C.-F., Chan, Y.-L. (2005). Inhibition of sars-cov replication by siRNA. *Antiviral Res.* 65 (1), 45–48.

35. Li, T., Zhang, Y., Fu, L., Yu, C., Li, X., Li, Y., Zhang, X., Rong, Z., Wang, Y., Ning, H.J. (2005). siRNA targeting the leader sequence of SARS-CoV inhibits virus replication. *Gene Ther.* 12 (9), 751–761.

36. Abbott, T.R., Dhamdhere, G., Liu, Y., Lin, X., Goudy, L., Zeng, L., Chemparathy, A., Chmura, S., Heaton, N.S., Debs, R.J. (2020). Development of CRISPR as an antiviral strategy to Combat SARS-CoV-2 and influenza. *Cell* 181 (4), 865–876. e12.

37. Nguyen, T.M., Zhang, Y., Pandolfi, P.P., Virus against virus: A potential treatment for 2019-nCov (SARS-CoV-2) and other RNA viruses. *Cell Res.* 2020. 30 (3), 189–190.

38. Tanaka, P., Santos, J., Oliveira, E., Miglioli, N., Assis, A., Monteleone-Cassiano, A., Ribeiro, V., Duarte, M., Machado, M., Mascarenhas, R. (2020). A CRISPR-Cas9 system designed to introduce point mutations into the human ACE2 gene to weaken the interaction of the ACE2 receptor with the SARS-CoV-2 S protein. *Preprints* doi:10.20944/preprints202005.0134.v1.

39. Tang, Z., Zhang, X., Shu, Y., Guo, M., Zhang, H., Tao, W.J. (2021). Insights from nanotechnology in COVID-19 treatment. *Nano Today* 36, 101019.

40. Ashton, S., Song, Y.H., Nolan, J., Cadogan, E., Murray, J., Odedra, R., Foster, J., Hall, P.A., Low, S., Taylor, P.J. (2016). Aurora Kinase Inhibitor nanoparticles target tumors with favorable therapeutic index in vivo. *Sci. Transl. Med.* 8 (325), 325ra17–325ra17.

41. LaBauve, A.E., Rinker, T.E., Noureddine, A., Serda, R.E., Howe, J.Y., Sherman, M.B., Rasley, A., Brinker, C.J., Sasaki, D.Y., Negrete, O.A.J., (2018). Lipid-coated mesoporous silica nanoparticles for the delivery of the ML336 antiviral to inhibit encephalitic alphavirus infection. *Sci. Rep.* 8 (1), 1–13.

42. Zhang, Y., Li, N., Suh, H., Irvine, D.J.J. (2018). Nanoparticle anchoring targets immune agonists to tumors enabling anti-cancer immunity without systemic toxicity. *Nat. Commun.* 9 (1), 1–15.

43. Hanley, B., Lucas, S.B., Youd, E., Swift, B., Osborn, M. (2020). Autopsy in suspected COVID-19 cases. *J. Clin. Pathol.* 73 (5), 239–242.

44. Kim, C.G., Kye, Y.-C., Yun, C.-H. (2019). The role of nanovaccine in cross-presentation of antigen-presenting cells for the activation of CD8+ T cell responses. *Pharmaceutics* 11 (11), 612.

45. Keech, C., Albert, G., Cho, I., Robertson, A., Reed, P., Neal, S., Plested, J.S., Zhu, M., Cloney-Clark, S., Zhou, H. (2020). Phase 1–2 trial of a SARS-CoV-2 recombinant spike protein nanoparticle vaccine. *N. Engl. J. Med.* 383 (24), 2320–2332.

46. Mahase, E. (2021). COVID-19: Novavax vaccine efficacy is 86% against UK variant and 60% against South African variant. *Br. Med. J.* 372, n296.

47. Sahin, U., Muik, A., Derhovanessian, E., Vogler, I., Kranz, L.M., Vormehr, M., Baum, A., Pascal, K., Quandt, J., Maurus, D. (2020). COVID-19 vaccine BNT162b1 elicits human antibody and TH 1 T cell responses. *Nature* 586 (7830), 594–599.

48. Jackson, L.A., Anderson, E.J., Rouphael, N.G., Roberts, P.C., Makhene, M., Coler, R.N., McCullough, M.P., Chappell, J.D., Denison, M.R., Stevens, L.J. (2020). An mRNA vaccine against SARS-CoV-2—preliminary report. *N. Engl. J. Med.* 83, 1920–1931.

49. Theobald, N. (2020). Emerging vaccine delivery systems for COVID-19: Functionalised silica nanoparticles offer a potentially safe and

effective alternative delivery system for DNA/RNA vaccines and may be useful in the hunt for a COVID-19 vaccine. *Drug Discov. Today.* 25, 1556–1558.

50. Wang, C., Zheng, X., Gai, W., Zhao, Y., Wang, H., Wang, H., Feng, N., Chi, H., Qiu, B., Li, N.

(2017). MERS-CoV virus-like particles produced in insect cells induce specific humoural and cellular imminity in rhesus macaques. *Oncotarget* 8 (8), 12686.

51. www.vbivaccines.com/wire/coronavirus-vaccineprogram-update/ (accessed on May 26, 2021).

Chapter 13 Vaccine Development Strategies and the Current Status of COVID-19 Vaccines

Mohsen Akbarian, Kenneth Lundstrom, Elrashdy M. Redwan, and Vladimir N. Uversky

13.1 INTRODUCTION

The global community found 2020 a very challenging year for health because of the COVID-19 pandemic. The SARS-CoV-2, first reported in late December 2019 in China, and then spreading worldwide, has become one of the most difficult human challenges in modern history. In addition to overshadowing global health, the virus has also had a significant impact on the world economy and caused geopolitical changes[1, 2]. Human coronaviruses, such as the severe acute respiratory syndrome coronavirus (SARS-CoV), and the Middle East respiratory syndrome coronavirus (MERS-CoV), are associated with severe respiratory failure that can cause death in the elderly and those with weakened immune systems [3]. Researchers have used the structural features and life cycle of the coronaviruses to find a variety of targets for vaccines. After exploring many available methods, vaccines remain the best choice to prevent and control the morbidity and mortality of endemic/pandemic emergent infectious diseases [4]. Since there is still much unknown about many aspects of the SARS-CoV-2 biology and pathology, and since new variants of the virus are identified on a regular basis (a crucial fact that adds to these ambiguities), extreme caution is needed when formulating a vaccine against this virus. We describe here some of the latest developments in combating SARS-CoV-2 infections. The classification of available vaccines will be discussed first, then strategies for the development of these biologics will be reviewed. Along with immune responses to vaccines, the efficacy of vaccines against novel SARS-CoV-2 variants are described. Finally, possible concerns about the use of these vaccines will be addressed.

13.2 VACCINE CATEGORIES AND ADJUVANTS

Vaccines designed to combat SARS-CoV-2 can be classified based on their function and the life cycle of the virus in infected human cells. SARS-CoV-2 vaccines are generally based on inactivated or attenuated viruses, protein subunits and peptides, viral vectors and nucleic acids [5, 6]. Nucleic acid–based vaccines, DNA and RNA vaccines, contain sequences that can encode the virus spike protein, which eventually induce immune responses. Adenovirus vector-based vaccines, because of the presence of viral proteins on their surface, can elicit immune responses, such as stimulation of toll-like receptors (TLR). Also, antigens, such as protein subunit vaccines, can provoke cell-dependent immune responses [7]. However, some vaccines are not able to produce adequate immune responses. Therefore, some adjuvants are used to enhance immune responses or the resulted responses to specific and desired pathways.

Adjuvants have commonly been applied for the increased stimulation of immune responses. There are generally three main types of adjuvants: aluminum-based, emulsions, and TLR agonists. Some other less commonly used adjuvants do not belong to these categories [8]. Affinity, magnitude, durability, and isotypes of antibodies are some of the criteria that should be considered when choosing an adjuvant for proper formulation of coronavirus vaccines [9]. Though numerous adjuvants have already been evaluated in preclinical studies of vaccine candidates, among all available adjuvants very few have been approved for human use, such as salt-based adjuvants (aluminum or calcium), and MF59. The excellent safety of these, and their ability to strengthen immune responses, have made them the most popular group of adjuvants [8]. For example, alum was used to formulate vaccines derived from the SARS-CoV spike (S) protein and its receptor-binding domain (RBD), which elicited increased humoral immune responses in animal models [10–12]. Enhanced high affinity viral neutralizing antibodies, higher titers of serum IgG_1, and the presence of long-lasting memory B and T cells were also demonstrated [10–12]. Moreover, it has been shown that using alum reduces the dose required for efficient vaccination. Aluminium hydroxide and aluminum hydroxide gels are used to formulate vaccines against the SARS-CoV-2 [8].

In addition to alum, emulsion adjuvants have also been successful in formulating vaccines. For example, AS03 and AS03 emulsion adjuvants are used to increase the immunogenicity of antigens in human vaccines. Compared to alum, AS03 and AS03 emulsion may result in more appropriate responses, probably by recruiting immune cells, improving antigen uptake, and promoting activation of antigen-presenting

DOI: 10.1201/9781003190394-13

cells (APCs) [13, 14]. In the case of CoV vaccines, emulsion adjuvants have been used at the pre-clinical level. For example, MF59 has been used in inactivated SARS and MERS vaccines and/or RBD vaccines for MERS-CoV. Emulsions such as MF59-like and alum stabilized Pickering emulsion (PAPE) have also been used to enhance the immune response of protein subunit vaccines against SARS-CoV-2 [8].

One more important player in innate immunity should be mentioned here, namely, the family of toll-like receptors (TLRs), which are essential for rapid activation of the immune system and efficient adaptive immunity. Therefore, agonists have been designed to activate TLRs. The poly I:C, CpG, resiquimod (R848), and glucopyranosyl lipid A (GLA) agonists for the TLR3, TLR9, TLR7/8, and TLR4, respectively, have been used for vaccine development against SARS-CoV [15, 16]. Recently, a combination of CpG and alum adjuvants in the formulation of SARS-CoV or MERS-CoV vaccines was shown to stimulate high production of neutralizing antibodies compared to alum alone, or even alum with other TLR agonists [12, 17]. However, because of a lack of detailed information on the mechanism of SARS-CoV-2 and its variants, the use of any adjuvants should be carefully evaluated.

Another interesting direction in the field of vaccine development is the use of nanomaterials as potential adjuvants and carriers. Many nanomaterials, such as liposomes, biopolymers, self-assembled proteins, quantum dots, and carbon-based nanomaterials have been designed for third generation vaccines. Vaccines based on nanomaterials have demonstrated efficacy against HIV and influenza virus, and many tropical diseases, such as malaria and toxoplasmosis, caused by parasites [18]. Lipid nanoparticle formulations have been developed for SARS-CoV-2 mRNA vaccines, as described below.

13.3 DEVELOPMENT STRATEGIES OF VACCINES AGAINST COVID-19

Today, development of an effective vaccine against the SARS-CoV-2 is a top global health priority, particularly because no efficient antiviral drugs are available, and vaccines are the only solution to stop the pandemic from spreading. There are different strategies for vaccine development depending on which stage of the viral life cycle is targeted. Ultimately, independent of the target, the vaccine should prevent viral infection (entry) or replication. It should also activate immune memory cells and increase immunity levels. Vaccines can be classified into three groups, where the first generation includes inactivated vaccines (based on killed or attenuated virus), the second generation includes protein subunit and viral vector-based vaccines, and the third generation encompasses nucleic acid vaccines [19]. Using vaccine development platforms, novel anti-SARS-CoV-2 vaccines have become a reality in less than a year, re-emphasizing that we are living in "the golden age of vaccinology".

When a vaccine enters the body, it triggers a series of immune reactions that are ultimately expected to increase the immunity [20]. However, depending on the type of vaccine used, the response may be different. This is illustrated in Figure 13.1 showing the stages of immune responses following vaccination. Related to immune reactions during vaccination, the intracellular pathway in myocytes varies depending on the type of vaccine applied. For example, for RNA-based vaccines, the mRNA of the viral antigen is translated in the cytoplasm and degraded into immunogenic peptides by the host cell proteasome [21]. In the case of DNA vaccines, the gene of interest has to enter the nucleus, where mRNA is transcribed and transported to the cytoplasm for translation of antigen [22]. Attenuated viruses replicate in infected cells, resulting in immune stimulation [23].

While the level and direction of natural or vaccine-induced immune responses in the body depend to some extent on racial and genetic diversity, a series of common immunological events can be classified. It is generally estimated that between 40% and 75% of people infected with the SARS-COV-2 have a mild syndrome or are even asymptomatic, with the development and severity of the infection correlating with time-dependent anti-S, anti-RBD IgG, and neutralizing antibody conversion kinetics [24]. Interestingly, people carry the virus in their bodies for a longer period than originally expected and serve as hidden carriers [25]. There is a consensus that protective immunity against virulent viruses should depend on both B- and T-cell-based immune responses, irrespectively of whether the immunity is built up during natural infection or post-vaccination. Various studies have shown that the immune responses to SARS-CoV, MERS-CoV, and SARS-CoV-2 are similar in several ways. As soon as symptoms appear in a patient one to two weeks post-infection, anti-CoV IgM and IgG will be detectable in the blood. Also, high levels of neutralizing antibodies have been observed, though no association between these and the IgM and IgG antibodies has been found. Fortunately, it has been shown that pre-existing antibodies produced by seasonal coronavirus infection are able to cross-neutralize the SARS-CoV-2, which depends on resting B- and T-cell memory [26]. In addition to

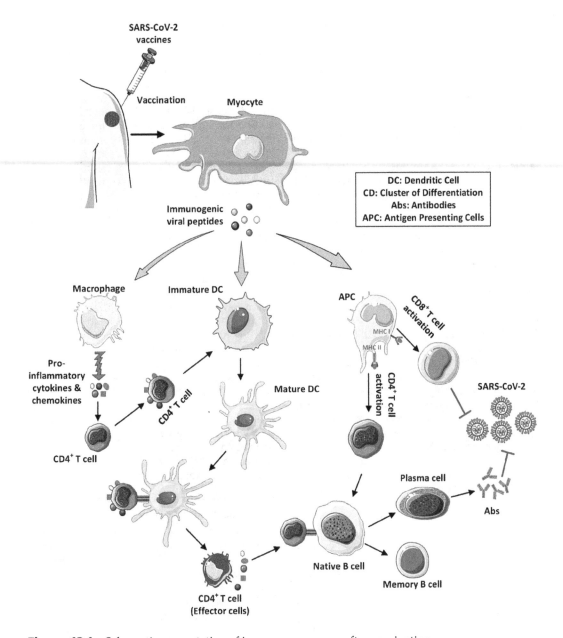

Figure 13.1 Schematic presentation of immune responses after vaccination.

the S protein and the RBD, high levels of neutralizing antibodies against the N protein have been shown to occur, though these antibodies are unlikely to be able to neutralize the virus. Since T cells are involved in many infections and play a key role in the production and secretion of cytokines, they are likely to be affected by the SARS-CoV-2. Recently, it has been observed that the number of T cells increases during SARS-CoV-2 infections.

Following vaccination, immunogenic agents (antigens) elicit innate immune responses at the injection site. Once viral antigens are produced, macrophage cells, dendritic cells, and APCs receive the antigens and trigger adequate responses. In macrophage cells, cytokines and chemokines are produced and secreted, which in turn, with the help of mature dendritic cells, eventually produce effective CD4+ T cells. On the other hand, APCs with two pathways, MHC I and II, respectively, lead to the activation of CD8+ and CD4+ T cells. Activation of the latter cells, native B cells develop into memory B cells and plasma cells. These events occur at four locations: the injection site, the lymph nodes, the blood, and finally the bone marrow.

Circulating follicular T helper cells, which play an important role in recalling antibodies against infection, have also been reported to develop during SARS-CoV-2 infection [4]. Regarding vaccination and subsequent immunity, most of the available vaccines need adjuvants to strengthen their responses. For example, an adjuvant such as alum can activate both systemic and mucosal immunity. Also, it has been observed that TLR agonists can activate APCs directly, and thus activate both humoral and cellular immunity [27].

While SARS-CoV-2 is considered a mucosal-borne virus (oral-nasal cavities), so far all approved vaccines against it have been delivered by intramuscular injection. However, both adenovirus- and influenza virus-based vaccine candidates, are under development for intranasal administration. As previously summarized [28], there are two main types of mucosal surfaces: (1) Stratified columnar epithelial surfaces (examples include lung, gut, and endocervix); and (2) Stratified squamous epithelial surfaces (found, for example, in the nose, eyes, vagina, and ectocervix). Both types of these epithelial layers use differential adaptive immune mechanisms for protection, which means that the vaccine must stimulate type-appropriate effector responses [28]. Notably, polymeric immunoglobulin receptors (pIgRs) are expressed on the former type of epithelial surfaces, and can transport dimeric IgA to the lumen, suggesting that they can neutralize incoming pathogens or toxins. On the contrary, however, the latter type of epithelial surface lacks pIgRs and relies on IgG for protection. In the upper respiratory tract, IgA protects the nasal cavity, whereas IgG protects the lower respiratory tract (lung). Both types of mucosal surfaces can host tissue-resident memory T cells. Mucosal immunity provides opportunities to block infection. Promising results were obtained in experimental animal models after immunization with the SARS-CoV vaccine candidates based on the RBD of SARS-CoV S protein, which elicited mucosal immunity, playing a central role in protection during virus challenge [29]. However, little or no information is currently available on the protective mucosal immunity stimulation by COVID-19 vaccines in humans.

The urgent need for the development of vaccines against SARS-CoV-2 has led to unprecedented cooperation between academia, industry, and governmental organizations. It has resulted in an accelerated strategy compared to traditional vaccine development (Figure 13.2) [30]. Normally, the traditional vaccine development process can take 10–15 years. The process usually starts with bioinformatics and computer modeling approaches for the identification and selection of suitable antigen candidates [31]. The vaccine candidates are then validated in vitro, and in preclinical animal models, followed by clinical phases I–III to evaluate safety, tolerability and immunogenicity of vaccine candidates, which explains the long time required from bench to bedside [32]. In the case of COVID-19 vaccine development, each step has been accelerated, particularly the clinical evaluation, where phase II trials were initiated while phase I trials were still in progress. Similarly, phase III trials commenced before phase II trials were finished. Most significantly, vaccine production started while the phase III trials were in progress and before vaccine approval had been received from the authorities.

The COVID-19 vaccine development process might have been seen to be too fast and risky, but all safety guidelines have been followed, and vaccines have been approved for emergency use authorization (EUA) without any compromises being made. The only gamble taken was the economic risk of manufacturing large quantities of vaccine before receiving EUA. The whole procedure, from basic research to the approval of several COVID-19 vaccines, took approximately one year, which is quite astonishing compared to the previous accelerated development of a vaccine against mumps virus, which took nearly five years to reach approval [33].

13.4 FIRST-GENERATION VACCINES

13.4.1 Inactivated Vaccine

Various methods of inactivation based on radiation (γ-radiation, X-ray, and UV) and chemicals (methanol, formalin, and β-propiolactone), have been used on viruses to preserve their antigenic properties while reducing or eliminating their infectivity. Inactivated vaccines have been used successfully to control the spread of viruses, such as polio, influenza, and hepatitis A. It should be emphasized here that these types of vaccines do not typically have problems, such as re-activation of a virus and/or mutation into new, more virulent variants [19]. However, unexpected or poor immune responses, the need for the administration of high and repeated vaccine doses, and in some cases, pulmonary inflammation have also been reported [34]. In addition to inactivated viral vaccines, attenuated viral vaccines have been developed. The advantages of these vaccines, which are relatively inexpensive, include long-lasting and strong immune responses. Furthermore, there is no need for adjuvant use. Nonetheless, they also show some

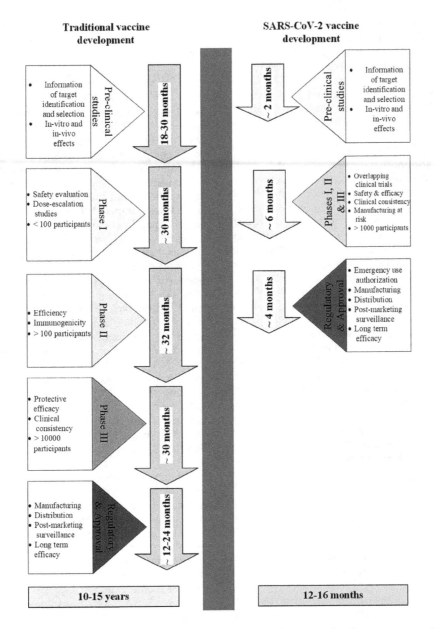

Figure 13.2 Comparison of the accelerated and traditional vaccine development strategies from the initial stage to the final use. The data were extracted from [30].

disadvantages, for example, potential reactivation of virus and reduced safety compared to inactivated viral vaccines.

13.5 SECOND-GENERATION VACCINES

13.5.1 Protein Subunit Vaccines

Protein subunit vaccines target viral or bacterial proteins as antigens. So far, these vaccines have been developed against hepatitis B, meningitis, and pneumonia viruses, as well as many bacterial pathogens, such as tetanus, diphtheria, pertussis (whooping cough), and meningitis caused by *Haemophilus influenzae* type b (Hib). In the case of SARS-CoV, different viral proteins, including nucleocapsid protein, the RBD of the S protein, and the full-length S protein have been used as antigens. These types of vaccines have attracted considerable attention because they can produce favourable immune responses without the presence of actual viral genetic material. However, since the virus components are no longer present in these vaccines, the responses are naturally accompanied by a significant delay, which has led to the use of these vaccines along with adjuvants [12, 35]. Protein subunit vaccines based on expression of the full-length or a truncated form of the SARS-COV-2 S protein in Drosophila S2 and *Spodoptera frugiperda* Sf9 insect cells has elicited neutralizing antibody responses in animal models [36].

13.5.2 Viral Vector–Based Vaccines

These vaccines have been developed, applying replication-deficient viral vectors for the expression of selected antigens. A number of adenovirus, lentivirus, rhabdovirus, measles virus, alphavirus, and poxvirus vectors have been used for vaccine development. Additionally, several types of replication-competent viral vectors, including vesicular stomatitis virus (VSV) against Ebola virus, and chimeric yellow fever virus/dengue virus (YFV/DENV) against DENV have been applied for vaccine development [37]. In the context of SARS-CoV-2 vaccines, adenoviruses [38, 39], modified vaccinia virus Ankara (MVA) [40], rhabdoviruses (vesicular stomatitis virus, VSV) [41], measles virus (MV) [42], Newcastle disease virus [43], and alphaviruses [44] have been used as delivery vectors. The strategy of prime-boost vaccination has generated robust long-lasting immune responses [45]. The chimpanzee adenovirus-based nCoV-19 vaccine has been subjected to several phase I–III clinical trials. Interim results from four randomized phase III trials showed good safety profiles, and 62% vaccine efficacy after two immunizations with 5×10^{10} ChAdOx1 nCoV-19 particles, and 90% efficacy after a prime dose of 2.2×10^{10} particles followed by boost with the standard dose [46]. The human Ad26-based vaccine candidate Ad26.COV2 S has been subjected to clinical trials showing good safety and strong immune responses in a phase I/II clinical trial [47]. The Ad26-based vaccine candidate needs only a single administration in contrast to other Ad-based vaccine candidates requiring a prime-boost regimen. In another approach, the efficacy of the prime-boost strategy has been enhanced by using an Ad26-based vector expressing the full-length SARS-CoV-2 S protein for the prime vaccination followed by a boost immunization with an Ad5-based vector [45]. In this approach, pre-existing immunity against adenoviruses affecting antigen expression and immunogenicity has been eliminated. Interim results from a phase III study with the rAd26-S/rAd5-S vaccine candidate Sputnik V showed 91.6% vaccine efficacy [45]. Recently, COVID-19 vaccine candidates based on adenovirus vectors have received EUA. The ChAdOx1 nCoV-19 vaccine and the Ad26.COV2.S have been approved for EUA in a number of countries, and the Russian Ad26/Ad5-based Sputnik V has received the authorization in Russia and some additional countries.

13.6 THIRD-GENERATION VACCINES

13.6.1 DNA-Based Vaccines

The first DNA-based vaccines were already developed in 1983. DNA vaccines are based on plasmid DNA expressing antigens for the vaccine targets in transfected host cells. DNA plasmids are relatively stable and can replicate independently in host cells. However, low transfection efficacy and the need for delivery to the nucleus has hampered their efficacy as vaccine vectors. To address these issues, electroporation, jet injection, gene gun, and nanoparticle technologies have been applied. Numerous types of nanoparticles, such as lipid and polymer nanoparticles, lipid-polymer hybrid nanoparticles, DNA-polymer complexes, nanoparticles coated with polymeric materials and gold, and protein-DNA complexed nanoparticles have been formulated for improved DNA delivery [48]. MERS-CoV S and N proteins have been expressed from DNA plasmid as vaccine antigens [49]. Effective and specific immunogenic responses, including the production of γ-interferon, IL-2, CD4+, CD8+, and IL-2, and the induction of cytotoxic T lymphocytes have been reported in animal studies. One of the most important advantages is that production of plasmid DNA in bacteria is rapid and inexpensive [50]. Other important advantages are the possibility of combining DNA-based vaccines with other vaccine platforms (such as first generation vaccines), excellent heat and shelf-life stability, ease of DNA sequence engineering and reduced safety risk compared to viral vectors [48]. However, limited immune responses caused by low transfection efficiency of DNA vaccines is a disadvantage [19].

In the context of DNA-based SARS-CoV-2 vaccines, a DNA vaccine candidate expressing the full-length SARS-CoV-2 S protein elicited neutralizing antibodies in immunized rhesus macaques [51]. Vaccinated monkeys developed both humoral and cellular immune responses, and were protected against challenges with SARS-CoV-2. In the context of clinical trials, a phase I with the full-length SARS-CoV-2 S DNA vaccine (INO-4800) study in 40 healthy volunteers demonstrated excellent safety and tolerability, and provided specific humoral and cellular immune responses in 100% of vaccinated subjects [52].

13.6.2 RNA-Based Vaccines

Vaccine candidates based on mRNA represent an attractive alternative, as mRNA molecules introduced into to the host cell cytoplasm can immediately start the translation of antigen, which will trigger immune responses. However, mRNA molecules are prone to degradation by host cell RNases because of their single-stranded structure. Modifications to the mRNA structure can improve stability. Moreover, encapsulation of mRNA in lipid nanoparticles (LNPs) provides further stability and improved delivery to host cells [49]. Two LNP-mRNA vaccine candidates expressing the full-length SARS-CoV-2 S protein from a stabilization-engineered mRNA have provided excellent vaccine efficacy in clinical trials. The Pfizer/BioNTech BNT162b2 vaccine candidate showed 95% efficacy in phase III trials [53]. Likewise, the Moderna mRNA-1273 vaccine candidate provided 94.1% protection in phase III trials [54]. Both mRNA vaccines have received EUAs and the BNT162b2 was approved on August 23, 2021 by the FDA. While the above-mentioned RNA-based vaccines have demonstrated good safety and efficacy, their formulation requires special storage and transportation conditions. For example, the BNT162b2 vaccine needs to be stored at −80°C, and the mRNA-1273 vaccine at −20°C, which generates extra demands for distribution and administration logistics.

Tables 13.1 and 13.2 summarize the efforts of the scientific community to develop vaccines against the SARS-CoV-2 showing a broad diversity of platforms used

13.7 COVID-19 VACCINES: CURRENT STATUS

As vaccines are most likely to present the best opportunity to conquer the pandemic, many academic institutions, pharmaceutical and biotech companies, and governmental organizations have cooperated for the development of safe vaccines. Any vaccine development requires the identification and selection of appropriate antigens, lab-scale production of antigens or engineering of antigen-expressing vectors, safety, immunogenicity and protection studies in animal models, and human clinical trials to determine vaccine safety and efficacy. Moreover, large-scale vaccine manufacturing and regulatory clearance are mandatory for vaccine approval. For all these steps, in particular the further the process advances, huge capital investment is needed. That is why the cooperation between academia, industry, and governmental organizations has been crucial for being able to develop COVID-19 vaccines at an unprecedented speed. One important factor relates to the route of vaccine administration, as it can affect the type of immune response [19]. So far, all COVID-19 vaccines, which have received EUAs are based on intramuscular administration, though studies applying intradermal, intranasal, intravenous, and subcutaneous injections are in progress. Several types of vaccines, including mRNA-based vaccines from Pfizer/BioNTech and Moderna, adenovirus-based vaccines from Oxford University/AstraZeneca, Janssen Pharmaceuticals, and Gamaleya Research Institute, and inactivated vaccines from Sinovac, Sinophram, and Covaxin have been approved for emergency use by national and/or international regulatory authorities (see Table 13.3). Moreover the BTN162b2 mRNA vaccine was approved by the FDA on August 23, 2021.

Despite the success so far, vaccine manufacture and distribution is still a global challenge. Regardless of the massive scale of vaccine production in several countries, the currently available quantities of doses are not sufficient for the vaccination of the whole global population. The limitation of vaccine availability is of concern to prevent the spread of new SARS-CoV-2 variants/mutations, and to provide a second dose for individuals already immunized with a prime dose. One question is whether the delay of the booster immunization will affect the efficiency of the prime immunization? Is there a time limitation on receiving the second dose? Can different vaccines be mixed and matched, as has been suggested for clinical trials on adenovirus- and RNA-based vaccines?

The standard immune response kinetics against vaccine (antigen) doses are already well-known (Figure 13.3). Of note, while the majority of the aforementioned COVID-19 vaccines are based on the e SARS-CoV-2 S protein, the sequences of the S proteins are different. Therefore, the expected immune responses

Table 13.1 SARS-CoV-2 vaccine candidates subjected to clinical trials as of April 2021

Platform	Vaccine Candidates	
	n	%
Protein subunit	28	33
Viral vector (non-replicating)	12	14
DNA	10	12
Inactivated virus	11	13
RNA	11	13
Viral vector (replicating)	4	5
Virus-like particles	4	5
Viral vector + APCs[a]	2	2
Live attenuated virus	2	2
Viral vector + APCs	1	1
Total	85	

[a] APCs, antigen-presenting cells.

Table 13.2 Characteristics of SARS-CoV-2 vaccine candidates

Vaccine Platform	Type of Vaccine Candidate	Number of Doses	Schedule	Route of Administration	Developer	Phase
Inactivated virus	CoronaVac SARS-CoV-2 vaccine (inactivated)	2	Day 0 + 14	IM	Sinovac Research and Development Co., Ltd	Phase IV
—	Inactivated SARS-CoV-2 vaccine (produced in Vero cells)	2	Day 0 + 21	IM	Sinopharm + China National Biotec Group Co + Wuhan Institute of Biological Products	Phase III
—	BBIBP-CorV Inactivated SARS-CoV-2 vaccine (produced in Vero cells)	2	Day 0 + 21	IM	Sinopharm + China National Biotec Group Co + Beijing Institute of Biological Products	Phase III
—	SARS-CoV-2 vaccine (produced in Vero cells)	2	Day 0 + 28	IM	Institute of Medical Biology + Chinese Academy of Medical Sciences	Phase III
—	QazCovid-in® - COVID-19 inactivated vaccine	2	Day 0 + 21	IM	Research Institute for Biological Safety Problems, Rep. of Kazakhstan	Phase III
—	Inactivated SARS-CoV-2 vaccine (produced in Vero cells)	1, 2 or 3	ND	IM	Beijing Minhai Biotechnology Co.	Phase II
—	ERUCOV-VAC Inactivated virus	2	Day 0 + 21	IM	Erciyes University	Phase II
—	COVID-19 Inactivated vaccine	2	Day 0 + 14	IM	Shifa Pharmed Industrial Co.	Phase II/III
—	FAKHRAVAC (MIVAC) Inactivated SARS-CoV-2 vaccine	2	Day 0 + 14 +/- 21	IM	Organization of Defensive Innovation and Research	Phase I
—	BBV152 Whole-Virion inactivated SARS-CoV-2 vaccine	2	Day 0 + 14	IM	Bharat Biotech International Limited	Phase III
—	VLA2001 Inactivated virus	2	Day 0 + 21	IM	Valneva, National Institute for Health Research, United Kingdom	Phase I/II
Viral vector (Non-replicating)	(Covishield) ChAdOx1-S – (AZD1222) Chimpanzee Adenovirus	1–2	Day 0 + 28	IM	AstraZeneca + University of Oxford	Phase IV

Platform	Name/Description	Doses	Schedule	Route	Developer	Phase
—	Ad5-nCoV Adenovirus type 5 vector Full-length S protein	1	Day 0	IM	CanSino Biological Inc./Beijing Institute of Biotechnology	Phase III
—	Gam-COVID-Vac Sputnik V Adenovirus-based (rAd26-S+rAd5-S)	2	Day 0 + 21	IM	Gamaleya Research Institute; Health Ministry of the Russian Federation	Phase III
—	Ad26.COV2.S Adenovirus 26 vector Full-length S protein	1–2	Day 0 or Day 0 + 56	IM	Janssen Pharmaceutical	Phase III
—	GRAd-COV2 Gorilla Adenovirus (GRAd) full-length S protein	1	Day 0	IM	ReiThera + Leukocare + Univercells	Phase II/III
—	VXA-CoV2-1 Ad5 adjuvanted oral vaccine platform	2	Day 0 + 28	Oral	Vaxart	Phase I
—	hAd5-S + N-ETSD Adenovirus type 5:S-Fusion + N-ETSD	1–2	Day 0 + 21	SC or Oral	ImmunityBio, Inc.	Phase I
—	AdCOVID, Adenovirus-based platform expressing the receptor-binding domain (RBD) of the S protein. E1, E2b and E3 - deleted Adenovirus	1–2	Day 0	IN	Altimmune, Inc.	Phase I
—	BBV154, Adenovirus vector COVID-19 vaccine	1	Day 0	IN	Bharat Biotech International Limited	Phase I
—	Chimpanzee Adenovirus serotype 68 (ChAd) and self-amplifying mRNA (SAM) vectors expressing S protein alone, or with additional SARS-CoV-2 T cell epitopes	2–3	Day 0 + 14 + 28 or Day 0 + 28 + 56 or Day 0 + 112	IM	Gritstone Oncology	Phase I
—	COH04S1 (MVA-SARS-2-S) - Modified vaccinia Ankara (sMVA) platform + synthetic SARS-CoV-2	1–2	Day 0 + 28	IM	City of Hope Medical Center + National Cancer Institute	Phase I
—	MVA-SARS-2-S Vaccinia virus Full-length S protein	2	Day 0 + 28	IM	University of Munich (Ludwig-Maximilians)	Phase I
Viral vector (Non-replicating) + APC	LV-SMENP-DC vaccine. Dendritic cells modified with lentivirus vectors expressing COVID-19 minigene SMENP and immune modulatory genes. CTLs are activated by LV-DC presenting COVID-19 specific antigens.	1	Day 0	SC & IV	Shenzhen Geno-Immune Medical Institute	Phase I/II

(Continued)

Table 13.2 (Continued) Characteristics of SARS-CoV-2 vaccine candidates

Vaccine Platform	Type of Vaccine Candidate	Number of Doses	Schedule	Route of Administration	Developer	Phase
Protein subunit	SARS-CoV-2 rS/Matrix M1-Adjuvant produced in insect cells) Full-length S protein nanoparticle vaccine	2	Day 0 + 21	IM	Novavax	Phase III
—	Recombinant SARS-CoV-2 vaccine (produced in CHO cells)	2–3	Day 0 + 28 or Day 0 + 28 + 56	IM	Anhui Zhifei Longcom Biopharmaceutical + Institute of Microbiology, Chinese Academy of Sciences	Phase III
—	KBP-COVID-19 RBD-based (produced tobacco plant cells)	2	Day 0 + 21	IM	Kentucky Bioprocessing Inc.	Phase I/II
—	VAT00002: SARS-CoV-2 S protein with adjuvant	2	Day 0 + 21	IM	Sanofi Pasteur + GSK	Phase III
—	SCB-2019 + AS03 or CpG 1018 adjuvant plus Alum adjuvant (Native like Trimeric subunit S Protein vaccine)	2	Day 0 + 21	IM	Clover Biopharmaceuticals Inc./GSK/Dynavax	Phase II/III
—	COVAX-19® Recombinant S protein + adjuvant	1	Day 0	IM	Vaxine Pty Ltd.	Phase I
—	SARS-CoV-2 S + MF59 adjuvant Molecular clamp-stabilized S protein	2	Day 0 + 28	IM	CSL Ltd. + Seqirus + University of Queensland	Phase II/III
—	MVC-COV1901 (S-2P protein + CpG 1018)	2	Day 0 + 28	IM	Medigen Vaccine Biologics + Dynavax + National Institute of Allergy and Infectious Diseases (NIAID)	Phase II
—	FINLAY-FR1 anti-SARS-CoV-2 Vaccine (RBD + adjuvant)	2	Day 0 + 28	IM	Instituto Finlay de Vacunas	Phase I/II
—	FINLAY-FR-2 anti-SARS-CoV-2 Vaccine (RBD chemically conjugated to tetanus toxoid plus adjuvant)	2	Day 0 + 28	IM	Instituto Finlay de Vacunas	Phase III
—	EpiVacCorona (EpiVacCorona vaccine based on peptide antigens	2	Day 0 + 21	IM	Federal Budgetary Research Institution State Research Center of Virology and Biotechnology "Vector"	Phase III
—	SARS-CoV-2 RBD (baculovirus production in Sf9 cells)	2	Day 0 + 28	IM	West China Hospital + Sichuan University	Phase II

Vaccine	No.	Schedule	Route	Developer	Phase
IMP CoVac-1 (SARS-CoV-2 HLA-DR peptides)	1	Day 0	SC	University Hospital Tuebingen	Phase I
UB-612 (Multitope peptide based S1-RBD-protein based vaccine)	2	Day 0 + 28	IM	COVAXX + United Biomedical Inc.	Phase II/III
AdimrSC-2f (recombinant RBD +/− aluminum)	ND	ND	ND	Ad immune Corporation	Phase I
CIGB-669 (RBD+AgnHB)	3	Day 0 + 14 + 28 or Day 0 +28 + 56	IN	Center for Genetic Engineering and Biotechnology (CIGB)	Phase I/II
CIGB-66 (RBD + aluminum hydroxide)	3	Day 0 + 14 + 28 or Day 0 +28 + 56	IM	Center for Genetic Engineering and Biotechnology (CIGB)	Phase III
BECOV2	2	Day 0 + 28	IM	Biological E. Limited	Phase I/II
Recombinant SARS-CoV-2 spike protein, aluminum adjuvanted	2	Day 0 + 21	IM	Nanogen Pharmaceutical Biotechnology	Phase I/II
Recombinant protein vaccine S-268019 (using baculovirus expression vector system)	2	Day 0 + 21	IM	Shionogi	Phase I/II
SARS-CoV-2-RBD-Fc fusion protein			SC or IM	University Medical Center Groningen + Akston Biosciences Inc.	Phase I/II
COVAC-1 and COVAC-2 sub-unit vaccine (spike protein) + SWE adjuvant	2	Day 0 + 28	IM	University of Saskatchewan	Phase I/II
GBP510, a recombinant surface protein vaccine with adjuvant AS03 (aluminum hydroxide)	2	Day 0 + 28	IM	SK Bioscience Co., Ltd. and CEPI	Phase I/II
Razi Cov Pars, recombinant spike protein	3	Day 0 + 21 +51	IM and IN	Razi Vaccine and Serum Research Institute	Phase I
SARS-CoV-2 S + MF59 adjuvant molecular clamp-stabilized S protein	2	Day 0 + 28	IM	The University of Queensland	Phase I
SK SARS-CoV-2 recombinant surface antigen protein subunit (NBP2001) + adjuvanted with alum	2	Day 0 + 28	IM	SK Bioscience Co., Ltd.	Phase I
SpFN (S ferritin nanoparticles) S protein with a liposomal formulation QS21 (ALFQ) adjuvant	2–3	Day 0 + 28 + 180	IM	Walter Reed Army Institute of Research (WRAIR)	Phase I
EuCorVac-19 S protein+ adjuvant	2	Day 0 + 21	IM	POP Biotechnologies and EuBiologics Co., Ltd	Phase I/II
ReCOV: Recombinant two-component S and RBD proteins (produced in CHO cells)	2	Day 0 + 21	IM	Jiangsu Rec-Biotechnology	Phase I

(Continued)

Table 13.2 (Continued) Characteristics of SARS-CoV-2 vaccine candidates

Vaccine Platform	Type of Vaccine Candidate	Number of Doses	Schedule	Route of Administration	Developer	Phase
RNA based vaccine	mRNA-1273 LNP-encapsulated full-length prefusion-stabilized S protein	2	Day 0 + 28	IM	Moderna + National Institute of Allergy and Infectious Diseases (NIAID)	Phase IV
—	Comirnaty BNT162b1 and b2 (LNP-encapsulated full-length S and RBD mRNAs)	2	Day 0 + 21	IM	Pfizer/BioNTech + Fosun Pharma	Phase IV
—	ChulaCov19 mRNA vaccine	2	Day 0 + 21	IM	Chulalongkorn University	Phase I
—	CVnCoV Vaccine	2	Day 0 + 28	IM	CureVac AG	Phase III
—	MRT5500, an mRNA vaccine candidate	2	Day 0 + 21	IM	Sanofi Pasteur and Translate Bio	Phase I/II
—	mRNA-1273.351. LNP-encapsulated full-length, prefusion stabilized S targeting the SARS-CoV-2 B.1.351 variant	3	Day 0 or Day 0 + 28 or Day 56	IM	Moderna + National Institute of Allergy and Infectious Diseases (NIAID)	Phase I
—	CoV2 SAM (LNP) self-amplifying mRNA (SAM) LNP platform + Spike antigen		Day 0 + 28	IM	GlaxoSmithKline	Phase I
—	PTX-COVID19-B, mRNA vaccine	2	Day 0 + 28	IM	Providence Therapeutics	Phase I
—	LNP-nCoVsaRNA	2	ND	IM	Imperial College London	Phase I
—	ARCoV Thermostable LNP.encapsulated SARS-CoV-2 S mRNA	2	Day 0 + 14 or Day 0 + 28	IM	Academy of Military Science (AMS), Walvax Biotechnology and Suzhou Abogen Biosciences	Phase II
—	ARCT-021 (single shot mRNA vaccine) The LUNAR-COV19 (ARCT-021) vaccines is comprised of a lipid-mediated delivery system called Lipid-enabled and Unlocked Nucleomonomer Agent modified RNA (LUNAR)	ND	ND	IM	Arcturus Therapeutics	Phase II

Category	Name / Description	Doses	Schedule	Route	Developer	Phase
DNA-based vaccine	INO-4800+electroporation The INO-4800 vaccine is a double-stranded DNA plasmid that encodes antigens found in SARS-CoV-2. It is delivered intradermally into the arm of patients using proprietary CELLECTRA technology, which uses a small pulse of electricity (called electroporation) to form small pores in the patient's cells which allows for easier uptake of the nucleic acid vaccine.	2	Day 0 + 28	ID	Inovio Pharmaceuticals + International Vaccine Institute + Advaccine (Suzhou) Biopharmaceutical Co., Ltd	Phase II/III
	AG0301-COVID19 AG0302-COVID19 is a DNA vaccine encoding antigens from SARS-CoV-2. It entered phase II/III clinical trials in Japan on December 7, 2020.	2	Day 0 + 14	IM	AnGes + Takara Bio + Osaka University	Phase II/III
	nCov vaccine The vaccine is being developed on a DNA platform using a non-replicating and non-integrating plasmid	3	Day 0 + 28 + 56	ID	Zydus Cadila	Phase III
	GX-19 GX-19 is a DNA vaccine expressing the SARS-CoV-2 S-protein antigen. On vaccination, host cells will take up the DNA and express the protein, which will then have an immune response made against it	2	Day 0 + 28	IM	Genexine Consortium	Phase I/II
	Covigenix VAX-001 - DNA vaccines + proteo-lipid vehicle (PLV) formulation	2	Day 0 + 14	IM	Entos Pharmaceuticals Inc.	Phase I
	CORVax - Spike S Protein Plasmid DNA Vaccine	2	Day 0 + 14	ID	Providence Health & Services	Phase I
	COVIGEN COVIGEN is a needle-free SARS-CoV-2 Recombinant DNA vaccine	2	Day 0 + 28	ID or IM	University of Sydney, Bionet Co., LtdTechnovalia	Phase I
	COVID-eVax, a candidate plasmid DNA vaccine of the S protein	2		IM	Takis + Rottapharm Biotech	Phase I/II

(Continued)

Table 13.2 (Continued) Characteristics of SARS-CoV-2 vaccine candidates

Vaccine Platform	Type of Vaccine Candidate	Number of Doses	Schedule	Route of Administration	Developer	Phase
–	bacTRL-Spike oral DNA vaccine. bacTRL-Spike-1 is an oral vaccine containing the live bacterium Bifidobacterium longum, which has been engineered to deliver plasmids containing synthetic DNA encoding spike protein from SARS-CoV-2 directly to human cells	1	Day 0	Oral	Symvivo Corporation	Phase I
–	GLS-5310 GLS-5310 is a DNA vaccine encoding the spike protein and a second antigenic target of SARS-CoV-2	2	Day 0 + 56 or Day 0 + 84	ID	GeneOne Life Science, Inc.	Phase I/II
Virus like particles	Coronavirus-like particle COVID-19 (CoVLP)	2	Day 0 + 21	IM	Medicago Inc.	Phase II/III
	SARS-CoV-2 VLP Vaccine. Virus-like particle vaccine adjuvanted with alum and CpGODN-K3	2	Day 0	SC	The Scientific and Technological Research Council of Turkey	Phase I
–	VBI-2902a Enveloped virus-like particle (eVLP) of SARS-CoV-2 spike S protein + aluminum phosphate adjuvant	2	Day 0 + 28	IM	VBI Vaccines Inc.	Phase I/II
–	RBD SARS-CoV-2 HBsAg VLP vaccine	2	Day 0 + 28	IM	Serum Institute of India + Accelagen Pty + SpyBiotech	Phase I/II
Viral vector (Replicating)	rVSV-SARS-CoV-2-S Vaccine A replication-competent rVSV expressing SARS-CoV-2 S by replacing the open-reading frame of the native VSV entry glycoprotein gene, G, with that of the SARS-CoV-2 S (Wuhan-Hu-1 isolate)	1	Day 0	IM	Israel Institute for Biological Research	Phase I/II
–	V591-001 – Measles-vector based (TMV-o38) SARS-CoV-2 Vaccine candidate uses a measles virus vector platform to deliver the antigens to the immune system to spur antibody production against the SARS-CoV-2 virus	1–2	Day 0 + 28	IM	Merck & Co. + Themis + Sharp & Dohme + Institute Pasteur + University of Pittsburgh	Phase I/II Study stopped

—	DelNS1-2019-nCoV-RBD-OPT1 (Intranasal flu-based-RBD)	1	Day 0	IN	University of Hong Kong, Xiamen University and Beijing Wantai Biological Pharmacy	Phase II
—	NDV-HXP-S, Newcastle disease virus (NDV) vector expressing the S protein of SARS–CoV-2, with or without the adjuvant CpG 1018	2	Day 0 + 28	IM	Mahidol University: The Government Pharmaceutical Organization (GPO); Icahn School of Medicine at Mount Sinai	Phase I/II
—	AdCLD-CoV19 (adenovirus vector). A replication-defective human adenovirus type 5/35 vector-based vaccine expressing the SARS–CoV-2 S protein	1	Day 0	IM	Cellid Co., Ltd.	Phase I/II
Viral vector (Replicating) + APC	Dendritic cell vaccine AV-COVID-19. A vaccine consisting of autologous dendritic cells loaded with antigens from SARS–CoV-2, with or without GM-CSF	1	Day 0	IM	Aivita Biomedical, Inc. National Institute of Health Research and Development, Ministry of Health, Republic of Indonesia	Phase I/II
—	COVID-19/aAPC vaccine. Lentivirus modification with immune modulatory genes and viral minigenes to artificial antigen presenting cells (aAPCs)	3	Day 0 + 14 + 28	SC	Shenzhen Geno-Immune Medical Institute	Phase I
Live attenuated virus	COVI-VAC A vaccine developed with Codagenix's Synthetic Attenuated Virus Engineering (SAVE) platform, which uses synthetic biology to re-code the genes of viruses into safe and stable vaccines	1–2	Day 0 or Day 0 + 28	IN	Codagenix/Serum Institute of India	Phase I
—	MV-014-212, a live attenuated vaccine that expresses the spike (S) protein of SARS–CoV-2	3	Day 0 +/– 35	IN	Meissa Vaccines, Inc.	Phase I

Abbreviations: IM: intramuscular; SC: subcutaneous; ID: intradermal; IN: intranasal; IV: intravenous.
Source: Data from DRAFT Landscape of COVID-19 Candidate Vaccines – April 15, 2021.

Table 13.3 List of the most advanced coronavirus vaccine candidates

Vaccines	Nature of the Vaccine	Common Side Effects	Efficacy (%)	Approval Status	Route of Administration	Doses (Each Vial)
Pfizer/BioNTech, (Germany/ United States)	LNP formulation-based mRNA vaccine that encodes full length S protein	♦	95	EUA by the FDA Approved by the FDA	Intramuscular	5
Pfizer/ BioNTech, Pfizer (Germany/ United States)	LNP formulation-based mRNA vaccine that encodes the S protein RBD	♦	95	Phase I/II	Intramuscular	5
Moderna (United States)		•	94.5	EUA by the FDA	Intramuscular	10
University of Oxford, AstraZeneca (United Kingdom)	Non-replicating simian adeno-virusvector encoding the S protein	♦	79	EUA by the by FDA	Intramuscular	10
CanSino biologics, AD5-nCOV (China)	Adenovirus type 5 vector expressing the S protein	♦	66	Phase III	Nasal spray	10
Inovio Pharmaceuticals, INO-4800 (United States)	DNA plasmid encoding the S protein	N/A	N/A	Phase III	Intramuscular	N/A
CoronaVac (China)	Inactivated virus	♦	50	Phase III	Intramuscular	600SU of inactivated SARS-CoV-2 virus
Sinopharm (China)	Inactivated virus	N/A	79	EUA by several countries	Intramuscular	6.5
Anhui Zhifei (China)	RBD-Dimer + adjuvant	N/A				
Novavax (United States)	Protein subunit (S protein including a saponin-based adjuvant)	♦	89	Phase III	Intramuscular	10
Zydus Cadila (India)	Plasmid DNA vaccine encoding the S protein	N/A	N/A	Phase III trial	Intramuscular	N/A
Sputnik V (Russia)	Adenovirus 26 and 5 serotype-based vector expressing the S protein	♦	91.6	EUA by several countries	Intramuscular	5
Covaxin (India)	Inactivated virus	•	80.6	Phase III trial	Intramuscular	10
Ad26.COV2.S (United States)	Adenonvirus 26 serotype-based vector expressing the S protein	♦	72	EUA by the FDA	Intramuscular	5

Abbreviations: ♦ pain, fatigue and headache. • pain, fatigue and chills. EUA, emergency use authorization, N/A = no answer, the company did not report; LNP, lipid nanoparticles; RBD: receptor-binding site; S: spike protein.
Source: Table adapted from (5, 6).

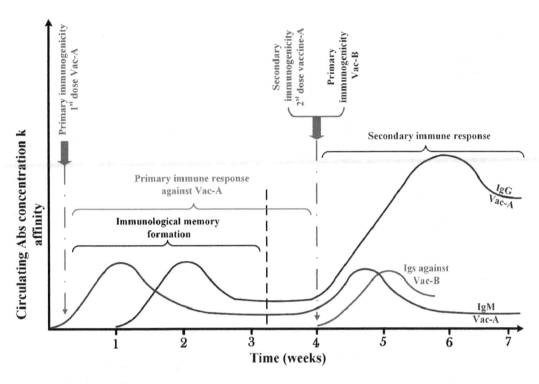

Figure 13.3   Profiles of immune responses elicited against single or combined COVID-19 vaccines.

would be variable between different vaccines, which complicates the use of two different COVID-19 vaccines for the immunization of the same patient. The vaccine mix and match approach will be evaluated in a human clinical trial with 800 participants. The first vaccination will be carried out with the adenovirus vector-based vaccine from the University of Oxford/ AstraZeneca, and 4–12 weeks later a second vaccination will take place with the Pfizer/BioNTech mRNA vaccine, or vice versa. Preliminary results of this combined vaccination indicated that potent immune responses were triggered and the strategy showed clear benefits [55].

Both B and T lymphocytes are involved in immune responses after primary and secondary immunizations. Kinetics of the IgM and IgG production show low affinity after the primary immunization, but after the second and/or every boosting dose with the same vaccine, the avidity of both increase exponentially. It remains to be seen whether vaccine combinations will increase pre-immunized immunity or initiate a new immune response profile.

13.8   COVID-19 VACCINES AND EMERGENCE OF NEW SARS-CoV-2 VARIANTS

In early April 2020, massive sequencing of the SARS-CoV-2 genome from hundreds of thousands of patients began in the UK. Analysis of these data identified a new SARS-CoV-2 variant VUI 202012/01 (B.1.1.7.), which carries 17 genetic changes [50]. Recent studies have shown that this new variant, while more transmissible, does not have a higher mortality rate than the original SARS-CoV-2, and can be neutralized by existing vaccines [56, 57]. Other variants have since been detected in South Africa and Brazil [58]. While the Pfizer/BioNTech (BNT162b2), Moderna (mRNA-1273), and the University of Oxford/AstraZeneca (ChAdOx1 n-Cov19) vaccines have demonstrated efficacy against the UK variant [51], a recent study indicated that the ChAdOx1 n-CoV19 vaccine did not provide protection against mild-to-moderate COVID-19 caused by the South African variant B.1.351 [59]. Therefore, because of the high mutation rate in coronaviruses there is a risk that new variants will spread and hamper the function and efficacy of present vaccines [60]. It is essential to quickly identify new variants and dedicate resources to develop vaccines that would efficiently target new mutations.

13.9   THE CREDIBILITY OF CONCERNS ABOUT COVID-19 VACCINES

The demand for mass vaccination to combat the COVID-19 pandemic has presented a number of challenges. The exceptionally rapid vaccine development has raised concerns about the vaccine's safety and efficacy, particularly among the general population [61]. This has led to vaccination hesitancy, which needs to be addressed repeatedly by the proper vaccine education at all levels of society [62]. Moreover, the initial clinical vaccine trials were conducted on healthy volunteers, typically 18–55 years of age. Only more recently have studies been expanded to include children and the elderly. Additionally, patients with pre-existing health conditions have not yet been evaluated. While serious adverse events related to vaccinations have been limited, recent cases of thrombosis and thrombocytopenia, though at extremely low rates, have been detected after vaccination with adenovirus- [62] and mRNA-based [63] vaccines. This has certainly been of concern and has paused vaccinations in certain countries. Among many exceptional benefits of vaccination with the currently available vaccines are (1) Reduction and/or limitation of the viral spreading; (2) Control of the disease development and minimization of moderate and severe consequences of infection; (3) Decrease in the pressure on medical care personnel and hospitals; and (4) Reduced mortality.

13.10 CONCLUSIONS

The rapid spread of SARS-CoV-2 was a wake-up call to make us aware of the limitations of human knowledge and technology progress. In this modern age, we can imagine that we are invincible. However, the reality is very different, leading to global medical, economic, and social hardships. Despite all, however, humanity is finding its way back, with much gratitude to the available knowledge and technological platforms for developing vaccines and therapeutics to fight the COVID-19 pandemic. A number of vaccine candidates against COVID-19 have been developed and a few of them have received EUA. The BNT162b mRNA was recently approved by the FDA. Mass vaccination is in progress in many countries. However, some challenges remain, such as vaccine availability related to issues with manufacturing and distribution, especially the prioritization of developed countries at the cost of developing nations. The vaccine efficacy, particularly in the context of novel variants, and the duration of protection are other issues of concern. Furthermore, vaccine-related adverse events need to be monitored closely, especially in the light of recent findings of post-vaccination cases of thrombosis and thrombocytopenia. In any case, lessons have been learnt from the COVID-19 pandemic. Changes in human behavior related to hygiene, travel, eating habits, and the relationship between humans and animals during the pandemic, will influence how our "new normal" will look. We need to be better prepared for novel SARS-CoV-2 variants and other emerging viruses, which may be less harmful or pathogenic to animals than to humans. In preparation we also need to establish the scientific readiness and financial resources by fruitful cooperation between academia, industry, and government organizations to guarantee that rapid action can be taken against emerging viral outbreaks. As many predict, it is not *if*, but *when* it will happen, and if we have learnt anything from COVID-19, now is the time to make sure we are well prepared!

REFERENCES

1. Setti, L., Passarini, F., De Gennaro, G. et al. (2020). Searching for SARS-COV-2 on particulate matter: A possible early indicator of COVID-19 epidemic recurrence. *Int. J. Environ. Res. Public Health* 17, 2986.

2. Padhan, R., Prabheesh, K. (2021). The economics of COVID-19 pandemic: A survey. *Econ. Anal. Policy* 70, 220–237.

3. Damas, J., Hughes, G.M., Keough, K.C. et al. (2020). Broad host range of SARS-CoV-2 predicted by comparative and structural analysis of ACE2 in vertebrates. *Proc. Natl. Acad. Sci. U.S.A.* 117(36), 22311–22322.

4. Tregoning, J.S., Brown, E.S., Cheeseman, H.M. et al. (2020). Vaccines for COVID-19. *Clin. Exp. Immunol.* 202(2), 162–192.

5. Chung, Y.H., Beiss, V., Fiering, S.N. et al. (2020). COVID-19 vaccine frontrunners and their nanotechnology design. *ACS Nano.* 14, 12522–12537.

6. Chauhan, G., Madou, M.J., Kalra, S. et al. (2020). Nanotechnology for COVID-19: Therapeutics and vaccine research. *ACS Nano.* 14(7), 7760–7782.

7. Saif, L.J. (2020). Vaccines for COVID-19: Perspectives, prospects, and challenges based on candidate SARS, MERS, and animal coronavirus vaccines. *Eur. Med. J.* doi:10.33590/emj/200324.

8. Liang, Z., Zhu, H., Wang, X. et al. (2020). Adjuvants for coronavirus vaccines. *Front. Immunol.* 11, 2896.

9. Iwasaki, A. and Yang, Y. (2020). The potential danger of suboptimal antibody responses in COVID-19. *Nat. Rev. Immunol.* 20(6), 339–341.

10. Spruth, M., Kistner, O., Savidis-Dacho, H. et al. (2006). A double-inactivated whole virus candidate SARS coronavirus vaccine stimulates neutralising and protective antibody responses. *Vaccine* 24(5), 652–661.

11. Coleman, C.M., Liu, Y.V., Mu, H. et al. (2014). Purified coronavirus spike protein nanoparticles induce coronavirus neutralizing antibodies in mice. *Vaccine* 32(26), 3169–3174.

12. Zakhartchouk, A.N., Sharon, C., Satkunarajah, M. et al. (2007). Immunogenicity of a receptor-binding

domain of SARS coronavirus spike protein in mice: Implications for a subunit vaccine. *Vaccine* 25(1), 136–143.

13. Shi, S., Zhu, H., Xia, X. et al. (2019). Vaccine adjuvants: Understanding the structure and mechanism of adjuvanticity. *Vaccine* 37(24), 3167–3178.

14. O'Hagan, D., Ottc, G.S., De Gregorio, E. et al. (2012). The mechanism of action of MF59: An innately attractive adjuvant formulation. *Vaccine* 30(29), 4341–4348.

15. Gai, W., Zou, W., Lei, L. et al. (2008). Effects of different immunization protocols and adjuvant on antibody responses to inactivated SARS-CoV vaccine. *Viral Immunol.* 21(1), 27–37.

16. Zhao, K., Wang, H., and Wu, C. (2011). The immune responses of HLA-A* 0201 restricted SARS-CoV S peptide-specific CD8+ T cells are augmented in varying degrees by CpG ODN, PolyI: C and R848. *Vaccine* 29(38), 6670–6678.

17. Lan, J., Deng, Y., Chen, H. et al. (2014).Tailoring subunit vaccine immunity with adjuvant combinations and delivery routes using the Middle East respiratory coronavirus (MERS-CoV) receptor-binding domain as an antigen. *PLoS One* 9(11), e112602.

18. Heinrich, M.A., Martina, B., and Prakash, J. (2020). Nanomedicine strategies to target coronavirus. *Nano Today* 100961.

19. Badgujar, K.C., Badgujar, V.C., and Badgujar, S.B. (2020). Vaccine development against coronavirus (2003 to present): An overview, recent advances, current scenario, opportunities and challenges. *Diab. Metab. Synd. Clin. Res. Rev.* 14(5), 1361–1376.

20. Basu, A., Sarkar, A., and Maulik, U. (2020). Strategies for vaccine design for corona virus using Immunoinformatics techniques. *bioRxiv*. doi:10.1101/2020.02.27.967422.

21. Zhang, C., Maruggi, G., Shan, H. et al. (2019). Advances in mRNA vaccines for infectious diseases. *Front. Immunol.* 10, 594.

22. Hobernik, D., Bros, M. (2018). DNA vaccines – How far from clinical use? *Int. J. Mol. Sci.* 19(11), 3605.

23. Mok, D.Z., Chan, K.R. (2020). The effects of pre-existing antibodies on live-attenuated viral vaccines. *Viruses* 12(5), 520.

24. Lucas, C., Klein, J., Sundaram, M. et al. (2020). Kinetics of antibody responses dictate COVID-19 outcome. *medRxiv*. doi:10.1101/2020.12.18.20248331.

25. Chau, N.V.V., Lam, V.T., Dung, N.T. et al. (2020). The natural history and transmission potential of asymptomatic SARS-CoV-2 infection. *Clin. Infect. Dis.* 71(10), 2679–2687.

26. Jeyanathan, M., Afkhami, S., Smaill, F. et al. (2020). Immunological considerations for COVID-19 vaccine strategies. *Nat. Rev. Immunol.* 20(10), 615–632.

27. Haque, A. and Pant, A.B. (2020). Efforts at COVID-19 vaccine development: Challenges and successes. *Vaccines* 8(4), 739.

28. Iwasaki, A., Omer, S.B. (2020). Why and how vaccines work. *Cell* 183(2), 290–295.

29. Du, L., He, Y., Zhou, Y. et al. (2009). The spike protein of SARS-CoV: A target for vaccine and therapeutic development. *Nat. Rev. Microbiol.* 7(3), 226–236.

30. von Linstow, M.-L., Winther, T.N., Eltvedt, A. et al. (2020). Self-reported immunity and opinions on vaccination of hospital personnel among paediatric healthcare workers in Denmark. *Vaccine* 38(42), 6570–6577.

31. Pagliusi, S., Jarrettb, S., Hayman, B. et al. (2020). Emerging manufacturers engagements in the COVID-19 vaccine research, development and supply. *Vaccine* 38(34), 5418–5423.

32. Hwang, A., Veira, C., Malvolti, S. et al. (2020). Global vaccine action plan lessons learned II: Stakeholder perspectives. *Vaccine* 38(33), 5372–5378.

33. Kashte, S., Gulbake, A., El-Amin Iii, S.F. et al. (2021). COVID-19 vaccines: Rapid development, implications, challenges and future prospects. *Human Cell* 34(3), 1–23.

34. Zhang, C.-H., Lu, J.-H., Wang, Y.-F. et al. (2005). Immune responses in Balb/c mice induced by a candidate SARS-CoV inactivated vaccine prepared from F69 strain. *Vaccine* 23(24), 3196–3201.

35. Deng, M.-P., Hu, Z.-H., Wang, H.-L. et al. (2012). Developments of subunit and VLP vaccines against influenza A virus. *Virol. Sin.* 27(3), 145–153.

36. Lundstrom, K. (2020). The current status of COVID-19 vaccines. *Front. Genome Edit.* 2(10), 579297.

37. Lundstrom, K. (2020). Application of viral vectors for vaccine development with a special emphasis on COVID-19. *Viruses* 12(11), 1324.

38. Wu, S., Zhong, G., Zhang, J. et al. (2020).A single dose of an adenovirus-vectored vaccine provides protection against SARS-CoV-2 challenge. *Nat. Commun.* 11(1), 1–7.

39. Feng, L., Wang, Q., Shan, C. et al. (2020). An adenovirus-vectored COVID-19 vaccine confers protection from SARS-COV-2 challenge in rhesus macaques. *Nat. Commun.* 11(1), 1–11.

40. Koch, T., Dahlke, C., Fathi, A. et al. (2020). Safety and immunogenicity of a modified vaccinia virus Ankara vector vaccine candidate for Middle East respiratory syndrome: An open-label, phase 1 trial. *Lancet Infect. Dis.* 20(7), 827–838.

41. Kurup, D., Wirblich, C., Ramage, H. et al. (2020). Rabies virus-based COVID-19 vaccine CORAVAX™ induces high levels of neutralizing antibodies against SARS-CoV-2. *NPJ Vac.* 5(1), 1–9.

42. Franklin, R., Young, A., Neumann, B. et al. (2020). Homologous protein domains in SARS-CoV-2 and measles, mumps and rubella viruses: Preliminary evidence that MMR vaccine might

provide protection against COVID-19. *medRxiv.* doi:10.1101/2020.04.10.2005320.

43. Shirvani, E. and Samal, S.K. (2020). Newcastle disease virus as a vaccine vector for SARS-CoV-2. *Pathogens* 9(8), 619.

44. Erasmus, J.H., Khandhar, A.P., O'Connor, M.A. et al. (2020). An alphavirus-derived replicon RNA vaccine induces SARS-CoV-2 neutralizing antibody and T cell responses in mice and nonhuman primates. *Sci. Transl. Med.* 12(555), eabc9396.

45. Logunov, D.Y., Dolzhikova, I.V., Zubkova, O.V. et al. (2020). Safety and immunogenicity of an rAd26 and rAd5 vector-based heterologous prime-boost COVID-19 vaccine in two formulations: Two open, non-randomised phase 1/2 studies from Russia. *Lancet* 396(10255), 887–897.

46. Voysey, M., Clemens, S.A.C., Madhi, S.A. et al. (2021). Safety and efficacy of the ChAdOx1 nCoV-19 vaccine (AZD1222) against SARS-CoV-2: An interim analysis of four randomised controlled trials in Brazil, South Africa, and the UK. *Lancet* 397(10269), 99–111.

47. Sadoff, J., Le Gars, M., Shukarev, G. et al. (2021). Interim results of a phase 1–2a trial of Ad26.COV2.S COVID-19 vaccine. *N. Engl. J. Med.* 384, 1824–1835.

48. Lim, M., Md Badruddoza, A.Z., Firdous, J. et al. (2020). Engineered nanodelivery systems to improve DNA vaccine technologies. *Pharmaceutics* 12(1), 30.

49. Chi, H., Zheng, X., Wang, X. et al. (2017). DNA vaccine encoding Middle East respiratory syndrome coronavirus S1 protein induces protective immune responses in mice. *Vaccine* 35(16), 2069–2075.

50. Vogel, F.R. and Sarver, N. (1995). Nucleic acid vaccines. *Clin. Microbiol. Rev.* 8(3), 406–410.

51. Yu, J., Tostanoski, L.H., Peter, L. et al. (2020). DNA vaccine protection against SARS-CoV-2 in rhesus macaques. *Science* 369(6505), 806–811.

52. Tebas, P., Yang, S.P., Boyer, J.D. et al. (2021). Safety and immunogenicity of INO-4800 DNA vaccine against SARS-CoV-2: A preliminary report of an open-label, Phase 1 clinical trial. *EClinicalMedicine* 31, 100689.

53. Polack, F.P., Thomas, S.J., Kitchin, N. et al. (2020). Safety and efficacy of the BNT162b2 mRNA COVID-19 vaccine. *N. Engl. J. Med.* 383(27), 2603–2615.

54. Baden, L.R., El Sahly, H.M., Essink, B. et al. (2020). Efficacy and safety of the mRNA-1273 SARS-CoV-2 vaccine. *N. Engl. J. Med.* 384(5), 403–416.

55. Callaway, E. (2021). Mixing COVID vaccines triggers potent immune response. *Nature* 593(7860), 491.

56. Mahase, E., (2020). What have we learnt from the new variant in the UK? *BMJ* 371, m4944.

57. Davies, N.G., Barnard, R.C., Jarvis, C.I. et al. (2021). Estimated transmissibility and severity of novel SARS-CoV-2 variant of concern 202012/01 in England. *medRxiv.* doi:10.1101/2020.12.24.20248822.

58. Sanches, P.R.S., Charlie-Silva, I., Braz, H.L.B. et al. (2021). Recent advances in SARS-CoV-2 Spike protein and RBD mutations comparison between new variants Alpha (B.1.1.7, United Kingdom), Beta (B.1.351, South Africa), Gamma (P.1, Brazil) and Delta (B.1.617.2, India). *J. Virus Erad.* 7(3), 100054.

59. Madhi, S.A., Baillie, V., Cutland, C.L. et al. (2021). Efficacy of the ChAdOx1 nCoV-19 COVID-19 vaccine against the B.1.351 variant. *N. Engl. J. Med.* 384, 1885–1898.

60. Rahimi, F., Abadi, A.T.B. (2021). Implications of the emergence of a new variant of SARS-CoV-2, VUI-202012/01. *Arch. Med. Res.* 384, 2124–2130.

61. Redwan, E.M. (2021). COVID-19 pandemic and vaccination build herd immunity. *Eur. Rev. Med. Pharm. Sci.* 25 (2), 577–579.

62. Schultz, N.H., Sørvoll, I.H., Michelsen, A.E. et al. (2021). Thrombosis and Thrombocytopenia after ChAdOx1 nCoV-19 vaccination. *N. Engl. J. Med.*

63. Lee, E.-J., Cines, D.B., Gernsheimer, T. et al. (2021). Thrombocytopenia following Pfizer and Moderna SARS-CoV-2 vaccination. *Am. J. Hematol.* 95, 534–537.

Chapter 14 Clinical Trials of COVID-19 Therapeutics and Vaccines

History, Current Status, and Limitations

Candan Hizel Perry, Havva Ö. Kılgöz, and Şükrü Tüzmen

14.1 INTRODUCTION

14.1.1 Novel Coronavirus (SARS-CoV-2): What We Know So Far

Over the past decade, three Coronaviruses from the Beta (β)-coronavirus genus have been discovered: Severe acute respiratory syndrome coronavirus (SARS-CoV) caused the SARS outbreak in 2002 [1], and the Middle East respiratory syndrome coronavirus (MERS-CoV) was identified in the 2012 MERS outbreak [2]. In 2019, following a cluster of pneumonia cases in Wuhan City, China, the novel zoonotic ("spill over" from animals to people) SARS-CoV-2 was identified as the causative agent of COVID-19 [3, 4]. Having 79.5% nucleotide identity with SARS-CoV, SARS-CoV-2 caused global health concern along with an unprecedented challenge to identify effective drugs and vaccines for prevention and treatment [5, 6]. SARS-CoV-2 is a highly contagious single-stranded RNA (ssRNA) virus, with almost 30,000 bases encoding four viral structural proteins including spike (S), envelope (E), membrane (M), and nucleocapsid (N) proteins, 16 non-structural proteins (NSP1-16), and various accessory proteins (ORF3a, ORF6, ORF7a, ORF7b, ORF 8 and ORF10) [7]. It has been revealed that primary transmission of SARS-CoV-2 is through person-to-person respiratory droplets/close contact and fomite transmission [8–10].

Since December 2019, the identification and rapid spread of the SARS-CoV-2 virus in China has turned into a global threat that was eventually declared pandemic by the World Health Organization (WHO) on March 11, 2020 [8]. As of April 20, 2021, the WHO confirmed that COVID-19 cases exceeded 141 million, including more than 3 million deaths globally [11].

Recently, evolving variants of SARS-CoV-2 identified in the United Kingdom, South Africa, Brazil, Japan, and India have become a growing concern worldwide for their higher transmission rates and ability to cause severe infection leading to more hospitalizations and deaths [12–14]. Accordingly, because of the escalating death toll and the devastating impact of the coronavirus on healthcare systems, considerable global research efforts from the pharmaceutical industry and academia have focused on the development of potential effective therapy options, such as vaccines and the repurposing of drug molecules already approved for the treatment of other diseases [4].

In this chapter, we aim to present a summary of authorized clinical trials on vaccine development and repurposed drugs against COVID-19. In this context, the approval of COVID-19 drugs and vaccines is also discussed. Additionally, we give a brief overview of the immunopathology and pathophysiology of COVID-19, which are crucial for understanding the rational of the potential clinical and therapeutic treatment modalities employed to combat the ongoing SARS-CoV-2 public health crises.

14.1.2 Immunopathology/Pathophysiology Underlying COVID-19 and Drug Targets

While SARS-CoV-2 infected individuals have been reported as experiencing symptoms including fever, shortness of breath, muscle pain, sore throat and cough in the first two weeks after exposure, some remain asymptomatic. General clinical features in moderate-to-severe and critical COVID-19 patients are usually characterized by viral pneumonia, which makes the disease pathology more challenging [15, 16]. To date, the majority of infections are reported to be mild or asymptomatic, while approximately 20% are severe infections requiring hospitalization with an estimated 2%–5% mortality [8].

Patients with severe COVID-19 infection have been shown to be characterized by irregular immune response because of compromised immune systems, which worsens disease outcomes, such as pulmonary disease with a variety of severity and pathology profiles [8, 17].

The innate immune system, known as the first line of defense, is stimulated on the recognition of pathogen-associated molecular patterns (PAMPs) induced by SARS-CoV-2 during the infection, which recruits dendritic cells (DCs), macrophages, and neutrophils with several inflammatory cytokines. While multiple immune response pathways are activated during the infection, a complete suppression of viral replication or total clearance of infection is reported in 80% of SARS-CoV-2 patients [8, 16, 18]. The overproduction of cytokines and chemokines is known as cytokine release syndrome (cytokine storm). This was considered to be the

DOI: 10.1201/9781003190394-14

main cause of tissue damage and the acute respiratory distress syndrome (ARDS) resulting from the infiltration of inflammatory cells into the lungs, causing further immunopathology [8, 17–19].

14.2 CLINICAL TRIALS IN THE COVID-19 ERA

The COVID-19 pandemic and rising death toll have sparked a surge in clinical research aimed at developing vaccines, new antibodies, and drugs to treat and prevent SARS-CoV-2 infections. Various forms of COVID-19 vaccines, including mRNA, adenovirus vector-based vaccines, and inactivated vaccines, have been approved for emergency use in various countries as a result of these clinical studies.

In this section we have summarized the therapeutic agents and vaccines currently being tested and approved for emergency use at unprecedented speed in the context of the global clinical trial landscape for COVID-19 [4, 20].

14.2.1 Immunization Strategies to Combat COVID-19 Pandemic at the Crossroads

Since the global spread of COVID-19, a number of vaccines against the SARS-CoV-2 have been evaluated in preclinical and clinical trials around the world. During the preparation of this manuscript, the WHO announced a list of 88 candidate vaccines in clinical phase

evaluation [11, 21], some of which have been approved for emergency use [4] (Figure 14.1). Selected clinical trials of SARS-CoV-2 vaccines are listed in Table 14.1. In addition, preclinical and clinical evidence from previous outbreaks of other coronaviruses, such as SARS-CoV (2003) and MERS-CoV (2012), have aided in the design of SARS-CoV-2 vaccines [16]. Until recently, the COVID-19 vaccines developed by Pfizer/ BioNTech, Moderna, and Janssen have been authorized for emergency use in the United States (USA) by the FDA while, the vaccines from Pfizer-BioNTech, Moderna, and the University of Oxford/AstraZeneca have been approved in the European Union (EU) by the European Medicines Agency (EMA) [14, 22, 23]. Moreover, the vaccine from Sinovac has been authorized in 22 countries to date, including China, Brazil, and Turkey [24]. Remarkably, as of April 18, 2021, more than 793 million vaccine doses have been administered globally [11]. In this section we have provided an overview of the major vaccine platforms and classification as potential effective tools against COVID-19 outbreak.

14.2.1.1 DNA Vaccines

Despite numerous DNA vaccine-based immunotherapeutic strategies against several diseases being under preclinical and clinical development, though approved in veterinary medicine, none have yet been approved for human use [8, 10, 5].

(A) (B)

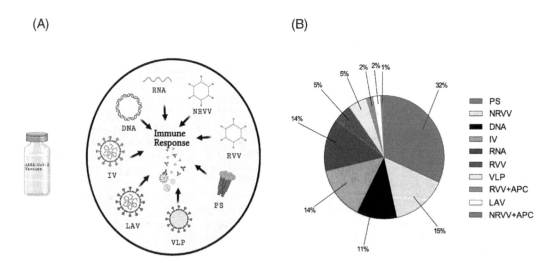

Figure 14.1 (A) The main vaccine development strategies for COVID-19; (B) The percentages of candidate vaccine platforms in clinical development. *Abbreviations:* PS: Protein subunit vaccines; NRVV: Non-replicating viral vector vaccines; IV: Inactivated virus vaccines; RVV: Replicating viral vector vaccines; VLP: Virus-like particle vaccines; APC: Antigen presenting cell; RNA: RNA-based vaccines; DNA: DNA-based vaccines; LAV: Live attenuated virus vaccines.

Source: Created with Biorender.com.

Table 14.1 Selected clinical trials of SARS-CoV-2 vaccines

Platform	Name/Description	Administration Route/Dose	Developer	Clinical Evaluation Stage/Registration #	FDA Licensed Example for Human Use
RNA	mRNA-1273	IM 2 doses (Day 0 + 28)	Moderna Inc./NIAID	Phase 3 NCT04470427	N/A
	BNT162 (3 LNP-mRNAs)	IM 2 doses (Day 0 + 21)	Pfizer/BioNTech/Fosun Pharma	Phase 3 NCT04368728 NCT04713553	
	CVnCOV vaccine	IM 2 doses (Day 0 + 28)	CureVac AG	Phase 3 NCT04674189	
DNA	INO-4800+EP	ID 2 doses (Day 0 + 28)	Inovio Pharmaceutical + International Vaccine Institute + Advaccine (Suzhou) Biopharmaceutical	Phase 2/3 NCT04642638	N/A
	AG0301-COVID19	IM 2 doses (Day 0 + 14)	AnGes + Takara Bio + Osaka University	Phase 2/3 NCT04655625	
	nCov vaccine	ID 3 doses (Day 0 + 28 + 56)	Zydus Cadila	Phase 3 CTRI/2020/07/026352	
PS	NVX-CoV2373 (Full length recombinant SARS-CoV-2 glycoprotein nanoparticle vaccine adjuvanted with Matrix M)	IM 2 doses (Day 0 + 21)	Novavax	Phase 3 NCT04611802 EUCTR2020-004123-16-GB NCT04583995	Shingrix™
	Recombinant SARS-CoV-2 vaccine (CHO Cell)	IM 2–3 doses (Day 0 + 28 or Day 0 + 28 + 56)	Anhui Zhifei Longcom Biopharmaceutical + Institute of Microbiology, Chinese Academy of Sciences	Phase 3 NCT04646590	
	SCB-2019 + AS03 or CpG 1018 adjuvant plus Alum adjuvant	IM 2 doses (Day 0 + 21)	Clover Biopharmaceuticals Inc./GSK/Dynavax	Phase 2/3 NCT04672395	

(Continued)

Table 14.1 (Continued) Selected clinical trials of SARS-CoV-2 vaccines

Platform	Name/Description	Administration Route/Dose	Developer	Clinical Evaluation Stage/Registration #	FDA Licensed Example for Human Use
IV	SARS-CoV-2 vaccine (CoronaVac)	IM 2 doses (Day 0 + 14)	Sinovac Research and Development Co. Ltd	Phase 3 NCT04456595 NCT04508075 NCT04582344 NCT04617483 NCT04651790	Influenza virus vaccine
	Inactivated SARS-CoV-2 vaccine (Vero cell)	IM 2 doses (Day 0 + 21)	Sinopharm + China National Biotec Group Co + Wuhan Institute of Biological Products	Phase 3 ChiCTR2000034780 ChiCTR2000039000 NCT04510207 NCT04612972	
	ChAdOx1-S - (AZD1222)	IM 1 or 2 dose(s) (Day 0 + 28)	AstraZeneca + University of Oxford	Phase 3 NCT04516746 NCT04536051 EUCTR2020-005226-28-DE	
NRVV	Recombinant novel corona-virus vaccine (Adenovirus type 5 –Ad5– vectored)	IM 1 dose (Day 0)	CanSino Biological Inc./ Beijing Institute of Biotechnology	Phase 3 NCT04526990 NCT04540419	Smallpox and Monkeypox vaccine
	Gam-COVID-Vac (Sputnik V) (rAd26-S+rAd5-S)	IM 2 doses (Day 0 + 21)	Gamaleya Research Institute; Health Ministry of the Russian Federation	Phase 3 NCT04530396 NCT04564716 NCT04642339 NCT04656613	
	Ad26.COV2.S	IM 1 or 2 dose(s) (Day 0 or Day 0 +56)	Janssen Pharmaceutical	Phase 3 NCT04505722 NCT04614948	
NRVV + APC	DelNS1-2019-nCoV-RBD-OPT1	IN 1 dose (Day 0)	University of Hong Kong, Xiamen University and Beijing Wantai Biological Pharmacy	Phase 2 ChiCTR2000039715	N/A

	Vaccine	Route/Dose	Phase / Trial No.	Developer	Comparator
RVV	rVSV-SARS-CoV-2-S vaccine	IM 1 dose (Day 0)	Phase 1/2 NCT04608305	Israel Institute for Biological Research	ERVEBO
	AdCLD-CoV19 (adenovirus vector)	IM 1 dose (Day 0)	Phase 1/2 NCT04666012	Cellid Co., Ltd.	
	NDV-HXP-S, NDV vector expressing the spike protein of SARS-CoV-2, with or without the adjuvant CpG 1018	IM 2 doses (Day 0 + 28)	Phase 1/2 NCT04764422	Mahidol University, The Government Pharmaceutical Organization, Icahn School of Medicine	
RVV + APC	AV-COVID-19. A vaccine consisting of autologous dendritic cells loaded with antigens from SARS-CoV-2, with or without GM-CSF	IM 1 dose (Day 0)	Phase 1/2 NCT04386252	Aivita Biomedical, Inc.	N/A
	COVI-VAC	IN 1–2 dose(s) (Day 0 or Day 0 + 28)	Phase 1 NCT04619628	Codagenix/Serum Institute of India	
LAV	RBD SARS-CoV-2 HBsAg VLP vaccine	IM 2 doses (Day 0 + 28)	Phase 1/2 ACTRN1262000817943 ACTRN1262000130898987	Serum Institute of India/ Accelagen Pty/SpyBiotech	M-M-R II
VLP	Coronavirus-Like Particle COVID-19 (CoVLP)	IM 2 doses (Day 0 + 21)	Phase 2/3 NCT04662697 NCT04636697	Medicago Inc.	GARDASIL
	VBI-2902a. An enveloped VLP of SARS-CoV-2 S glycoprotein and aluminum phosphate adjuvant.	IM 2 doses (Day 0 + 21)	Phase 1/2 NCT04773665	VBI Vaccines Inc.	

Abbreviations: ID: Intradermal; IM: Intramuscular; IN: Intranasal; PS: Protein subunit; IV: Inactivated virus; NRVV: Non-replicating viral vector; RVV: Replicating viral vector; LAV: Live attenuated virus; VLP: Virus like particle; APC: Antigen presenting cell; DC: Dendritic cell; RBD: Recombinant SARS-CoV-2 S1 subunit protein; EP: Electroporation; ERVEBO: Ebola Zaire Vaccine; M-M-R II: Measles, Mumps, and Rubella Virus Vaccine Live; GARDASIL: Human Papillomavirus Quadrivalent (Types 6, 11, 16, and 18) Vaccine; Shingrix™: Zoster Vaccine Adjuvanted; N/A: Not available.

The DNA-based vaccine platform was introduced in the 1990s/2000s, and several preclinical studies have shown its potential for treating various viral infections [17, 25]. In DNA-based vaccine strategies, the antigen of interest is introduced into plasmid DNA administered to host cells for antigen expression and eventually secretion from cells [26]. Antigens are then processed and presented by immune cells to elicit humoral and cell-mediated immune responses specific to the expressed antigen [8, 17, 19, 27].

Currently, there are 10 DNA-based SARS-CoV-2 candidate vaccines in clinical development [21]. In a Phase I clinical trial, the INO-4800 DNA plasmid-based vaccine candidate targeting the SARS-CoV-2 full length spike (S) glycoprotein, has shown good safety, tolerance, and immunogenicity in all of the 38 vaccinated subjects. All participants were reported to generate anti-spike humoral and cellular immune responses following the second dose of the vaccine, with no serious side effects [28]. Currently, an INO-4800 plasmid-based vaccine candidate is being evaluated in Phase II/III trials.

Even though there are several advantages of the DNA-based vaccine platform, including good biocompatibility of plasmid DNA, and inexpensive and rapid mass production with a long shelf life, challenges remain to be addressed [8]. These may include the poor immunogenicity compared to RNA and conventional vaccines, the need for specialized delivery techniques such as electroporation (EP), and the necessity of molecular adjuvants for increased efficacy and enhanced immune response [8, 25]. One drawback compared to RNA vaccines is that DNA needs to be delivered to the nucleus, which reduces its efficacy.

14.2.1.2 RNA Vaccines

RNA-based candidate vaccines have been subjected to preclinical and clinical evaluation aiming to provide prolonged immunity against various pathogens, including influenza, and Zika viruses [29]. However, until recently none of the RNA-based vaccines have found any applications in humans prior to SARS-CoV-2 RNA vaccine trials [26, 27]. In the case of COVID-19, there are 12 RNA-based SARS-CoV-2 candidate vaccines in use in clinical evaluation [21].

The RNA-based strategy might be deployed on either self-amplifying RNA (saRNA) derived from alphaviruses or conventional messenger RNA (mRNA) [27]. These RNA molecules are transfected into host cells, where immediate translation of the protein of interest takes place in the cytoplasm [25, 27].

The mRNA-1273 vaccine, encoding the full-length SARS-CoV-2 S protein encapsulated in lipid nanoparticles (LNPs) [22], was developed by Moderna. It has shown 94.1% efficacy at preventing COVID-19 after two intra-muscular (IM) injections 28 days apart in Phase III clinical evaluation. No safety issues have been reported except for minor transient reactogenicity. Furthermore, the BNT162b2 mRNA vaccine developed by Pfizer/BioNTech has been evaluated in Phase III trials. BNT162b2 is an LNP-encapsulated mRNA vaccine encoding the nucleoside-modified full-length S protein of SARS-CoV-2. In placebo-controlled clinical trials, the test subjects received prime and booster IM injections of the vaccine 21 days apart. The interim results from Phase II/III have shown good tolerability of the BNT162b2 vaccine candidate with 95% efficacy in people 16 years of age and older [30].

On December 11, 2020, the FDA issued the first emergency use authorization (EUA) for the BNT162b2 mRNA vaccine developed by Pfizer/BioNTech in individuals 16 years of age and older. A week later, on December 18, the FDA granted an EUA for the mRNA-1273 vaccine manufactured by Moderna, for individuals 18 years of age and older.

14.2.1.3 Viral Vector Vaccines

In the context of viral vector vaccine strategies, the gene of interest is incorporated into the genome of a recombinant or modified viral vector to express specific antigens as a delivery platform [8]. The gene coding for an antigen can be controlled by a specific promoter integrated into the vector and elicit both T cell and high-titer antibody responses as it mimics the natural infection even without the need of an adjuvant [8, 25]. Because of their distinct features, different types of viral vectors have been used for antigen-specific immunization strategies. Nevertheless, some viral vectors can induce low immunogenicity through pre-existing immunity [17, 25, 27]. Viral vaccine vectors can be further classified as two main groups, depending on their ability of replication in host cells: replicating viral vectors (RVV) and non-replicating viral vectors (NRVV) [19]. NRVVs are still capable of infecting/transducing host cells, promoting the expression of desired antigens [8]. At the time of writing there are 20 viral vector candidate vaccines for SARS-CoV-2 in clinical phase assessment, including 6 RVV and 14 NRVV vaccine candidates [21].

14.2.1.4 Replicating Viral Vector (RVV)

In December 2019, ERVEBO, a recombinant replicating vaccine based on the vesicular stomatitis virus (VSV) vector expressing the EBOV glycoprotein (GP) gene, was the first FDA-approved vaccine for the prevention of Ebola virus disease (EVD) [31]. Various candidate vaccines for SARS-CoV-2 using attenuated viral vector platforms are being tested in preclinical and clinical studies [21]. In this approach, relatively low doses of virus need to be used, since the vector has the ability to elicit strong immune responses because of its replication at the site of vaccination [8, 27]. Among five candidate vaccines in clinical evaluation, an influenza virus vector is used for the expression of the SARS-CoV-2 S RBD (DelNS1-2019-nCoV-RBD-OPT1) for establishment of long-term immunity against SARS-CoV-2. In a Phase II clinical evaluation, DelNS1-2019-nCoV-RBD-OPT1 is a RVV vaccine candidate administered as a single dose intranasal spray [32].

14.2.1.5 Non-Replicating Viral Vector (NRVV)

In September 2019, the FDA authorized the first live NRVV vaccine developed for the prevention of both smallpox and monkeypox diseases [33] (fda.gov). NRVV vaccines have been subjected to preclinical and clinical evaluation in order to deliver the designed cargo against several diseases [21, 27]. The simian adenovirus vector-based ChAdOX1 nCoV-19 (also AZD1222) vaccine expressing the full-length SARS-CoV-2 S protein has been evaluated in Phase II/III clinical trials. Even though both cellular and humoral responses were generated against SARS-CoV-2 after a single dose of ChAdOx1 nCoV-19, a booster dose seemed to be important for improved neutralizing antibody profiles [34]. In the interim analysis of Phase II/III trials, ChAdOx1 nCoV-19 was found to be well tolerated, with improved immunogenicity in all age groups following booster immunization [23]. Interim results from four clinical trials demonstrated a vaccine efficacy of 62.1% to 90% [35].

Another vaccine candidate, the Gam-COVID-Vac (Sputnik V) is based on heterologous prime-boost vaccination with two nonreplicating human adenovirus vector serotypes, Ad26 and Ad5, both incorporating the full-length SARS-CoV-2 S protein [36]. The strategy of using two serotypes was to avoid preexisting immunity against Ad-vectors for the second immunization. Clinical assessment of the vaccine profile was carried out by an initial rAd26-S vaccine dose administered to healthy adults, followed by a second dose of rAd5-S on day 21. Initial validation showed good safety and strong immunogenicity in healthy adults. Interim results from the Phase III trial showed over 90% vaccine efficacy in healthy volunteers. The Sputnik V vaccine administration is authorized in 65 countries including Egypt, Albania, Zimbabwe, and Jordan [24].

The Ad26.COV2.S candidate vaccine (Janssen Pharmaceuticals), encoding the full-length SARS-CoV-2 S protein was developed by using the recombinant adenovirus type 26 (Ad26) vector. In contrast to other COVID-19 vaccine candidates, Ad26.COV2.S has been administered as a single-dose vaccine providing good safety and robust efficacy in animal models. AD26.COV2.S has been subjected to the Phase III ENSEMBLE trial on several continents in up to 60,000 volunteers over 18 years of age with or without comorbidities. The FDA issued an EUA for AD26-COV2.S for use in people 18 years of age and older [37].

14.2.1.6 Inactivated/Live Attenuated Virus Vaccines

Inactivated or live attenuated viruses represent a type of traditional viral vaccine platform that uses viruses as a whole, or as subunits, to provoke immune responses. Viral vaccines can be divided into two types: inactivated virus, and attenuated virus vaccines, which rely on different processes in development [16, 27]. There are 14 SARS-CoV-2 vaccine candidates using viruses as a whole, or as subunits, in clinical development [21]. Among these, 12 are based on inactivated virus (IV), and 2 are live attenuated virus (LAV) vaccines.

14.2.1.6.1 Inactivated Virus (IV)

Progress in the development of different inactivation strategies has contributed to the success of several IV vaccines [16, 19, 27]. The first IV vaccine was the human influenza virus vaccine. Depending on purification procedure, IV vaccines can comprise either whole virus or subunit vaccines [27]. The IV platform has been shown to be safer than live-attenuated vaccines (LAV); however, it often requires an adjuvant for enhanced immunogenicity [16]. For SARS-CoV-2 vaccine development efforts, 12 candidate IV vaccines have been reported to be in clinical evaluation, of which six are in Phase III [21].

Sinovac has developed CoronaVac, an IV vaccine with Aluminum hydroxide (Alum) adjuvant, which has been investigated in Phase III trials. This vaccine, applied as a two-dose IM regimen, has demonstrated good safety, tolerability, and immunogenicity against SARS-CoV-2 in healthy subjects aged 18–59 years. Only mild or moderate side effects, including 9% of participants complaining about temporary injection site pain, have been reported [38]. Furthermore, another IV SARS-CoV-2 vaccine candidate BBIBP-CorV developed by Sinopharm, was evaluated in Phase I/II in healthy individuals aged 18–80 years. Interim clinical trial results of this vaccine have shown its safety and tolerability in all subjects as a two-dose regimen. The most frequent side effect reported was fever. All participants receiving the vaccine, generated humoral responses on day 42 and seroconversion was observed after the administration of two doses of 4 μg. Currently, there are several conducted or ongoing Phase III studies in different countries, including Argentina, Peru, United Arab Emirates, Jordan, and Egypt [24]. Last but not least, the whole-virion inactivated SARS-CoV-2 vaccine, BBV152, developed by Bharat Biotech in India, is in Phase III clinical evaluation. The vaccine was formulated with TLR 7/8 agonist adsorbed to Alum, which resulted in high tolerability and improved virus-specific immune response.

14.2.1.6.2 Live Attenuated Virus

One of the well-known live attenuated virus (LAV) (weakened) vaccines is MMR, developed for the prevention of mumps, measles and rubella [27]. LAV vaccines are produced by attenuating the wild type virus, which still can replicate after administration, but usually do not cause a disease [25]. Even if it does, it is often significantly milder than the actual symptoms of the disease. The immune response to a LAV vaccine is very similar to natural infection, therefore a small dose of virus could be enough to provoke immune response [16]. There are only two LAV vaccine candidates reported to be at the stage of clinical evaluation for SARS-CoV-2 [21]. The LAV vaccine candidate COVI-VAC, developed by Codagenix (India) and MV-014-212, developed by Meissa Vaccines, Inc. are currently in Phase I clinical assessment, administered through the intranasal route (no published data available).

14.2.1.7 Recombinant Protein Subunit Vaccines

While protein subunit (PS) vaccines have limitations regarding the low immunogenicity, the use of immunostimulatory adjuvants often can overcome this issue, providing sufficient protective immunity [16, 27]. In addition, carrier nanoparticles can be conjugated in order to enhance multi-meric antigenic presentation, which results in increased immunogenicity [19]. Traditional subunit vaccines relied on purification of viral surface proteins. The advent of recombinant protein expression technologies has facilitated the production significantly, and has allowed the purification of large quantities of protein subunits for immunization.

In the context of the COVID-19 pandemic, there are 28 PS SARS-CoV-2 vaccine candidates being explored in clinical trials. The Matrix-M1

adjuvanted recombinant S protein nanoparticle vaccine candidate NVX-CoV2373 was produced in the established baculovirus *Spodoptera frugiperda* (Sf9) insect cell expression system. Phase I results showed robust humoral and cellular immune responses against SARS-CoV-2, with high viral neutralizing activity [27, 39]. Additionally, the NVX-CoV2373 vaccine developed by Novavax, showed 89.3% vaccine efficacy in a Phase III trial [40].

Moreover, the SCB-2019 vaccine candidate comprising S-Trimer protein formulated with either AS03 or CpG/Alum adjuvants is currently under Phase II/III clinical investigation [41]. Interim Phase I results for SCB-2019 showed promising neutralizing antibody responses with either of the adjuvants. On immunization, the vaccine successfully promoted SARS-CoV-2 specific humoral and Th1-biased CD4+ T cell responses [41].

14.2.1.8 Virus-Like Particle Vaccines

Virus-like particle (VLP) vaccines are noninfectious, engineered from viral proteins assembled as multimers to mimic the structure of wildtype virus, but containing no viral genetic material [8]. Moreover, these empty viral shells exhibit high immunogenicity because of the similar structure and size of native virions [17, 25]. Recently, four SARS-CoV-2 vaccine candidates using VLP technology have entered the stage of clinical trials [21].

A subunit VLP vaccine, RBD SARS-CoV-2 HBsAg, is currently under Phase I/II evaluation, where the hepatitis B surface antigen (HBsAg) is fused with the RBD antigen, aiming to promote prolonged immune response against SARS-CoV-2 infection. A second VLP-based vaccine candidate, CoVLP was formulated with a squalene-based adjuvant AS03, and is in Phase II/III clinical assessment. Moreover, another VLP-based vaccine candidate has been developed by Bilkent and Middle East Technical Universities in Turkey, and is evaluated in combination with alum and CpGODN-K3 adjuvants in a Phase I study [21].

14.2.2 Insights into Repurposing Drugs as Therapeutic Options for COVID-19

Despite the importance of vaccines for preventing and eradicating COVID-19, as the massive task of vaccinating the whole global populations remains challenging there is an urgent need for alternative therapeutic approaches. Additionally, given that *de novo* development of drugs against SARS-CoV-2 takes a long time, rigorous and adequate clinical trials focusing on drug repurposing can be crucial to discovering effective treatments against COVID-19 in a shorter time frame [6, 42, 43]. Repurposing of existing approved drugs can present a practical approach during the emergent pandemic because of the available data on the safety of repurposing drugs. Hence, from the beginning, the COVID-19 pandemic has prompted the repurposing of a plethora of existing approved drugs by conducting over 200 Phase II/III clinical trials to evaluate the safety and efficacy of repurposed drugs against SARS-CoV-2, previously developed against viral and parasitic infections such as HIV, Influenza, Ebola and Malaria (Table 14.2) [6, 42, 43].

As for the treatment mechanism against SARS-CoV-2 of repurposed drugs, principally two distinct approaches have been explored: prevention of virus entry into host cells by blocking virus–cell membrane fusion (e.g. hydroxychloroquine (HCQ)/chloroquine), and suppression of different intracellular steps of virus replication by inhibiting the RNA-dependent RNA polymerase (RdRp), an enzyme that plays a key role in the replication of an extensive range of viruses, including SARS-CoV-2 (for example, favipiravir and remdesivir). Additionally, mechanisms related to the inhibition of viral proteases (for example, lopinavir/ritonavir), the inhibition of cytokine release and anti-inflammatory responses (for example, dexamethasone, tocilizumab and colchicine) have also been explored [42, 44, 45] (Figure 14.2) (Table 14.2). For comprehensive reviews related to mechanisms of the repurposed drugs, the reader is referred to Chapter 7.

In keeping with drug repurposing investigations, several drugs, including remdesivir, HCQ, Kaletra (lopinavir/ritonavir) [46], favipiravir [47], ivermectin, (TCZ) tocilizumab, dexamethasone, and colchicine [48] have been studied in different multi-national and multi-armed trials, to assess their clinical efficacy for COVID-19 treatment, and can be found at ClinicalTrials.gov with National Clinical Trial (NCT) identifiers. While some of these clinical trials are already completed, others are still ongoing and recruiting. Selected compelling examples of repurposed drugs in clinical trials are listed in Table 14.2. Among these repurposed drugs, in particular remdesivir and HCQ, have been the center of attention. However, the SOLIDARITY trial (NCT04315948) is one of the largest international randomized trials launched by the WHO and partners, enrolling almost 12,000 patients at 500 hospital sites across 30 countries. This trial evaluated the clinical effectiveness of remdesivir/lopinavir/ritonavir/HCQ together with Interferon β-1A on three important outcomes: mortality, need for assisted ventilation, and duration of hospital

stay. The outcome was that all four evaluated treatments showed little or no effect on overall mortality, initiation of ventilation, or duration of hospital stay in hospitalized patients, as presented in an interim report [46].

To overcome the pandemic crisis and to identify effective treatment against SARS-CoV-2, the repurposing of existing FDA approved antiviral drugs is given high priority. Accordingly, the RdRp inhibitor remdesivir received an EUA from the FDA in May 2020 [49], and the FDA approved remdesivir for patients aged 12 years and older in October 2020 [50] on the basis of clinical trial data (NCT04280705) which demonstrated better clinical benefit than placebo in shortening the recovery time of adult patients with COVID-19 [46, 50]. Another clinical study (NCT04292730) examined the effect of remdesivir on patients with moderate COVID-19 disease and found no benefit at the end of the 10-day treatment, while a 5-day treatment showed statistically significant but modest improvement of clinical status versus standard of care [51]. However, a recent update of the WHO clinical trial (NCT04315948) has failed to demonstrate any beneficial therapeutic effect of remdesivir, (HCQ), lopinavir, and interferon regimens on hospitalized patients with COVID-19 [46].

The other promising example is an Influenza virus drug, favipiravir, which interferes with viral replication by inhibiting RdRp [44]. Though favipiravir has not been approved by the FDA it has received an EUA in Italy, and currently is in use in different countries, such as Japan, China, Russia, India, Kazakhstan, and Turkey. Approval has also recently been granted in Saudi Arabia [52].

HCQ and chloroquine phosphate (CQ) are two other disputed repurposed drugs. They have been developed as antimalarial drugs that interfere with the viral endosomal entry pathway, and some experts considered HCQ as one of the most promising COVID-19 drugs [53].

Recently, the randomized TOGETHER clinical trial conducted in Brazil with 1,476 adult diagnosed with respiratory symptoms caused by SARS-CoV-2 infections failed to show any significant benefit of HCQ and lopinavir/ritonavir in hospitalized patients [45].

Overall, despite the fact that several clinical trials have been completed and others are still ongoing, no clinical research has demonstrated efficacy of any repurposed drug that could cure COVID-19. For this reason, there is an urgent need for a concerted and sustained clinical research effort. Since the efficacy of many repurposed drug treatment modalities tested in preclinical studies and/or clinical trials have often

Table 14.2 Selected repurposed drug and related clinical trials

Drug Candidate	Drug Class/ Disease Indication	Proposed Mode of Action	Possible Drug–Drug Interaction	Selected Clinical Trials
Colchicine	Anti-inflammatory (inflammatory arthritis and gout, pericarditis and coronary disease)	▪ Anti-inflammatory response through NLRP3 inflammasome and cytokine storm suppression	Substrate for: **CYP3A4** *Attention for co-administration with moderate and strong inhibitors of these CYP3A4	▪ COLCORONA (NCT0432268)/ NCT04472611/ NCT04539873/ NCT04667780/ NCT04510038 *ClinicalTrials.gov*
Dexamethasone	Corticosteroids	▪ Inhibition of release of cytokines		▪ RECOVERY NCT04381936 *ClinicalTrials.gov*
Favipiravir (T-705)		▪ Inhibition of RNA-dependent RNA polymerase (RdRp)	Inhibitor for: **CYP2C8**	▪ NCT04358549/ NCT04346628/ NCT04319900/ NCT04474457/ NCT04501783/ NCT04358549/ NCT04333589/ NCT04356495/ NCT0446440/ NCT04464408/ EUCTR2020-002106-68-GB/JPRN-jRCTs041200025/ JapicCTI-205238/ EUCTR2020-001528-32-IT *ClinicalTrials.gov*
Hydroxychloroquine/ chloroquine	Antimalarials/ Antirheumatic	▪ Blockade viral entry into cells by inhibiting the glycosylation of host receptors ▪ Immunomodulatory effects through reduction of cytokine production and inhibition of autophagy and lysosomal activity in host cells	Substrate for: **CYP2C8/CYP2D6/ CYP3A4/CYP3A5** *Attention for co-administration with moderate and strong inhibitors of these CYPs	▪ WHO SOLIDARITY trial (trial of treatments for COVID-19 in hospitalized adults) (NCT04315948) ▪ NCT04325893/ NCT04340544/ NCT04333732/ NCT0434172 NCT04403100 (together trial) *ClinicalTrials.gov*
Ivermectin	Anti-helmintic (anti-parasitic agent)	▪ Reported to inhibit the in vitro replication of SARS-CoV-2 by inhibiting of the IMP α/β receptor responsible for viral protein transmission into host cell nucleus	Substrate for CYP3A4 *Attention for co-administration with moderate and strong inhibitors of these CYP3A4	▪ NCT04510233/ NCT04343092/ NCT04381884 *ClinicalTrials.gov*
Kaletra (Lopinavir/ ritonavir)	Antiviral – HIV protease inhibitors	▪ Inhibition of 3-chymotrypsin-like protease	Substrate and inhibitor for **CYP3A4**	▪ WHO SOLIDARITY trial (trial of treatments for COVID-19 in hospitalized adults) (NCT04315948) *ClinicalTrials.gov* ▪ NCT04292899/ NCT04252664/ NCT042576/ NCT04280705/ NCT04276688/ NCT04403100 (Together Trial) *ClinicalTrials.gov*

Drug Candidate	Drug Class/ Disease Indication	Proposed Mode of Action	Possible Drug–Drug Interaction	Selected Clinical Trials
Remdesivir (GS-5734)	Antiviral for HIV for Hepatitis C and Ebola	■ Inhibition of RNA-dependent RNA polymerase (RdRp)	**N/A** for CYP inhibitors and inducers	■ WHO SOLIDARITY trial (trial of treatments for COVID-19 in hospitalized adults) (NCT04315948) ■ ADAPTIVE Trial (ACTT) NCT04280705 ■ NCT04252664/ NCT04257656/ NCT04292730 *ClinicalTrials.gov*
Tocilizumab	Monoclonal antibody	■ Inhibition of *Interleukin 6 (IL-6)* and reduction in cytokine storm	May decrease blood concentration of **CYP1A2/ CYP2C9/ CYP2C19/ CYP3A4**	■ NCT04356937/ NCT04445272/ NCT04403685 *ClinicalTrials.gov*

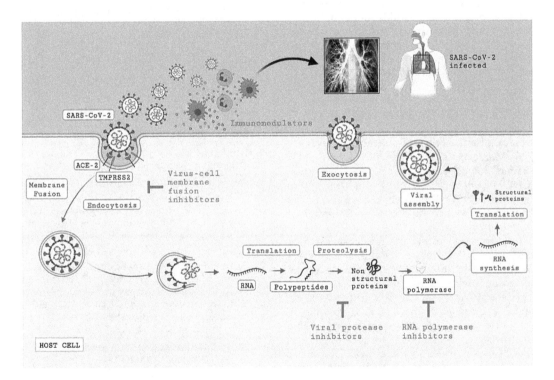

Figure 14.2   Representation of SARS-CoV-2 life cycle and major therapeutic strategies for COVID-19.
Source: Created with Biorender.com.

ended with mixed results or failure to demonstrate clinical efficacy against the SARS-CoV-2 virus, more clinical studies are urgently needed to evaluate the efficacy of the new repurposed drugs alone or in combination with other drugs for COVID-19 treatment [4, 26].

14.3 CONCLUSION

The COVID-19 pandemic has claimed millions of lives since its emergence in Wuhan and its rapid spread across the world. Despite the fact that scientific research has explained COVID-19 through the elucidation of SARS-CoV-2 pathogenesis, there is still much to learn, especially about the dynamic and complex interactions between SARS-CoV-2 and the immune response of the host [3, 4]. The COVID-19 pandemic has had a significant effect on clinical research, resulting in a crowded clinical pipeline of more than 4,000 studies linked to COVID-19 (*ClinicalTrials.gov*), including approximately 1,500 trials involving drugs or vaccines [48]. Hundreds of trials for other diseases were suspended as a result of this extraordinary situation. Despite the fact that many COVID-19 vaccines have been approved by various regulatory authorities in different countries, no drug has been officially approved, so far, with the exception of remdesivir and favipiravir. As a result, clinical studies on COVID-19 related to novel therapeutic methods should continue to focus on low-hanging fruits in the fight against SARS-CoV-2 infection [6].

Integration of genomic approaches, such as pharmacogenomics (PGx), into clinical trials for repurposed drugs would undoubtedly add a significant dimension to achieving successful dosing and reducing drug-induced adverse events [54]. Another important concern is the lack of information on different responses to SARS-CoV-2 infections in males and females. So, in future clinical trials, much needed resources should be dedicated to this type of research in order to investigate gender-specific discrepancies in pharmacotherapies against COVID-19 [55]. Moreover, despite the fact that the US Centers for Disease Control and Prevention (CDC) recommend that pregnant women can receive the COVID-19 vaccine, there is still not enough evidence to support the vaccination of pregnant women [56].

In summary, despite the fact that the pandemic has not yet been silenced, a new wave of SARS-CoV-2 infections has begun, with an increased number of new SARS-CoV-2 variants. The task at hand is to deal with these variants, and these mutations have spread so quickly across the globe that we are unlikely to be able to fully eradicate them in the near future. A crucial factor relates to the efficacy of current vaccines against the new SARS-CoV-2 variants and the need for reengineering of existing vaccines. Moreover, a similar strategy to the one applied for influenza virus vaccines could be of interest. Research efforts for a pandemic vaccine development that targets both the influenza virus and the SARS-CoV-2 would be equally interesting [57]. Another issue related to the adenovirus-based vaccines (ChAdOx1 nCoV-19 and Ad26.COV2.S), and the mRNA-based vaccines (BNT162b2 and mRNA-1273), has been their association with rare cases of thrombocytopenia [58, 59], which should be thoroughly investigated, and caution should be used when individuals with a preexisting susceptibility to thrombocytopenia are vaccinated.

Needless to say, the current COVID-19 vaccines will not be the last ones needed. While, for the time being, they are most essential as they can slow down the progression of the pandemic and reduce the severity of disease, we have been dealing with since December 2019. However, in the long run we need novel drugs and vaccines to eradicate COVID-19 once and for all.

REFERENCES

1. Li, W., Wong, S.K., Li, F., Kuhn, J.H., Huang, I.C., Choe, H., Farzan, M. (2006). Animal origins of the severe acute respiratory syndrome coronavirus: Insight from ACE2-S-Protein interactions. *J. Virol.* 80(9), 4211–4219. https://doi.org/10.1128/jvi.80.9.4211-4219.2006.

2. Memish, Z.A., Perlman, S., Van Kerkhove, M.D., Zumla, A. (2020). Middle East respiratory syndrome. *Lancet* 395(10229), 1063–1077. https://doi.org/10.1016/s0140-6736(19)33221-0.

3. Dhama, K., Khan, S., Tiwari, R., et al. (2020). Coronavirus disease 2019–COVID-19. *Clin. Microbiol. Rev.* 33(4). https://doi.org/10.1128/cmr.00028-20.

4. Chilamakuri, R., Agarwal, S. (2021). COVID-19: Characteristics and therapeutics. *Cells* 10(2), 206. https://doi.org/10.3390/cells10020206.

5. Hu, T., Liu, Y., Zhao, M., Zhuang, Q., Xu, L., He, Q. (2020). A comparison of COVID-19, SARS and MERS. *PeerJ* 8, e9725. https://doi.org/10.7717/peerj.9725.

6. Sanders, J.M., Monogue, M.L., Jodlowski, T.Z., Cutrell, J.B. (2020). Pharmacologic treatments for coronavirus disease 2019 (COVID-19). *JAMA.* https://doi.org/10.1001/jama.2020.6019.

7. Alexandersen, S., Chamings, A., Bhatta, T.R. (2020). SARS-CoV-2 genomic and subgenomic RNAs in diagnostic samples are not an indicator of active replication. *Nat. Commun.* 11(1), 6059. https://doi.org/10.1038/s41467-020-19883-7.

8. Flanagan, K.L., Best, E., Crawford, N.W., et al. (2020). Progress and pitfalls in the quest for effective SARS-CoV-2 (COVID-19) vaccines. *Front. Immunol.* 11, 579250. https://doi.org/10.3389/fimmu.2020.579250.

9. Tu, Y.F., Chien, C.S., Yarmishyn, A.A., et al. (2020). A review of SARS-CoV-2 and the ongoing clinical trials. *Int. J. Mol. Sci.* 21(7), 2657. https://doi.org/10.3390/ijms21072657.

10. Rabaan, A.A., Al-Ahmed, S.H., Sah, R., et al. (2020). SARS-CoV-2/COVID-19 and advances in developing potential therapeutics and vaccines to counter this emerging pandemic. *Ann. Clin. Microbiol. Antimicrob.* 19(1), 40. https://doi.org/10.1186/s12941-020-00384-w.

11. WHO | World Health Organization. (2021, May 10). World Health Organization. https://www.who.int/.

12. Fontanet, A., Autran, B., Lina, B., Kieny, M.P., Karim, S.S.A., Sridhar, D. (2021). SARS-CoV-2 variants and ending the COVID-19 pandemic. *Lancet* 397(10278), 952–954. https://doi.org/10.1016/s0140-6736(21)00370-6.

13. Madhi, S.A., Baillie, V., Cutland, C.L., et al. (2021). Safety and efficacy of the ChAdOx1 nCoV-19 (AZD1222) COVID-19 vaccine against the B.1.351 variant in South Africa. *medRxiv*. https://doi.org/10.1101/2021.02.10.21251247.

14. Sahin, U., Muik, A., Derhovanessian, E., et al. (2020). COVID-19 vaccine BNT162b1 elicits human antibody and TH1 T cell responses. *Nature* 586(7830), 594–599. https://doi.org/10.1038/s41586-020-2814-7.

15. Liu, X., Liu, C., Liu, G., Luo, W., Xia, N. (2020). COVID-19: Progress in diagnostics, therapy and vaccination. *Theranostics* 10(17), 7821–7835. https://doi.org/10.7150/thno.47987.

16. Jain, S., Batra, H., Yadav, P., Chand, S. (2020). COVID-19 vaccines currently under preclinical and clinical studies, and associated antiviral immune response. *Vaccines* 8(4), 649. https://doi.org/10.3390/vaccines8040649.

17. Rawat, K., Kumari, P., Saha, L. (2021). COVID-19 vaccine: A recent update in pipeline vaccines, their design and development strategies. *Eur. J. Pharmacol.*, 892, 173751. https://doi.org/10.1016/j.ejphar.2020.173751.

18. Hussen, J., Kandeel, M., Hemida, M.G., Al-Mubarak, A.I.A. (2020). Antibody-based immunotherapeutic strategies for COVID-19. *Pathogens* 9(11), 917. https://doi.org/10.3390/pathogens9110917.

19. Poland, G.A., Ovsyannikova, I.G., Crooke, S.N., Kennedy, R.B. (2020). SARS-CoV-2 vaccine development: Current status. *Mayo Clin. Proc.* 95(10), 2172–2188. https://doi.org/10.1016/j.mayocp.2020.07.021.

20. Ahamad, S., Branch, S., Harrelson, S., Hussain, M.K., Saquib, M., Khan, S. (2021). Primed for global coronavirus pandemic: Emerging research and clinical outcome. *Eur. J. Med. Chem.* 209, 112862. https://doi.org/10.1016/j.ejmech.2020.112862.

21. Draft landscape and tracker of COVID-19 candidate vaccines. [cited 2021 Mar 13]. Retrieved from: https://www.who.int/publications/m/item/draft-landscape-of-covid-19-candidate-vaccines.

22. Baden, L.R., El Sahly, H.M., Essink, B., et al. (2021). Efficacy and safety of the mRNA-1273 SARS-CoV-2 vaccine. *N. Engl. J. Med.* 384(5), 403–416. https://doi.org/10.1056/nejmoa2035389.

23. Ramasamy, M.N., Minassian, A.M., Ewer, K.J., et al. (2020). Safety and immunogenicity of ChAdOx1 nCoV-19 vaccine administered in a prime-boost regimen in young and old adults (COV002): A single-blind, randomised, controlled, Phase 2/3 trial. *Lancet* 396(10267), 1979–1993. https://doi.org/10.1016/s0140-6736(20)32466-1.

24. COVID19 Vaccine Tracker. [cited 2021 May 21]. Retrieved from: https://covid19.trackvaccines.org/.

25. Li, Y.D., Chi, W.Y., Su, J.H., Ferrall, L., Hung, C.F., Wu, T.C. (2020). Coronavirus vaccine development: From SARS and MERS to COVID-19. *J. Biomed. Sci.* 27(1), 104. https://doi.org/10.1186/s12929-020-00695-2.

26. Das, G., Ghosh, S., Garg, S., et al. (2020). An overview of key potential therapeutic strategies for combat in the COVID-19 battle. *RSC Advances* 10(47), 28243–28266. https://doi.org/10.1039/d0ra05434h.

27. Chakraborty, S., Mallajosyula, V., Tato, C.M., Tan, G.S., Wang, T.T. (2021). SARS-CoV-2 vaccines in advanced clinical trials: Where do we stand? *Adv. Drug Deliv. Rev.* 172, 314–338. https://doi.org/10.1016/j.addr.2021.01.014.

28. Tebas, P., Yang, S., Boyer, J.D., et al. (2021). Safety and immunogenicity of INO-4800 DNA Vaccine against SARS-CoV-2: A preliminary report of an open-label, Phase 1 clinical trial. *EClinicalMedicine* 31, 100689. https://doi.org/10.1016/j.eclinm.2020.100689.

29. Jeyanathan, M., Afkhami, S., Smaill, F., Miller, M.S., Lichty, B.D., Xing, Z. (2020). Immunological considerations for COVID-19 vaccine strategies. *Nat. Rev. Immunol.* 20(10), 615–632. https://doi.org/10.1038/s41577-020-00434-6.

30. Polack, F.P., Thomas, S.J., Kitchin, N., et al. (2020). Safety and efficacy of the BNT162b2 mRNA COVID-19 vaccine. *N. Engl. J. Med.* 383(27), 2603–2615. https://doi.org/10.1056/nejmoa2034577.

31. Ollmann Saphire, E. (2020). A vaccine against Ebola virus. *Cell* 181(1), 6. https://doi.org/10.1016/j.cell.2020.03.011.

32. Turvey, S.E., Broide, D.H. (2010). Innate immunity. *J. Allergy Clin. Immunol.* 125(2), S24–S32. https://doi.org/10.1016/j.jaci.2009.07.016.

33. Simpson, K., Heymann, D., Brown, C.S., et al. (2020). Human Monkeypox: After 40 years, an unintended consequence of smallpox eradication. *Vaccine* 38(33), 5077–5081. https://doi.org/10.1016/j.vaccine.2020.04.062.

34. Barrett, J.R., Belij-Rammerstorfer, S., Dold, C., et al. (2020). Phase 1/2 trial of SARS-CoV-2 vaccine ChAdOx1 nCoV-19 with a booster dose induces multifunctional antibody responses. *Nat. Med.* 27(2), 279–288. https://doi.org/10.1038/s41591-020-01179-4.

35. Voysey, M., Clemens, S.A., Madhi, S.A., et al. (2021). Safety and efficacy of the ChAdOx1 nCoV-19 vaccine (AZD1222) against SARS-CoV-2: An interim analysis of four randomised controlled

trials in Brazil, South Africa, and the UK. *Lancet* 397(10269), 99–111. https://doi.org/10.1016/s0140-6736(20)32661-1.

36. Logunov, D.Y., Dolzhikova, I.V., Shcheblyakov, D.V., et al. (2021). Safety and efficacy of an rAd26 and rAd5 vector-based heterologous prime-boost covid-19 vaccine: An interim analysis of a randomised controlled Phase 3 trial in Russia. *Lancet* 397(10275), 671–681. https://doi.org/10.1016/s0140-6736(21)00234-8.

37. Sadoff, J., Le Gars, M., Shukarev, G., et al. (2021). Interim results of a Phase 1–2a trial of Ad26. COV2.S COVID-19 vaccine. *N. Engl. J. Med.* 384(19), 1824–1835. https://doi.org/10.1056/nejmoa2034201.

38. Zhang, Y., Zeng, G., Pan, H., et al. (2021). Safety, tolerability, and immunogenicity of an inactivated SARS-CoV-2 vaccine in healthy adults aged 18–59 years: A randomised, double-blind, placebo-controlled, Phase 1/2 clinical trial. *Lancet Infect. Dis.* 21(2), 181–192. https://doi.org/10.1016/s1473-3099(20)30843-4.

39. Keech, C., Albert, G., Cho, I., et al. (2020). Phase 1–2 trial of a SARS-CoV-2 recombinant spike protein nanoparticle vaccine. *N. Engl. J. Med.* 383(24), 2320–2332. https://doi.org/10.1056/nejmoa2026920.

40. Mahase, E. (2021). COVID-19: Novavax vaccine efficacy is 86% against UK variant and 60% against South African variant. *BMJ* n296. https://doi.org/10.1136/bmj.n296.

41. Richmond, P., Hatchuel, L., Dong, M., et al. (2021). Safety and immunogenicity of S-Trimer (SCB-2019), a protein subunit vaccine candidate for COVID-19 in healthy adults: A phase 1, randomised, double-blind, placebo-controlled trial. *Lancet* 397(10275), 682–694. https://doi.org/10.1016/s0140-6736(21)00241-5

42. Ravi, S., Jadhav, S., Vaidya, A., Ghooi, R. (2021). Repurposing drugs during the COVID-19 pandemic and beyond. *Pharm. Pat. Anal.* 10(1), 9–12. https://doi.org/10.4155/ppa-2020-0031.

43. Shaffer, L. (2020). 15 drugs being tested to treat COVID-19 and how they would work. *Nat. Med.* https://doi.org/10.1038/d41591-020-00019-9.

44. Bosaeed, M., Alharbi, A., Hussein, M., et al. (2021). Multicentre randomised double-blinded placebo-controlled trial of Favipiravir in adults with mild COVID-19. *BMJ Open* 11(4), e047495. https://doi.org/10.1136/bmjopen-2020-047495.

45. Reis, G., Moreira Silva, E.A.D.S., Medeiros Silva, D.C., et al. (2021). Effect of early treatment with Hydroxychloroquine or Lopinavir and Ritonavir on risk of hospitalization among patients with COVID-19. *JAMA Netw. Open* 4(4), e216468. https://doi.org/10.1001/jamanetworkopen.2021.6468.

46. WHO Solidarity Trial Consortium. (2021). Repurposed antiviral drugs for COVID-19: Interim WHO solidarity trial results. *N. Engl. J. Med.* 384(6), 497–511. https://doi.org/10.1056/nejmoa2023184.

47. Joshi, S., Parkar, J., Ansari, A., Vora, A., Talwar, D., Tiwaskar, M., Patil, S., Barkate, H. (2021). Role of Favipiravir in the treatment of COVID-19. *Int. J. Infect. Dis.* 102, 501–508. https://doi.org/10.1016/j.ijid.2020.10.069.

48. Recovery Trial. Randomized evaluation of COVID-19 therapy. [cited 2021, Apr 21]. Retrieved from: https://www.recoverytrial.net/.

49. FDA. Coronavirus (COVID-19) update: FDA issues emergency use authorization for potential COVID-19 treatment. [cited 2021, May 6]. Retrieved from: https://www.fda.gov/news-events/press-announcements/coronavirus-covid-19-update-fda-issues-emergency-use-authorization-potential-covid-19-treatment

50. Rubin, D., Chan-Tack, K., Farley, J., Sherwat, A. (2020). FDA approval of Remdesivir: A step in the right direction. *N. Engl. J. Med.* 383(27), 2598–2600. https://doi.org/10.1056/nejmp2032369.

51. Spinner, C.D., Gottlieb, R.L., Criner, G.J., et al. (2020). Effect of Remdesivir vs standard care on clinical status at 11 days in patients with moderate COVID-19. *JAMA* 324(11), 1048. https://doi.org/10.1001/jama.2020.16349.

52. Ghasemnejad-Berenji, M., Pashapour, S. (2020). Favipiravir and COVID-19: A simplified summary. *Drug Res.* 71(03), 166–170. https://doi.org/10.1055/a-1296-7935.

53. Khuroo, M. S. (2020). Chloroquine and Hydroxychloroquine in Coronavirus Disease 2019 (COVID-19). Facts, fiction and the hype: A critical appraisal. *Int. J. Antimicrob. Agents* 56(3), 106101. https://doi.org/10.1016/j.ijantimicag.2020.106101.

54. Badary, O.A. (2021). Pharmacogenomics and COVID-19: Clinical implications of human genome interactions with repurposed drugs. *Pharmacogenomics J.* 21(3), 275–284. https://doi.org/10.1038/s41397-021-00209-9.

55. Schiffer, V.M., Janssen, E.B., van Bussel, B.C., et al. (2020). The "sex gap" in COVID-19 trials: A scoping review. *EClinicalMedicine* 29–30, 100652. https://doi.org/10.1016/j.eclinm.2020.100652.

56. Bianchi, D.W., Kaeser, L., Cernich, A.N. (2021). Involving pregnant individuals in clinical research on COVID-19 vaccines. *JAMA* 325(11), 1041. https://doi.org/10.1001/jama.2021.1865.

57. Lurie, N., Saville, M., Hatchett, R., Halton, J. (2020). Developing COVID-19 vaccines at pandemic speed. *N. Engl. J. Med.* 382(21), 1969–1973. https://doi.org/10.1056/nejmp2005630.

58. Greinacher, A., Thiele, T., Warkentin, T.E., Weisser, K., Kyrle, P.A., Eichinger, S. (2021). Thrombotic thrombocytopenia after ChAdOx1 nCov-19 vaccination. *N. Engl. J. Med*. 384, 2092–2101. https://doi.org/10.1056/nejmoa2104840.

59. Muir, K.L., Kallam, A., Koepsell, S.A., Gundabolu, K. (2021). Thrombotic thrombocytopenia after Ad26.COV2.S vaccination. *N. Engl. J. Med*. 384(20), 1964–1965. https://doi.org/10.1056/nejmc2105869.

Chapter 15 Lessons Learned from COVID-19 and Their Implementations for Future Pandemics

Mauricio Corredor, Debmalya Barh, and Kenneth Lundstrom

15.1 INTRODUCTION

The 2009 Swine flu outbreak raised serious concern about an imminent pandemic [1]. The relatively short outbreaks of SARS (2002–2003) [2] and MERS (2012) [3]. did not reach the level of a global pandemic. Today, more than a year after the onset of the biggest pandemic in history, many scientific, medical, economic, and social questions remain. In this final chapter, we will evaluate the lessons learned from the COVID-19 pandemic so far. Social, economic, and political aspects will be considered, but not analyzed, because the point of view of science and medicine is always that of self-assessment, not that of the judgment of other disciplines.

Scientific and medical monitoring and follow-up have been crucial from the beginning of the pandemic, and the essential elements have been analyzed with scientific tools in epidemiology, viral pathology, diagnostics, and therapy [4]. On the other hand, much attention has been dedicated to fundamental aspects such as molecular virology [5] and vaccine development [6].

Organizations such as the World Health Organization (WHO), governmental funding, and even philanthropic foundations [7], have contributed to SARS-CoV-2 research to rapidly support research activities in laboratories and to provide practical solutions in hospitals. Hundreds of scientific publications and web postings have emerged through various international partnerships between thousands of scientists and clinicians worldwide. Using the words "COVID-19 and/or SARS-CoV-2", as search entries, bioRxiv alone reported 3,834 hits, arXiv 3,833 hits, medRxiv 10,122 hits, PubMed 85,527 hits, of which 5,694 corresponded to NIH grants, ScienceDirect 24,141 hits, and Google Scholar 628,000 hits. For "COVID-19" alone, Google Scholar found 3,710,000 hits. Though we have not reached the end of the pandemic, many questions regarding SARS-CoV-2 and COVID-19 remain open. For example, there are still a number of unsolved issues related to vaccines and future novel drugs.

This chapter and the book do not represent the end of the story, rather the beginning of the end. It is an opportunity to further analyze results and find out what has been learned since the beginning of the COVID-19 pandemic and what can be achieved in the future. Today, we have access to more advanced technologies and tools at the scientific, clinical, and pharmaceutical levels. None the less, we had to stop our own research, and even the treatment of patients with other diseases for a few months, to focus our resources on COVID-19.

At the onset of the pandemic in 2020, some health managers may have considered that the COVID-19 outbreak would have passed quickly like other epidemics and never reach pandemic levels. However, history taught us other lessons. A reductionist view of the problem can lead to underestimating the consequences, but a holistic vision will provide more rapid and effective solutions (https://ipbes.net/sites/default/files/2020-12/IPBES%20Workshop%20on%20Biodiversity%20and%20Pandemics%20Report_0.pdf). By remembering what happened and critically evaluating the actions taken will allow us to reflect on lessons learned for the future so as not to repeat mistakes made. This chapter highlights a range of successes and discusses some failures.

15.2 ARRIVAL OF SARS-CoV-2 AND THE COVID-19 PANDEMIC

Influenza A, AIDS, and COVID-19 were the three most recent human pandemics, caused by Influenza virus H1N1, human immunodeficiency virus (HIV), and SARS-CoV-2, respectively. The epidemics caused by Ebola, Swine flu virus H1N1 (2009–2010), SARS-Cov, MERS-CoV, and avian influenza virus H5N1 never reached pandemic levels. It was essential for the WHO to define COVID-19 as a pandemic, though terminology among the general public includes "corona", "coronavirus", "SARS-CoV-2", "virus", "pathogen", and "COVID-19". In the context of the Influenza A virus and AIDS pandemics, it was essential to distinguish the names of pandemics from the names of the viruses, which was not the case for the Ebola epidemic. Why is this important? To outline a pandemic as: "simply defining a pandemic as a large epidemic may make ultimate sense in terms of comprehensibility and consistency" [8]. In the context of earlier outbreaks, descriptions of catastrophic consequences of emerging epidemics were considered alarming, potentially creating panic in the society [9, 10]. During those outbreaks the warnings issued by scientists were not

DOI: 10.1201/9781003190394-15

communicated very well to the general public. Therefore, importantly, Dr Thedros Adhanom Gebreyesus, Director-General of the WHO, officially declared the outbreak a pandemic on March 11, 2020 by spelling out the name "COVID-19". This was the first time a multilateral organization has declared the start of a pandemic.

15.3 SCIENCE AND MEDICAL SUPPORT

In addition to the cautionary messages in the 2019 article entitled "Neglecting major health problems and broadcasting minor, uncertain issues in lifestyle science" the "war" was announced, but "not properly heard" [11]. In the first pandemic of modern times (there were pandemics in the fifteenth and sixteenth centuries too) in the twentieth century, scientific and technological resources were quite limited. In the First and Second World Wars, much scientific collaboration was devoted to weapon manufacture. However, medical development did not stop, which led to the exceptional discovery of antibiotics. These three great crises of humanity are not comparable, either socially or economically. Despite COVID-19 vaccine availability, we still face difficulties we have not been able to overcome, whether because of a lack of resources, technological tools, or their application [12]. In any case, science and medicine are definitely at stake. Never before has a disease, epidemic, or pandemic unleashed so much scientific, medical, administrative, and political effort, and resources at such a scale as for COVID-19. The unprecedented effort by scientists, engineers, and clinicians has been dedicated to investigating the causes, spread, function, and pathogenesis of SARS-CoV-2 to be able to eradicate the COVID-19 pandemic.

15.4 INTERNET AND COMPUTATIONAL TECHNOLOGIES

During the first six months of the pandemic, internet use and applications increased by more than two-fold in both developed and developing countries [13]. The global network was unprepared for such unanticipated expansion [14], and new networking models were needed. The COVID-19 pandemic created a new scenario for network providers to accelerate computing capacity sufficiently to be able to cope with massive user traffic demands [15]. The use of social networks, video conferencing, virtual meetings, online courses, and other types of communication from home have increased. WhatsApp, Telegram, Facebook, and other services have replaced face-to-face communication. The movie industry, for example, has replaced screening at cinemas with

Netflix and other services. It was a challenge for companies and network designers, as not all countries were planning to expand their coverage. Instead, cellphones have become the big platform for C++, Java, and HTML for Android developers. Hundreds of apps have been designed to survey, control, and trace the spread of infections, and identify individuals who have been in contact with persons who have tested positive for SARS-CoV-2. Today, it is not known whether apps can prevent or slow down the spread of COVID-19, but epidemiological models suggest that apps can be useful in changing the course of the pandemic [16].

Big data (BD), cloud computing (CC), machine learning (ML) [17], and artificial intelligence (AI) [18] were the massive computational areas for the development of networking and informatics science. For the analysis of the number of COVID-19 cases and deaths, new databases were created worldwide to facilitate the handling of new daily data. BD was assembled from the information collected in each country, related to infections, transmission, incidence curves, R naught, Ro (how contagious is an infectious disease), and the logarithm scale plots with their daily death and cumulative patient numbers. Numerous databases such as "COVID-19 Dashboard by the Center for Systems Science and Engineering" were crucial [19, 20] (Figure 15.1).

15.5 PROGRAMS, SOFTWARE, AND PLATFORMS

New or existing tools were enhanced or adapted to address the entire epidemic of the COVID-19 pandemic in real time. It will be impossible to describe the hundreds of software and platforms available for COVID-19. For example, the WHO electronic data collection platforms were established in the context of the COVID-19 outbreak (Figure 15.1). Another example is "The Guide to Global Digital Tools for COVID-19 Response" from the CDC website (https://www.cdc.gov/coronavirus/2019-ncov/global-covid-19/compare-digital-tools.html), which presents an overview of the main software packages used in the pandemic (Table 15.1). This resource compiles and compares various tools such as the District Health Information Software DHIS2 [21], the Surveillance Outbreak Response Management and Analysis System (SORMAS) [22], "GoData" [23], Open Data Kit ODK [24], Epi Info [25], CommCare [26], KoboToolbox [27], and as mentioned, the CDC database, the most practical and well-known resources available online in Excel, MS Office, and Paper formats. Different software packages are used in several countries, and the DHIS2 and SORMAS are used in the USA by national surveillance. For the software,

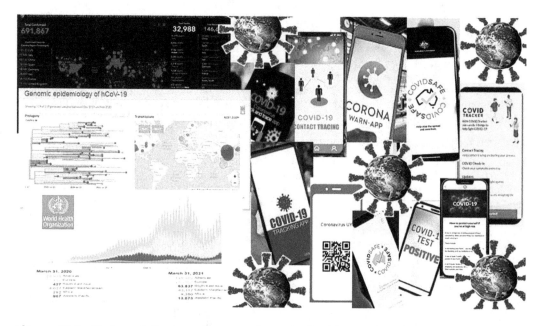

Figure 15.1   Various platforms, software, and apps for the COVID-19 pandemic. From left to right: Dashboard by the Center for Systems Science and Engineering (DCSSE), GISAID SARS-CoV-2 genome (https://www.epicov.org/epi3/frontend#3d1646) [20], the WHO database (https://COVID-19.who.int/region/amro/country/us), and nine global Coronavirus cellphone apps (https://covid-tracing.app/).

package, and cellphone apps for COVID-19, it was concluded in an excellent review that: "The significant technological advances and lessons learned can be adopted or adapted by other countries to ensure public health preparedness for future waves of COVID-19 and other pandemics" [28].

Table 15.1   Examples of tools listed in *The Guide to Global Digital Tools for COVID-19 Response* from the CDC

Tool	Web Site	References
DHIS2	https://www.mn.uio.no/ifi/english/research/networks/hisp/external	[21]
SORMAS	https://sormasorg.helmholtz-hzi.de/History_SORMAS.html	[22]
GoData	https://www.who.int/godataexternal)	[23]
ODK	https://www.cdc.gov/epiinfo/index.html	[24]
Epi Info	https://www.cdc.gov/epiinfo/index.html	[25]
CommCare	https://www.commcarehq.org/accounts/login/	[26]

15.6 EPIDEMIOLOGY, MATHEMATICS, AND STATISTICS

The epicenter of the onset of the COVID-19 outbreak was in China [29], then it spread to Europe [30], later reaching the USA [31], and at the present time it is prominent in Latin America and India [32, 33]. Epidemiologic strategies have been applied to follow the developments in these regions very closely, analyzing data, and producing rapid results. In a systematic review and meta-analysis pooled estimates for clinical characteristics and outcomes in COVID-19 patients were determined [34]. A databank comprising 6,007 publications and 207 studies from 11 countries/regions outlined the epidemiology of the COVID-19 pandemic.

15.7 GENOMICS AND BIOINFORMATICS

One year after the onset of the pandemic, the GISAID database reported more than 1.5 million genomes (1,541,111 on May 13, 2021) and the NCBI genome database 0.4 million (420,778 on May 10, 2021). In the first publication on the SARS-CoV-2 genome, the phylogenetic analysis showed strong diversity [35]. This trait is deeper than amino acid changes from the three – A, B, and C – variants. None the less, variant A is probably the ancestral type according to the isolate of the bat coronavirus outgroup [36]. SARS-CoV-2 is the seventh known coronavirus, which replicates in human cells. Apart from SARS-CoV and MERS-CoV, the other human coronaviruses, HKU1, NL63, OC43, and 229E, cause 15%–30% of common colds, and are not associated with severe symptoms [37]. The evolutionary origin of SARS-CoV-2 is not clear, but it has been postulated to stem from pangolins or bats [38–42]. The search for the origin is continuing, though both pangolins and bats are reservoirs for human coronavirus.

The sequencing of the SARS-CoV-2 genome has been crucial for the determination of the origin, transmissibility, and identification of novel mutants/variants of the virus. Moreover, sequence information has enhanced the understanding of the diagnostics, pathology, etiology, immunology, drug and vaccine development, and epidemiology [43]. Bioinformatics and systems biology have also gained from sequence information of the SARS-CoV-2 genome [44] and has been crucial in immunology and vaccine development [45–47]. A Google Scholar search for "bioinformatics" and "COVID-19" generated 143,000 hits. Furthermore, the user-friendly Genome Detective Coronavirus web-based software application was designed for rapid identification and characterization of novel coronavirus genomes [48].

15.8 SPIKE MUTATIONS

Extensive SARS-CoV-2 genome sequencing identified novel mutations in the SARS-CoV-2 S, M, and E proteins. In particular, mutations in the S protein caught the attention of researchers as some isolates from the UK, South Africa, Brazil, and India showed enhanced transmissibility. Mutations are frequent in RNA viruses and, for example for the E protein, the smallest of the SARS-CoV-2 structural proteins, mutations have been identified in most of its 75 amino acids. However, the association between mutations at amino acid positions 417, 484, 501, and 614 in the S protein and transmissibility (Figure 15.2; Table 15.2) has raised some concerns, which has been outlined by the CDC (https://www.cdc.gov/coronavirus/2019-ncov/cases-updates/variant-surveillance/variant-info.html).

The SARS-CoV-2 B.1.1.7 UK variant has been associated with potentially enhanced transmissibility and lethality [50–52]. Another concern

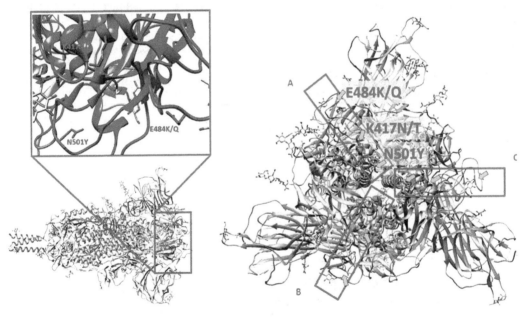

Figure 15.2   The Spike protein 6xr8 structure (from the RCSB PDB database) is highly glycosylated [49]. The upper left square shows the sites of some of the most frequent mutations at positions K417N/T, E484K/Q, and N501Y. These mutations bind to the ACE2 host cell receptor. The lower square shows the side view of the S protein where these mutations appear. The P681R and F888L mutations (see Table 15.2) are distal from these previously described mutation sites but are closer to the membrane. The figure on the right corresponds to part of the S protein that binds to the ACE2 receptor, showing the locations of K417N/T, E484K/Q, and N501Y mutations that form a triangular symmetry between A, B, and C subunits. The amino acids are only labeled in subunit A; subunits B and C, are marked with arrows.

Table 15.2 The latest mutations from the UK, South Africa, Brazil, and India which are of concern

Non synonymous Detected	Country	Isolate PAGO Linage	Virulence	Transmissibility	Antigenicity
K417N, E484K, N501Y, **D614G,** A701V	South Africa	B.1.351	As others, no difference	Close to 50% (20%–113%) higher	Substantial reduction in neutralization by antibodies
L452R, **E484Q,** P681R	India	B.1.617	In progress	In progress	Insignificant reduction in effective neutralization
L18F, T20N, P26S, D138Y, R190S, **K417T,** **E484K, N501Y, D614G,** H655Y, T1027I	Brazil	P.1	Close 45% (50% CrI, 10%–80%) More lethal	Close to 161% (145%–176%) higher	Total reduction in effective neutralization
E484K, S494P, **N501Y,** A570D, **D614G,** P681H, T716I, S982A, D1118H (K1191N)	United Kingdom	B.1.1.7	Increased	~50% increased transmission	Minimal impact on neutralization by convalescent and post-vaccination sera

In bold type, mutations occurring at the same position in different variants. PAGO Lineage is a database (https://cov-lineages.org). The references are in https://www.cdc.gov/coronavirus/2019-ncov/cases-updates/variant-surveillance/variant-info.html.

relates to whether current COVID-19 vaccines still show efficacy against the new variants. Application of pseudoviruses expressing wild-type and B.1.1.7 S protein for testing of sera from individuals vaccinated with the mRNA based BNT162b2 vaccine demonstrated modestly reduced titers against the B.1.1.7 variant [53]. In another study, the BNT162b2 vaccine showed 89.5% efficacy against the B.1.1.7 variant and 75.0% efficacy against the B.1.351 variant [54]. Moreover, the vaccine effectiveness against severe, critical, or fatal COVID-19 disease in Qatar with the presence of the predominant B.1.1.7 and B.1.351 variants was 97.4% [54]. However, the adenovirus-based ChAdOx1 nCoV-19 vaccine did not provide protection against the B.1.351 variant in adults in South Africa, indicating that the efficacy of existing COVID-19 vaccines needs to be evaluated against emerging SARS-CoV-2 variants and if necessary reengineered [55].

15.9 PATHOLOGY AND AGE

SARS-CoV-2 mainly targets the lungs, and lung damage is the leading cause of death in COVID-19 patients [56]. High viral load, lymphopenia, massive secretion of pro-inflammatory cytokines (cytokine storm), and thrombotic and thromboembolic events characterize the early stages of severe COVID-19. In the later stages the virus load and cytokine levels decrease, and tissue repair prevails. Moreover, lung injury is associated with comorbidity such as hypertension (52%), heart disease (38%), and diabetes mellitus (32%) [56]. Other physiological systems

such as the cardiovascular, urinary, gastrointestinal, reproductive (testes not ovary), and nervous systems are also affected by COVID-19 [57]. The phenotypic expression of various SARS-CoV-2 proteins in specific pulmonary microenvironments have been associated with pathological findings in COVID-19 patients, which has been important knowledge for a better understanding of the pathophysiology [58, 59]. Furthermore, significant attention has been dedicated to studies on histopathological changes in different organs after autopsy of COVID-19 patients [60]. The differences in SARS-CoV-2 lung invasion observed between adults and children will further be supported by physiology, biochemistry, and molecular biology research implementing bioinformatics and various omics approaches [61].

15.10 IMMUNOLOGY

Immunology and immunological responses against SARS-CoV-2 play a central role in COVID-19. For example, it has been documented that some individuals show T cell reactivity against other coronaviruses [62]. On the other hand, nobody had been exposed to SARS-CoV-2 before the onset of the pandemic. It has therefore been of great importance to try to understand the immune responses in COVID-19 patients against SARS-CoV-2 in the lungs and other organs. As the virus targets mainly the respiratory tract, eliciting both adaptive and innate immune responses from the immune system, it is also important to investigate differences between children and adults, and in particular, the inferior responses seen in elderly patients [63].

A search using "immunology" and "COVID-19" in Google Scholar, found 2.310.000 hits. SARS-CoV-2 infections elicit multiple antibody responses with neutralizing activity, demonstrated in animal models and human clinical trials [64]. These responses allow the identification of SARS-CoV-2 in infected, re-infected, or future patients. Today, viral immunology is useful to diagnose and determine the viral charge, allowing the development of immunological tests. The most relevant achievement in COVID-19 immunology so far, of course, has been the successful development of several vaccines [65]. The discovery of neutralizing antibody responses to SARS-CoV-2 in recovered COVID-19 patients, and their implications, are also important immunological findings [66].

15.11 RAPID DETECTION AND DIAGNOSTICS

Rapid identification of COVID-19 is essential for choosing the most effective treatment option. Moreover, the diagnostic method needs to be both fast and accurate. The desirable gold standard should also be able to rule out both false positives and false negatives. The classic approach was based on antigen tests, but with extraordinary technology development reverse transcriptase-polymerase chain reaction (RT-PCR) has been widely accepted, especially in the early stages of the pandemic. While some concern has been raised related to poor performance, especially in regard to its sensitivity, RT-PCR has been considered as the gold standard for COVID-19 diagnosis [67]. While continuous technology progress takes place for COVID-19 test development, it is appropriate to have several tests available in parallel to be able to exclude false positives or false negatives more efficiently [68]. As the term "gold standard" is frequently used in the context of diagnostic tests, it should be pointed out that it does not refer to a perfect test, but to the available one, which can be replaced by any test approved to demonstrated superiority. Today, there is a large spectrum of COVID-19 tests available, ranging from DNA-based technologies such as PCR, RT-PCR, and Next Generation Sequencing (NGS) as well as different immunological tests [69].

In many countries around the world, less attention is paid to individuals who are asymptomatic but still can spread the SARS-CoV-2. This is a key issue for COVID-19 but also for future pandemics. The central question is how to identify a disease that does not manifest itself. The initial approach is to conduct rapid testing, applying RT-PCR and NGS. However, this strategy is expensive, and requires qualified personnel and specific equipment. In contrast, accurate and inexpensive immunological self-testing kits allow for rapid diagnosis without the need for more sophisticated laboratory tests and results available only after several days.

15.12 COVID-19 VACCINES

The definite highlight of confronting COVID-19 is certainly the success in developing several vaccines against SARS-CoV-2. This involves all aspects of the process from bioinformatics, genetics, and genomics to identify SARS-CoV-2, the design of vaccine candidates showing immune response against SARS-CoV-2 in in silico modelling, which has then been confirmed in animal models. Furthermore, after the demonstration of protection against challenges with lethal doses of SARS-CoV-2 in animal models, vaccine candidates have been subjected to thorough evaluation in clinical trials in healthy volunteers. The extraordinary strategy developed for COVID-19 vaccines included the risk taken by moving into Phase II trials before Phase I results were available, as well as to Phase III without having confirmation of efficacy in Phase II. Another major risk was the start of vaccine production while Phase III trials were ongoing, and without vaccine approval by the authorities. This approach was only possible through the unprecedented co-operation between academic institutions, pharmaceutical companies and governmental organizations, which made it possible to develop ready-to-use vaccines in less than year, a process known generally to take 8–15 years. The current status of the development of COVID-19 vaccines is summarized in Table 15.3 and in Chapter 13 [70–76].

As indicated in Table 15.3, the adverse events observed after vaccinations seem to be similar with all types of COVID-19 vaccines comprising pain at the injection site, fever, and muscle aches. However, rare cases of thrombosis and thrombocytopenia have been detected in more than 423 million fully vaccinated individuals (as of May 31, 2021). While this issue needs to be addressed, the low frequency of incidences outweighs the risk of thrombocytopenia in COVID-19 patients and therefore strongly supports vaccination on a large scale. However, the issue with blood clots after vaccination is an important lesson learned from our experience with the COVID-19 pandemics. It should be taken into account when designing new vaccines. Another important point is that the scale of vaccination with almost half a billion people fully vaccinated, and a total number of 1.87 billion doses administered, rare events such as thrombocytopenia will remain undetected even in large clinical trials with thousands of people.

Table 15.3 SARS-CoV-2 vaccines approved by national FDAs (the US FDA; EMA in Europe) or currently subjected to clinical evaluations

Vaccines	Efficacy (%)	Approval	Doses	Side Effects
Pfizer/BioNTech (LNP-mRNA)	95	Yes	2	Fatigue, headache, fever, chills, muscle aches, pain or redness at injection site
Moderna (LNP-mRNA)	95	Yes	2	Fatigue, headache, fever, chills, muscle aches, pain or redness at the injection site
University of Oxford/ AstraZeneca (Adenovirus vector)	79	Yes	2	Tenderness, pain, warmth, redness, itching, swelling or bruising at injection site Generally feeling unwell, feeling tired (fatigue), chills or feeling feverish, headache, feeling sick (nausea), joint pain or muscle ache
Sputnik V (Adenovirus vector)	91	Yes	2	Small complaints of weakness, muscle pain for 24 hours
Johnson & Johnson/Janssen (Adenovirus vector)	72	Yes	1	Pain at the injection site, headache, fatigue, muscle ache, nausea
Sinovac (Inactivated virus)	65	Yes	2	Increase in blood pressure, pain at injection site, rashes, headache, and nausea.
Novavax (recombinant protein subunit)	86	No	2	Fever, small complaints
CureVac (LNP-mRNA)	Not available	No	2	Fever and/or headache, side effects resolved in 24–48 hours

One major issue with the current approved COVID-19 vaccines relates to their storage and transportation prior to mass vaccinations of the global population. For example, the LNP-mRNA BNT162b2 vaccine requires storage at −80°C, whereas the mRNA-1273 vaccine can be stored at −20°C. The adenovirus vector-based vaccines can be stored at +4°C for weeks. However, a lesson learned is that for next generation COVID-19 vaccines and vaccines targeting emerging viruses and other pathogens that in addition to reengineering vaccines to guarantee efficacy against novel mutants/variants or totally new strains or species, considerable efforts should be dedicated to more storage- and user-friendly vaccine formulations. To make sure that we shall be able to eradicate pandemics, we need to provide access to all humans across the globe. To achieve that we need to address the logistics problem we currently face for storage, transport, and administration of COVID-19 vaccines.

We can also learn from the history of RNA to quote Dr Isaacs [77]:

The history of immunization is full of heroes but also full of villains, and our successes are tempered by tragedies. Despite the urgent need for a vaccine against SARS-CoV-2, we should not neglect the lessons of history. These include ethical issues relating to vaccine safety, such as the possible risks of vaccine-induced enhancement witnessed with Dengue vaccine in the Philippines, and how our decisions may be represented by the anti-vaccine movement.

Indeed, while the large number of vaccines developed have shown excellent safety and efficacy, and saved millions of lives, vaccine-induced enhancement has been described for feline coronaviruses, Dengue virus, and feline immunodeficiency virus through the mechanism of antibody-dependent enhancement [78]. It is necessary to find a good balance between the induction of protective immunity and enhanced susceptibility to infection.

15.13 COVID-19 DRUGS

Perhaps one of the biggest concerns at the beginning and even during the first year of the pandemic was the lack of drugs for the treatment of COVID-19 patients. For this reason, antiviral and anti-parasitic drugs developed for other indications were quickly repurposed for COVID-19 treatment. In some cases, such as for chloroquine (CQ) and hydroxychloroquine (HCQ), the drugs were administered directly to COVID-19 patients without prior clinical evaluation [79]. Despite the large number of drugs repurposed for COVID-19, very few positive results have been obtained. The list is long, including a number of monoclonal antibodies, but also lopinavir, ritonavir, remdesivir, and interferon β 1A have been evaluated [80]. The FDA approved remdesivir, an inhibitor of viral RNA polymerase, in October 2020 in adults and pediatric patients for the treatment of COVID-19 patients requiring hospitalization [81].

In comparison of drug and vaccine development against SARS-CoV-2, the success rate has been significantly higher for vaccines, which has been explained as superior contributions (Figure 15.3). This is not a big surprise, as the success of eliciting antibody responses and providing protection against SARS-CoV-2 seems like a clearly easier challenge than the development of novel antiviral drugs. A relevant question is whether more resources dedicated to antivirals would have produced a functional COVID-19 drug. In that case we might have been able to save many more lives. On the other hand, there was an urgent need for a vaccine which could be administered to as many people as possible to generate herd immunity.

15.14 CONCLUSIONS, OR LESSONS LEARNED?

In summary, the extraordinary technology development has made it possible to forecast more quickly and accurately storms, earthquakes, and potential pandemics than ever before. So, in the case of the COVID-19 pandemic, the question is what we have learned that can help us to be better prepared if or when a new pandemic strikes. It is obvious that we can, and should, learn lessons on many levels. Obviously, the scientific progress has been enormous and while the mRNA-based approach had already been developed more than a decade ago, the breakthrough seen for COVID-19 mRNA vaccines has confirmed it as a major technology for vaccine development. However, despite this success, two lessons have been learned the hard way. Not surprisingly, SARS-CoV-2 as a typical RNA virus is prone to generating mutants, which we have certainly discovered since the end of 2020 [50–54]. The critical question has been whether the developed vaccines could provide protection against the novel SARS-CoV-2 variants, also how long the immunity lasts, and whether additional booster immunizations are necessary. Another issue is the recent detection of rare cases of thrombosis and thrombocytopenia in individuals vaccinated with COVID-19 vaccines. Initially, vaccine-induced thrombotic thrombocytopenia (VITT) was associated with adenovirus vector-based vaccines [82, 83], but later also mRNA-based vaccines caused rare cases of VITT were detected [84]. While VITT occurs at low frequency, their presence is not unexpected after mass vaccinations, but it is another lesson learned to also deal with severe adverse events and potentially to be addressed by vaccine reformulations.

In the case of COVID-19 drug discovery, much has been learned about the relatively modest achievements for repurposed drugs. Only rare examples of success have been seen, such as the approval of remdesivir for the treatment of hospitalized COVID-19 patients [81]. The discovery of novel COVID-19 specific antiviral drugs has not been successful either, the exception being

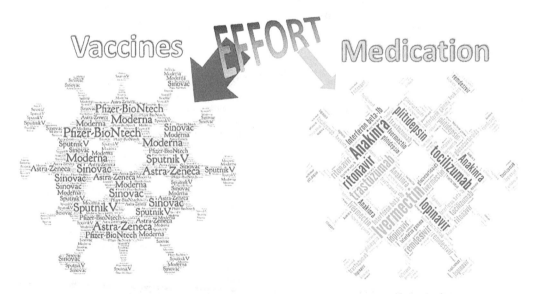

Figure 15.3 There is no doubt that the greatest effort has been devoted to obtaining vaccines. Would we have been able to obtain a drug at the same time as the vaccines for COVID-19? We will never know, but another year of the pandemic continues. This is the new challenge.

the combination therapy of the monoclonal antibodies casirivimab and imdevimab, which has been approved by the FDA for the treatment of non-hospitalized COVID-19 patients who are at high risk of developing serious disease [85]. It is difficult to pinpoint what could be improved for increasing the success rate for COVID-19 drugs, or in the case of future outbreaks, but clearly technology development and alertness and readiness to face new outbreaks are essential assets.

Perhaps the area where most lessons have been learned comprises the management of seriously ill COVID-19 patients. Moreover, the availability of ICU medical devices and personal protection equipment (PPE) has been guaranteed through appropriate enhanced production capacity and stockpiling.

Finally, we can all learn lessons from the COVID-19 pandemic. Wearing masks and washing hands have substantially contributed to the reduced spread of SARS-CoV-2, but also, significantly, other viral infections. Travel restrictions have also taught us a "new way of life" and while we might be able to return to the normal life we knew before the pandemic, we need to stay alert to be able to face new outbreaks better prepared than we were for COVID-19.

In a recent editorial in *Science*, Dr Collins, Director of the National Institutes of Health (NIH) in the USA, summarized the lessons learned from COVID-19 [86], "In the past, the world has rallied to confront new pandemics, only to lapse into complacency as the risk faded. Having now experienced the worst pandemic in 103 years, we must not make that mistake again."

ACKNOWLEDGEMENTS

MC wants to thank the COVID-19 researchers at in the GEBIOMIC group at the University of Antioquia, Medellin, Colombia.

REFERENCES

1. Gatherer, D. (2009). The 2009 H1N1 influenza outbreak in its historical context. *J. Clin. Virol.* 45, 174–178.

2. Cherry, J.D. (2004). The chronology of the 2002–2003 SARS mini pandemic. *Paediatr. Respir. Rev.* 5, 262–269.

3. Zaki, A.M., Van Boheemen, S., Bestebroer, T.M. et al. (2012). Isolation of a novel coronavirus from a man with pneumonia in Saudi Arabia. *N. Engl. J. Med.* 367, 1814–1820.

4. Li, H., Liu, Z., Ge, J. (2020). Scientific research progress of COVID-19/SARS-CoV-2 in the first five months. *J. Cell. Mol. Med.* 24, 6558–6570.

5. Hartenian, E., Nandakumar, D., Lari, A. et al. (2020). The molecular virology of coronaviruses. *J. Biol. Chem.* 295, 12910–12934.

6. Le, T.T., Andreadakis, Z., Kumar, A. et al. (2020). The COVID-19 vaccine development landscape. *Nat. Rev. Drug Discov.* 19, 305–306.

7. Gates, B. (2020). Pandemic I: The first modern pandemic. www.gatesnotes.com/Health/Pandemic-Innovation.

8. Morens, D.M., Folkers, G.K., Fauci, A.S. (2009). What is a pandemic? *J. Infect. Dis.* 200, 1018–1021.

9. de Jong, J.D., Claas, E.C.J., Osterhaus, A.D. et al. (1997). A pandemic warning? *Nature* 389, 554.

10. Osterholm, M.T. (2017). Preparing for the next pandemic. In *Global Health* (Ed. J.J. Kirton), pp. 225–238. Taylor & Francis Group, Routledge.

11. Ioannidis, J.P. (2019). Neglecting major health problems and broadcasting minor, uncertain issues in lifestyle science. *JAMA* 322, 2069–2070.

12. Cohen, J., Kupferschmidt, K. (2020). Countries test tactics in 'war' against COVID-19. *Science* 367, 1287–1288.

13. Feldmann, A., Gasser, O., Lichtblau, F. et al. (2021). *Implications of the COVID-19 pandemic on the internet traffic.* In *Broadband Coverage in Germany; 15th ITG-Symposium* (pp. 1–5). VDE.

14. Hossain, M.S., Muhammad, G., Guizani, N. (2020). Explainable AI and mass surveillance system-based healthcare framework to combat COVID-I9 like pandemics. *IEEE Network* 34, 126–132.

15. Abdulsalam, Y., Hossain, M.S. (2020). COVID-19 networking demand: An auction-based mechanism for automated selection of edge computing services. *IEEE Trans. Netw. Sci. Eng.* doi:10.1109/TNSE.2020.3026637.

16. Servick, K. (2020). Can phone apps slow the spread of the coronavirus? *Science* 368, 1296–1297.

17. Tuli, S., Tuli, S, Tuli, R. et al. (2020). Predicting the growth and trend of COVID-19 pandemic using machine learning and cloud computing. *Internet of Things* 11, 100222.

18. Allam, Z., Dey, G., Jones, D.S. (2020). Artificial intelligence (AI) provided early detection of the coronavirus (COVID-19) in China and will influence future urban health policy internationally. *AI* 1, 156–165.

19. Dong, E., Du, H., Gardner, L. (2020). An interactive web-based dashboard to track COVID-19 in real time. *Lancet Inf. Dis.* 20, 533–534.

20. Velazquez, A., Bustria, M., Ouyang, Y. et al. (2020). An analysis of clinical and geographical metadata of over 75,000 records in the GISAID COVID-19 database. *medRxiv.* doi:10.1101/2020.09.22.20199497.

21. Amarakoon, P., Braa, J., Sahay, S. et al. (2020). *Building agility in health information systems to*

respond to the COVID-19 pandemic: The Sri Lankan experience. In *IFIP Joint Working Conference on the Future of Digital Work: The Challenge of Inequality* (pp. 222–236). Springer, Cham.

22. Tom-Aba, D., Silenou, B.C., Doerrbecker, J. et al. (2020). The surveillance outbreak response management and analysis system (SORMAS): Digital health global goods maturity assessment. *JMIR Publ. Health Surveil* 6, e15860.

23. Ahmed, K., Bukhari, M.A., Mlanda, T. et al. (2020). Novel approach to support rapid data collection, management, and visualization during the COVID-19 outbreak response in the World Health Organization African region: Development of a data summarization and visualization tool. *JMIR Publ. Health Surveil* 6, e20355.

24. Mersha, A., Shibiru, S., Girma, M. et al. (2021). Health professionals practice and associated factors towards precautionary measures for COVID-19 pandemic in public health facilities of Gamo zone, southern Ethiopia: A cross-sectional study. *PLoS One* 16, e0248272.

25. Majiya, H., Aliyu-Paiko, M., Balogu, V.T. et al. (2020). Seroprevalence of COVID-19 in Niger State. *medRxiv.* doi:10.1101/2020.08.04.20168112.

26. Braithwaite, I., Callender, T., Bullock, M. et al. (2020). Automated and partly automated contact tracing: A systematic review to inform the control of COVID-19. *Lancet Dig. Health* 2, e607–e621.

27. Eniade, O.D., Agbana, D.E., Afam, B.O. (2021). Knowledge, attitude and prevention practices towards infection by severe acute respiratory syndrome-CoV-2 among residents of Kogi State during the COVID-19 pandemic. *J. Adv. Med. Medical Res.* 32, 36–46.

28. Nageshwaran, G., Harris, R.C., Guerche-Seblain, C.E. (2021). Review of the role of big data and digital technologies in controlling COVID-19 in Asia: Public health interest vs. privacy. *Digit. Health* 7. doi:10.1177/20552076211002953.

29. Tian, S., Hu, N., Lou, J. et al. (2020). Characteristics of COVID-19 infection in Beijing. *J. Infect.* 80, 401–406.

30. Velicu, M.A., Furlanetti, L., Jung, J. et al. (2021). Epidemiological trends in COVID-19 pandemic: Prospective critical appraisal of observations from six countries in Europe and the USA. *Br. Med. J.* 11, e045782.

31. Bendavid, E., Mulaney, B., Sood, N. et al. (2021). COVID-19 antibody seroprevalence in Santa Clara County, California. *Int. J. Epidemiol.* 50, 410–419.

32. Jakhmola, S., Baral, B., Jha, H.C. (2021). A comparative analysis of COVID-19 outbreak on age groups and both the sexes of population from India and other countries. *J. Infect. Dev. Countries* 15, 333–341.

33. Kanagarathinam, K., Sekar, K. (2020). Estimation of the reproduction number and early prediction of the COVID-19 outbreak in India using a statistical computing approach. *Epidemiol. Health* 42, 2020028.

34. Li, J., Huang, D.Q., Zou, B., Yang, H. et al. (2021). Epidemiology of COVID-19: A systematic review and meta-analysis of clinical characteristics, risk factors, and outcomes. *J. Med. Virol.* 93, 1449–1458.

35. Koyama, T., Platt, D., Parida, L. (2020). Variant analysis of Sars-CoV-2 genomes. *Bull. WHO* 98, 495.

36. Forster, P., Forster, L., Renfrew, C. et al. (2020). Phylogenetic network analysis of Sars-CoV-2 genomes. *Proc. Natl. Acad. Sci. USA* 117, 9241–9243.

37. Andersen, K.G., Rambaut, A., Lipkin, W.I. et al. (2020). The proximal origin of Sars-CoV-2. *Nat. Med.* 26, 450–452.

38. Zhang, S., Qiao, S., Yu, J. et al. (2021). Bat and pangolin coronavirus spike glycoprotein structures provide insights into Sars-CoV-2 evolution. *Nat. Commun.* 12, 1–12.

39. Tang, X., Wu, C., Li, X. et al. (2020). On the origin and continuing evolution of Sars-CoV-2. *Natl. Sci. Rev.* 7, 1012–1023.

40. Zhang, T., Wu, Q., Zhang, Z. (2020). Probable pangolin origin of Sars-CoV-2 associated with the COVID-19 outbreak. *Curr. Biol.* 30, 1346–1351.

41. Lam, T.T.Y., Jia, N., Zhang, Y.W. et al. (2020). Identifying Sars-CoV-2-related coronaviruses in Malayan pangolins. *Nature* 583, 282–285.

42. Han, G.Z. (2020). Pangolins harbor Sars-CoV-2-related coronaviruses. *Trends Microbiol.* 28, 515–517.

43. Rodríguez-Morales, A.J., Balbin-Ramon, G.J., Rabaan, A.A. et al. (2020). Genomic Epidemiology and its importance in the study of the COVID-19 pandemic. *Genomics* 1, 3.

44. Nashiry, A., Sarmin Sumi, S., Islam, S. et al. (2021). Bioinformatics and system biology approach to identify the influences of COVID-19 on cardiovascular and hypertensive comorbidities. *Brief Bioinform.* 22, 1387–1401.

45. Sumon, T.A., Hussain, M., Hasan, M.T. et al. (2020). A revisit to the research updates of drugs, vaccines and bioinformatics approaches in combating COVID-19 pandemic. *Front. Mol. Biosci.* 7, 493.

46. Ishack, S., Lipner, S.R. (2021). Bioinformatics and immunoinformatics to support COVID-19 vaccine development. *J. Med. Virol.* doi:10.1002/jmv.27017.

47. Cannataro, M., Harrison, A. (2021). Bioinformatics helping to mitigate the impact of COVID-19–editorial. *Brief Bioinform.* 22, 613–615.

48. Cleemput, S., Dumon, W., Fonseca, V. et al. (2020). Genome detective coronavirus typing tool for rapid identification and characterization of novel coronavirus genomes. *Bioinformatics* 36, 3552–3555.

49. Cai, Y., Zhang, J., Xiao, T. et al. (2020). Distinct conformational states of SARS-CoV-2 spike protein. *Science* 369, 1586–1592.

50. Davies, N.G., Jarvis, C.I., Edmunds, W.J., et al. (2021). Increased mortality in community-tested cases of SARS-CoV-2 lineage B. 1.1. 7. *Nature*, 593, 270–274.

51. Tegally, H., Wilkinson, E., Giovanetti, M. et al. (2021). Emergence of a SARS-CoV-2 variant of concern with mutations in spike glycoprotein. *Nature* 592, 438–443.

52. Natarajan, M.A., Javali, P.S., Pandian, C.J. et al. (2021). Computational investigation of increased virulence and pathogenesis of SARS-CoV-2 lineage B. 1.1. 7. *bioRxiv*. doi:10.1101/2021.01.25.428190.

53. Collier, D.A., De Marco, A., Ferreira, I.A.T.M. et al. (2021). Sensitivity of SARS-CoV-2 B.1.1.7 to mRNA vaccine-elicited antibodies. *Nature* 593, 136–141.

54. Abu-Raddad, L.J., Chemaitelly, H., Butt, A.A. et al. (2021). Effectiveness of the BNT162b2 COVID-19 vaccine against the B.1.1.7 and B.351 variants. *N. Engl. J. Med.* doi:10.1056/NEJMc2104974.

55. Madhi, S.A., Baillie, V., Cutland, C.L. et al. (2021). Efficacy of the ChAdOx1 nCoV-19 vaccine against the B.1.351 variant. *N. Engl. J. Med.* doi:10.1056/NEJMoa2102214.

56. Borczuk, A.C. (2021). Pulmonary pathology of COVID-19: A review of autopsy studies. *Curr. Opin. Pulm. Med.* 27, 184–192.

57. Batah, S.S., Fabro, A.T. (2020). Pulmonary pathology of ARDS in COVID-19: A pathological review for clinicians. *Resp. Med.* 176, 106239.

58. Bösmüller, H., Matter, M., Fend, F. et al. (2021). The pulmonary pathology of COVID-19. *Virchows Archiv.* 478, 137–150.

59. Yuki, K., Fujiogi, M., Koutsogiannaki, S. (2020). COVID-19 pathophysiology: A review. *Clin. Immunol.* 215, 108427.

60. Deshmukh, V., Motwani, R., Kumar, A. et al. (2021). Histopathological observations in COVID-19: A systematic review. *J. Clin. Pathol.* 74, 76–83.

61. V'kovski, P., Kratzel, A., Steiner, S. et al. (2021). Coronavirus biology and replication: Implications for Sars-CoV-2. *Nat. Rev. Microbiol.* 19, 155–170.

62. Sette, A., Crotty, S. (2020). Pre-existing immunity to Sars-CoV-2: The knowns and unknowns. *Nat. Rev. Immunol.* 20, 457–458.

63. Dhochak, N., Singhal, T., Kabra, S.K. et al. (2020). Pathophysiology of COVID-19: Why children fare better than adults? *Indian J. Pediatrics* 87, 537–546.

64. Gaebler, C., Wang, Z., Lorenzi, J.C. et al. (2021). Evolution of antibody immunity to Sars-CoV-2. *Nature* 591, 639–644.

65. Lundstrom, K. (2021) Viral vectors for COVID-19 vaccine development. *Viruses* 13, 317.

66. Wu, F., Liu, M., Wang, A. et al. (2020). Evaluating the association of clinical characteristics with neutralizing antibody levels in patients who have recovered from mild COVID-19 in Shanghai, China. *JAMA Intern. Med.* 180, 1356–1362.

67. Dramé, M., Tabue Teguo, M., Proye, E. et al. (2020). Should RT-PCR be considered a gold standard in the diagnosis of COVID-19? *J. Med. Vir.* 92, 2312–2313.

68. Versi, E. (1992). "Gold standard" is an appropriate term. *Br. Med. J.* 305, 187.

69. Xu, M., Wang, D., Wang, H. et al. (2020). COVID-19 diagnostic testing: Technology perspective. *Clin. Transl. Med.* 10, e158.

70. Meo, S.A., Bukhari, I.A., Akram, J. et al. (2021). COVID-19 vaccines: Comparison of biological, pharmacological characteristics and adverse effects of Pfizer/BioNTech and Moderna Vaccines. *Eur. Rev. Med. Pharmacol. Sci.* 25, 1663–1669.

71. Knoll, M.D., Wonodi, C. (2021). Oxford–AstraZeneca COVID-19 vaccine efficacy. *Lancet* 397, 72–74.

72. Jones, I., Roy, P. (2021). Sputnik V COVID-19 vaccine candidate appears safe and effective. *Lancet* 397, 642–643.

73. Sadoff, J., Gray, G., Vandebosch, A. et al. (2021). Safety and efficacy of single-dose Ad26. COV2. S vaccine against COVID-19. *N. Engl. J. Med.* doi:10.1056/NEJMoa2101544.

74. Shinde, V., Bhikha, S., Hoosain, Z. et al. (2021). Efficacy of NVX-CoV2373 COVID-19 vaccine against the B. 1.351 variant. *N. Engl. J. Med.* 384, 1899–1909.

75. Palacios, R., Patiño, E.G., de Oliveira Piorelli, R. et al. (2020). Double-blind, randomized, placebo-controlled Phase III clinical trial to evaluate the efficacy and safety of treating healthcare professionals with the adsorbed COVID-19 (inactivated) vaccine manufactured by Sinovac–PROFISCOV: A structured summary of a study protocol for a randomised controlled trial. *Trials* 21, 1–3.

76. Baraniuk, C. (2021). What do we know about China's COVID-19 vaccines? *Br. Med. J.* 373, n912.

77. Isaacs, D. (2020). What history teaches us about vaccines and pandemics. *Microbiol. Australia* 41, 168–171.

78. Huisman, W., Martina, B.E.E., Rimmelzwaan, R.A. et al. (2009). Vaccine-induced enhancement of viral infections. *Vaccine* 27, 505–512.

79. Hoffmann, M., Mösbauer, K., Hofmann-Winkler, H. et al. (2020). Chloroquine does not inhibit infection of human lung cells with Sars-CoV-2. *Nature* 585, 588–590.

80. Tarighi, P., Eftekhari, S., Chizari, M. et al. (2021). A review of potential suggested drugs for coronavirus disease (COVID-19) treatment. *Eur. J. Pharmacol.* 895, 173890.

81. Rubin, D., Chan-Tack, K., Farley, J. et al. (2020) FDA approval of Remdesivir: A step in the right direction. *N. Engl. J. Med.* 383, 2598–2600.

82. Greinacher, A., Thiele, T., Warkentin, T.E. et al. (2021). Thrombotic Thrombocytopenia after ChAdOx1 nCoV-19 vaccination. *N. Engl. J. Med.* doi:10.1056/NEJMoa2104840.

83. Muir, K.-L., Kallam, A., Koepsell, S.A. et al. (2021). Thrombotic Thrombocytopenia after Ad26. COV.S vaccination. *N. Engl. J. Med.* doi:10.1056/ NEJMc2105869.

84. Lee, E.-J., Cines, D.B., Gernsheimer, T. et al. (2021). Thrombocytopenia following Pfizer and Moderna SARS-CoV-2 vaccination. *Am. J. Hematol.* doi:10.1002/ajh.26132.

85. Fact sheet for health care providers emergency use authorization (EUA) of casirivimab and imdevimab. (2021). Accessed May 31 2021 https://www.fda.gov/media/143892/ download.

86. Collins, F.S. (2021). COVID-19 lessons for research. *Science* 371, 1081.

Index

Page numbers in **bold** indicate tables and page numbers in *italic* indicate figures.

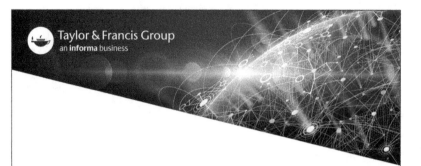